PRENATAL AND CHILDHOOD NUTRITION

Evaluating the Neurocognitive Connections

PRENATAL AND CHILDHOOD NUTRITION

Evaluating
the Neurocognitive
Connections

Edited by
Cindy Croft

AAP APPLE
ACADEMIC
PRESS

Apple Academic Press Inc. | Apple Academic Press Inc.
3333 Mistwell Crescent | 9 Spinnaker Way
Oakville, ON L6L 0A2 | Waretown, NJ 08758
Canada | USA

© 2015 by Apple Academic Press, Inc.

First issued in paperback 2021

Exclusive worldwide distribution by CRC Press, a member of Taylor & Francis Group

No claim to original U.S. Government works

ISBN 13: 978-1-77463-241-3 (pbk)
ISBN 13: 978-1-77188-094-7 (hbk)

Library of Congress Control Number: 2014948302

Library and Archives Canada Cataloguing in Publication

Prenatal and childhood nutrition: evaluating the neurocognitive connections/edited by Cindy Croft.

Includes bibliographical references and index.
ISBN 978-1-77188-094-7 (bound)
1. Children--Nutrition. 2. Pregnancy--Nutritional aspects. 3. Brain--Growth. 4. Cognition disorders in children--Nutritional aspects. I. Croft, Cindy, editor

RJ216.P68 2015   618.92'8   C2014-905749-0

Apple Academic Press also publishes its books in a variety of electronic formats. Some content that appears in print may not be available in electronic format. For information about Apple Academic Press products, visit our website at **www.appleacademicpress.com** and the CRC Press website at **www.crcpress.com**

ABOUT THE EDITOR

CINDY CROFT

Cindy Croft, MA in Education, is Director of the Center for Inclusive Child Care, Concordia University, St. Paul, Minnesota. She teaches for the Center for Early Education and Development at the University of Minnesota and in the early childhood program at Concordia University. She has authored two books, *The Six Keys: Promoting Children's Mental Health* and *Children and Challenging Behavior: Making Inclusion Work*, and she provides training and consultation to educators of children with various disabilities. She is a member of the National Association for the Education of Young Children, the Early Childhood and School-Age Trainers Association, the Minnesota Association for Children's Mental Health, and the Minnesota Association for Infant and Early Childhood Mental Health Division.

CONTENTS

ACKNOWLEDGMENT AND HOW TO CITE

The editor and publisher thank each of the authors who contributed to this book, whether by granting their permission individually or by releasing their research as open source articles or under a license that permits free use, provided that attribution is made. The chapters in this book were previously published in various places in various formats. To cite the work contained in this book and to view the individual permissions, please refer to the citation at the beginning of each chapter. Each chapter was read individually and carefully selected by the editor; the result is a book that provides a nuanced study of prenatal and childhood nutrition. The chapters included examine the following topics:

- Chapter 1 provides a good summary of current research endeavors on this topic.
- Chapter 2 argues that the differing food patterns between socioeconomic groups allow a better understanding of the effects of nutrition on learning outcomes.
- Other research has investigated individual aspects of nutrition's effects on development, but Chapter 3 provides a more general overview from which to build this book.
- The researchers in Chapter 4 make the connection between early nutrition and lifelong neurological health.
- Chapter 5 describes how we often think of nutrition as a "nurture" only variable, when in fact "nature" is also in play when it comes to neurocognitive development, with nutrition and genetics interacting with each other.
- Where other articles focus on particular aspects of nutrition, Chapter 6 investigates particular aspects of the neurological outcomes, breaking them down into a range of categories helpful to educational professionals.
- The serious neurodevelopment consequences of severe iodine deficiency have been well researched and document, but Chapter 7 investigates the effects of even mild iodine deficiencies on learning outcomes.
- Simplistic connections between diet and ADHD are often made in popular mainstream publications. Chapter 8 provides a more factual perspective based on solid research rather than anecdotal evidence.

- Again, there is a popular tendency to connect diet to autism, just as to ADHD. Chapter 9 investigates the reality of this and provides suggestions for researched-based nutritional counseling.
- The effects of iron deficiency on mental health are well-established and yet are often ignored. Chapter 10 reminds mental health professionals to investigate all angles when considering mental health treatment options.
- Vitamin D deficiency has reached epidemic proportions but is often overlooked as a serious consideration in mental health. Chapter 11 underlines the connections between Vitamin D deficiency and psychiatric disorders in the adolescent population.
- Chapter 12 broadens the foundation already offered in the previous chapter, providing a more detailed summary of the supporting research behind the breakfast-school performance connection.
- By this point, the connection between nutrition and neurocognitive development has been firmly established. Chapter 13 directs attention to a very particular dietary factor with a very particular effect on brain function.
- Although camel milk may not be considered a widely available intervention option for children with neurocognitive difficulties, the chemical investigations within Chapter 14 have dietary implications that can also be achieved within the Western diet.
- Chapter 15 provides a good overview of the various issues considered in this book, making the connection to positive and active intervention.

LIST OF CONTRIBUTORS

Amina Abubakar
KEMRI/Wellcome Trust Research Programme, Kilifi, Kenya, Department of Child and Adolescent Studies, Utrecht University, Utrecht, Netherlands, and Department of Cross-Cultural Psychology, Tilburg University, Tilburg, Netherlands

Katie Adolphus
Human Appetite Research Unit, Institute of Psychological Sciences, University of Leeds, Leeds, UK

Laila Y. AL-Ayadhi
Department of Physiology, Faculty of Medicine, King Saud University, P.O. Box 2925, Riyadh 11461, Saudi Arabia

Ya-Mei Bai
Department of Psychiatry, Taipei Veterans General Hospital, Taipei, Taiwan and Department of Psychiatry, College of Medicine, National Yang-Ming University, Taipei, Taiwan

John R. Burgess
School of Medicine, University of Tasmania, Sandy Bay, Tasmania 7005, Australia; and Department of Endocrinology, Royal Hobart Hospital, Hobart, Tasmania 7000, Australia

Laurie T. Butler
School of Psychology and Clinical Language Sciences, University of Reading, Reading, United Kingdom

Kecia N. Carroll
Department of Pediatrics, Vanderbilt University Medical Center, 2200 Children's Way, Nashville, TN 37232, USA

Wen-Han Chang
Department of Psychiatry, Taipei Veterans General Hospital, Taipei, Taiwan

Mu-Hong Chen
Department of Psychiatry, Taipei Veterans General Hospital, Taipei, Taiwan

Tzeng-Ji Chen
Department of Family Medicine, Taipei Veterans General Hospital, Taipei, Taiwan and Institute of Hospital and Health Care Administration, National Yang-Ming University, Taipei, Taiwan

Ying-Sheue Chen
Department of Psychiatry, Taipei Veterans General Hospital, Taipei, Taiwan

Byeong Moo Choe
Department of Psychiatry, College of Medicine, Dong-A University, Dong-A University Hospital, 26 Daesingongwon-ro, Seo-gu, Busan 602-715, Korea

Hee Won Chueh
Department of Pediatrics, College of Medicine, Dong-A University, Dong-A University Hospital, 26 Daesingongwon-ro, Seo-gu, Busan 602-715, Korea

Kevin Connolly
Department of Psychology, University of Sheffield, Sheffield, UK

Tina A. Crook
Department of Dietetics and Nutrition, University of Arkansas for Medical Sciences, Little Rock, AR 72202, USA

Sarah Cusick
Harold and Margaret Milliken Hatch Laboratory of Neuroendocrinology, The Rockefeller University, New York, New York

Margaret Joy Dauncey
Wolfson College, University of Cambridge, Barton Road, Cambridge, CB3 9BB, UK

Kathryn G. Dewey
Department of Nutrition, University of California at Davis, Davis, CA, USA and SUMMIT Institute of Development, Mataram, Nusa Tenggara Barat, Indonesia

Louise Dye
Human Appetite Research Unit, Institute of Psychological Sciences, University of Leeds, Leeds, UK

Nadra Elyass Elamin
Autism Research and Treatment Center, Shaik AL-Amodi Autism Research Chair, Faculty of Medicine, King Saud University, P.O. Box 2925, Riyadh 11461, Saudi Arabia

Teresa L. Finucane
Clinical Research Coordinator, University of Rochester Medical Center, Department of Psychiatry, 300 Crittenden Boulevard, Rochester, New York, 14642, USA

Jonathan Foster
Centre for Child Health Research, Telethon Institute for Child Health Research, The University of Western Australia, Perth, WA, Australia, School of Psychology and Speech Pathology, Curtin University, Perth, WA, Australia, Neurosciences Unit, Health Department of Western Australia, Perth, WA, Australia, and School of Paediatrics and Child Health, The University of Western Australia, Perth, WA, Australia

Meriel Friedman-Campbell
Psychiatric Nurse Practitioner, Irwin Army Community Hospital Behavioral Health, 600 Caisson Hill Road, Fort Riley, KS, 66442, USA

Michael Georgieff
Department of Pediatrics, University of Minnesota Medical School, Minneapolis, Minnesota

Barbara L. Gracious
Center for Innovation in Pediatric Practice, The Research Institute at Nationwide Children's Hospital and The Ohio State University, Columbus, OH, USA and Nationwide Children's Hospital 700 Children's Drive, Columbus, OH, 43205, USA

Joanna C. Hamlin
Department of Dietetics and Nutrition, University of Arkansas for Medical Sciences, Little Rock, AR 72202, USA

Marion E. Hare
Department of Preventive Medicine, University of Tennessee Health Science Center, 66 N. Pauline, Memphis, TN 38163, USA and Department of Pediatrics, University of Tennessee Health Science Center, 50 N. Dunlap, Memphis, TN 38103, USA

Ian Hay
Faculty of Education, University of Tasmania, Sandy Bay, Tasmania 7005, Australia; and Department of Endocrinology

Siobhan Hickling
Centre for Child Health Research, Telethon Institute for Child Health Research, The University of Western Australia, Perth, WA, Australia and School of Population Health, The University of Western Australia, Perth, WA, Australia

Penny Holding
KEMRI/Wellcome Trust Research Programme, Kilifi, Kenya, Department of Research and Training, International Centre for Behavioural Studies, Mombasa, Kenya, and Case Western Reserve University, Cleveland, OH, USA

Young-Seoub Hong
Department of Preventive Medicine, College of Medicine, Dong-A University, Dong-A University Hospital, 26, Daesingongwon-ro, Seo-gu, Busan 602-715, Korea and Heavy Metal Exposure Environmental Health Center, Dong-A University, 32, Daesingongwon-ro, Seo-gu, Busan 602-714, Korea

Ju-Wei Hsu
Department of Psychiatry, Taipei Veterans General Hospital, Taipei, Taiwan

Kai-Lin Huang
Department of Psychiatry, Taipei Veterans General Hospital, Taipei, Taiwan

Kristen L. Hynes
Menzies Research Institute Tasmania, University of Tasmania, Sandy Bay, Tasmania 7005, Australia; and Department of Endocrinology

S. Jill James
Department of Pediatrics, University of Arkansas for Medical Sciences, Little Rock, AR 72202, USA and Department of Pediatrics, University of Arkansas for Medical Sciences, Arkansas Children's Hospital Research Institute, 13 Children's Way Slot 512-41B, Little Rock, AR 72202, USA

Je-Wook Kang
Department of Child and Adolescent Psychiatry, College of Medicine, Inje University Busan Paik Hospital, 75 Bokji-ro, Busanjin-gu, Busan 614-735, Korea

Dong Woo Kim
Molecular Epidemiology Branch, National Cancer Center, 323 Ilsan-ro, Ilsandong-gu, Goyang-si, Gyeonggi-do 410-769, Korea

Jeongseon Kim
Molecular Epidemiology Branch, National Cancer Center, 323 Ilsan-ro, Ilsandong-gu, Goyang-si, Gyeonggi-do 410-769, Korea

Yu-Mi Kim
Department of Preventive Medicine, College of Medicine, Dong-A University, Dong-A University Hospital, 26, Daesingongwon-ro, Seo-gu, Busan 602-715, Korea and Heavy Metal Exposure Environmental Health Center, Dong-A University, 32, Daesingongwon-ro, Seo-gu, Busan 602-714, Korea

Patricia Kitsao-Wekulo
KEMRI/Wellcome Trust Research Programme, Kilifi, Kenya, Department of Publications and Ethics, International Centre for Behavioural Studies, Nairobi, Kenya, and Discipline of Psychology, School of Applied Human Sciences, University of KwaZulu-Natal, Durban, South Africa

Jane Kvalsvig
Discipline of Public Health Medicine, School of Nursing and Public Health, University of KwaZulu-Natal, Durban, South Africa

Min Jung Kwak
Department of Pediatrics, Pusan National University Hospital, Pusan National University School of Medicine, 179, Gudeok-ro, Seo-gu, Busan 602-739, Korea

Clare L. Lawton
Human Appetite Research Unit, Institute of Psychological Sciences, University of Leeds, Leeds, UK

Jung Hyun Lee
Department of Pediatrics, Kosin University Gospel Hospital, 262, Gamcheon-ro, Seo-gu, Busan 602-702, Korea

Jianghong Li
Centre for Child Health Research, Telethon Institute for Child Health Research, The University of Western Australia, Perth, WA, Australia, Centre for Population Health Research, Curtin Health Innovation Research Institute, Curtin University, Perth, WA, Australia, and Social Science Research Center, Berlin, Germany

Bruce S. McEwen
Harold and Margaret Milliken Hatch Laboratory of Neuroendocrinology, The Rockefeller University, New York, New York

Stepan Melnyk
Department of Pediatrics, University of Arkansas for Medical Sciences, Little Rock, AR 72202, USA

Jean Michel Mérillon
University de Bordeaux, ISVV, Groupe d'Etude des Substances Végétales à Activité Biologique, Villenave d'Ornon, France

Susan Messing
Clinical Research Coordinator, University of Rochester Medical Center, Department of Psychiatry, 300 Crittenden Boulevard, Rochester, New York, 14642, USA and Senior Research Associate, Department of Biostatistics and Computational Biology, University of Rochester Medical Center

Anett Nyaradi
Centre for Child Health Research, Telethon Institute for Child Health Research, The University of Western Australia, Perth, WA, Australia and School of Population Health, The University of Western Australia, Perth, WA, Australia

Wendy H. Oddy
Centre for Child Health Research, Telethon Institute for Child Health Research, The University of Western Australia, Perth, WA, Australia

Petr Otahal
Menzies Research Institute Tasmania, University of Tasmania, Sandy Bay, Tasmania 7005, Australia; and Department of Endocrinology

Jae Hong Park
Department of Psychiatry, College of Medicine, Dong-A University, Dong-A University Hospital, 26 Daesingongwon-ro, Seo-gu, Busan 602-715, Korea

Melissa N. Parkhurst
Clinical Research Coordinator, University of Rochester Medical Center, Department of Psychiatry, 300 Crittenden Boulevard, Rochester, New York, 14642, USA

Margaret Pauly
Department of Pediatrics, University of Arkansas for Medical Sciences, Little Rock, AR 72202, USA

Oleksandra Pavliv
Department of Pediatrics, University of Arkansas for Medical Sciences, Little Rock, AR 72202, USA

Chandrika Piyathilake
Department of Nutrition Sciences, University of Alabama at Birmingham, 326 Webb Nutrition Sciences Building, 1675 University Blvd., AL 35294, USA

Elizabeth L. Prado
Department of Nutrition, University of California at Davis, Davis, CA, USA and SUMMIT Institute of Development, Mataram, Nusa Tenggara Barat, Indonesia

Marcus Rattray
Reading School of Pharmacy, University of Reading, Reading, United Kingdom

Catarina Rendeiro
Molecular Nutrition Group, School of Chemistry, Food and Pharmacy, University of Reading, Reading, United Kingdom and School of Psychology and Clinical Language Sciences, University of Reading, Reading, United Kingdom

Karen Ringwald-Smith
St. Jude Children's Research Hospital, 262 Danny Thomas Place, Memphis, TN 38105, USA

Andrew B. Scholey
Centre for Human Psychopharmacology, Swinburne University of Technology, Melbourne, VIC, Australia

Ju-Hee Seo
Heavy Metal Exposure Environmental Health Center, Dong-A University, 32, Daesingongwon-ro, Seo-gu, Busan 602-714, Korea

Michael A. Smith
Department of Psychology, Faculty of Health and Life Sciences, Northumbria University, Newcastle upon Tyne, UK

Jeremy P. E. Spencer
Molecular Nutrition Group, School of Chemistry, Food and Pharmacy, University of Reading, Reading, United Kingdom

William Starrett
Department of Pediatrics, University of Arkansas for Medical Sciences, Little Rock, AR 72202, USA

Tung-Ping Su
Department of Psychiatry, Taipei Veterans General Hospital, Taipei, Taiwan and Department of Psychiatry, College of Medicine, National Yang-Ming University, Taipei, Taiwan

H. Gerry Taylor
Department of Pediatrics, Case Western Reserve University, Rainbow Babies and Children's Hospital, University Hospitals Case Medical Center, Cleveland, OH, USA

Frances A. Tylavsky
Department of Preventive Medicine, University of Tennessee Health Science Center, 66 N. Pauline, Memphis, TN 38163, USA

David Vauzour
Molecular Nutrition Group, School of Chemistry, Food and Pharmacy, University of Reading, Reading, United Kingdom

Eszter Völgyi
Department of Preventive Medicine, University of Tennessee Health Science Center, 66 N. Pauline, Memphis, TN 38163, USA

Theodore D. Wachs
Department of Psychological Sciences, Purdue University, West Lafayette, Indiana

Pierre Waffo-Téguo
University de Bordeaux, ISVV, Groupe d'Etude des Substances Végétales à Activité Biologique, Villenave d'Ornon, France

Claire M. Williams
School of Psychology and Clinical Language Sciences, University of Reading, Reading, United Kingdom

Hae Dong Woo
Molecular Epidemiology Branch, National Cancer Center, 323 Ilsan-ro, Ilsandong-gu, Goyang-si, Gyeonggi-do 410-769, Korea

Jae-Ho Yoo
Department of Pediatrics, College of Medicine, Dong-A University, Dong-A University Hospital, 26 Daesingongwon-ro, Seo-gu, Busan 602-715, Korea

Wonsuk Yoo
Department of Preventive Medicine, University of Tennessee Health Science Center, 66 N. Pauline, Memphis, TN 38163, USA

INTRODUCTION

Research on early brain development has exploded during the two last decades. Today, the architecture of the infant brain is known to be influenced by emotional, biological, and environmental factors that can inhibit or enhance potential in the developing child. External stressors including poor nutrition or neurotoxins can suppress neurocognitive function and even change actual brain structure, causing developmental delays, social emotional disorders, and contributing to overall developmental dysfunction. At the same time, interventions that mitigate early biological or environmental stressors on the developing infant brain can change the trajectory of a negative outcome to a more positive one.

Nutrition is not only a basic need that all humans have to sustain life but it is critical to successful early development. This compendium of research lends deeper insights to the links between nutrition and healthy brain function—and from the reverse perspective, between nutrition and neurocognitiive disorders. This research is critically important to parents, early educators, and interventionists, as well as health professionals who are invested in healthy outcomes for infants. Practitioners and policymakers need research-based approaches in order to provide successful interventions for young children, both in prevention and ongoing services for children with disabilities.

Finally, *Prenatal and Childhood Nutrition: Evaluating the Neurocognitive Connections* provides a research context for policymakers, educators, and families. The link between academics and nutrition should play a key role in decisions regarding education. If we know that we can give children a strong start by improving prenatal and early childhood nutrition, that knowledge should inform our actions and policies regarding prenatal and early childhood health.

Cindy Croft

Chapter 1, by Smith and Scholey, provides a background for recent research on nutrition and developmental growth, as well as an argument for why these topics are so vital to study.

Dietary patterns are sensitive to differences across socio-economic strata or cultural habits and may impact programing of diseases in later life. The purpose of Chapter 2 was to identify distinct dietary patterns during pregnancy in the Mid-South using factor analysis. Furthermore, Völgyi and colleagues aimed to analyze the differences in the food groups and in macro- and micronutrients among the different food patterns. The study was a cross-sectional analysis of 1155 pregnant women (mean age 26.5 ± 5.4 years; 62% African American, 35% Caucasian, 3% Other; and pre-pregnancy BMI 27.6 ± 7.5 kg/m2). Using food frequency questionnaire data collected from participants in the Conditions Affecting Neurocognitive Development and Learning in Early Childhood (CANDLE) study between 16 and 28 weeks of gestation, dietary patterns were identified using factor analysis. Three major dietary patterns, namely, Healthy, Processed, and US Southern were identified among pregnant women from the Mid-South. Further analysis of the three main patterns revealed four mixed dietary patterns, i.e., Healthy-Processed, Healthy-US Southern, Processed-US Southern, and overall Mixed. These dietary patterns were different ($p < 0.001$) from each other in almost all the food items, macro- and micro nutrients and aligned across socioeconomic and racial groups. The study describes unique dietary patterns in the Mid-South, consumed by a cohort of women enrolled in a prospective study examining the association of maternal nutritional factors during pregnancy that are known to affect brain and cognitive development by age 3.

Chapter 3, by Nyaradi and colleagues, examines the current evidence for a possible connection between nutritional intake (including micronutrients and whole diet) and neurocognitive development in childhood. Earlier studies which have investigated the association between nutrition and cognitive development have focused on individual micronutrients, including omega-3 fatty acids, vitamin B12, folic acid, choline, iron, iodine, and zinc, and single aspects of diet. The research evidence from observational studies suggests that micronutrients may play an important role in the cognitive development of children. However, the results of intervention trials utilizing single micronutrients are inconclusive. More generally, there is evidence that malnutrition can impair cognitive development, whilst breastfeeding appears to be beneficial for cognition. Eating breakfast is also beneficial for cognition. In contrast, there is currently inconclusive evidence regarding the association between obesity and cognition. Since individuals consume combinations of foods, more recently researchers have become interested in the cognitive impact of diet as a composite measure. Only a few studies to date have investigated the associations between dietary patterns and cognitive development. In future research, more well designed intervention trials are needed, with special consideration given to the interactive effects of nutrients.

In Chapter 4, Prado and Dewey present an overview of the pathway from early nutrient deficiency to long-term brain function, cognition, and productivity, focusing on research from low- and middle-income countries. Animal models have demonstrated the importance of adequate nutrition for the neurodevelopmental processes that occur rapidly during pregnancy and infancy, such as neuron proliferation and myelination. However, several factors influence whether nutrient deficiencies during this period cause permanent cognitive deficits in human populations, including the child's interaction with the environment, the timing and degree of nutrient deficiency, and the possibility of recovery. These factors should be taken into account in the design and interpretation of future research. Certain types of nutritional deficiency clearly impair brain development, including severe acute malnutrition, chronic undernutrition, iron deficiency, and iodine deficiency. While strategies such as salt iodization and micronutrient powders have been shown to improve these conditions, direct evidence of their impact on brain development is scarce. Other strategies also require further research, including supplementation with iron and other micronutrients, essential fatty acids, and fortified food supplements during pregnancy and infancy.

Considerable evidence links many neuropsychiatric, neurodevelopmental and neurodegenerative disorders with multiple complex interactions between genetics and environmental factors such as nutrition. Mental health problems, autism, eating disorders, Alzheimer's disease, schizophrenia, Parkinson's disease and brain tumours are related to individual variability in numerous protein-coding and non-coding regions of the genome. However, genotype does not necessarily determine neurological phenotype because the epigenome modulates gene expression in response to endogenous and exogenous regulators, throughout the life-cycle. Studies using both genome-wide analysis of multiple genes and comprehensive analysis of specific genes are providing new insights into genetic and epigenetic mechanisms underlying nutrition and neuroscience. Chapter 5, by Dauncy, provides a critical evaluation of the following related areas: (1) recent advances in genomic and epigenomic technologies, and their relevance to brain disorders; (2) the emerging role of non-coding RNAs as key regulators of transcription, epigenetic processes and gene silencing; (3) novel approaches to nutrition, epigenetics and neuroscience; (4) gene-environment interactions, especially in the serotonergic system, as a paradigm of the multiple signalling pathways affected in neuropsychiatric and neurological disorders. Current and future advances in these four areas should contribute significantly to the prevention, amelioration and treatment of multiple devastating brain disorders.

Adequate nutrition is fundamental to the development of a child's full potential. However, the extent to which malnutrition affects developmental and cognitive outcomes in the midst of co-occurring risk factors remains largely understudied. In Chapter 6, Kitsao-Wekulo and colleagues sought to establish if the effects of nutritional status varied according to diverse background characteristics as well as to compare the relative strength of the effects of poor nutritional status on language skills, motor abilities, and cognitive functioning at school age. This cross-sectional study was conducted among school-age boys and girls resident in Kilifi District in Kenya. The authors hypothesized that the effects of area of residence, school attendance, household wealth, age and gender on child outcomes are experienced directly and indirectly through child nutritional status. The use of structural equation modeling (SEM) allowed the disaggregation of the total effect of the explanatory variables into direct effects (effects that go directly from one variable to another) and indirect effects. Each of the models tested for the four child outcomes had a good fit. However, the effects on verbal memory apart from being weaker than for the other outcomes, were not mediated through nutritional status. School attendance was the most influential predictor of nutritional status and child outcomes. The estimated models demonstrated the continued importance of child nutritional status at school-age.

Severe iodine deficiency (ID) during gestation is associated with neurocognitive sequelae. The long-term impact of mild ID, however, has not been well characterized. Hynes and colleagues attempted in Chapter 7 to determine whether children born to mothers with urinary iodine concentrations (UICs) <150 µg/L during pregnancy have poorer educational outcomes in primary school than peers whose mothers did not have gestational ID (UIC ≥150 µg/L). This was a longitudinal follow-up (at 9 years old) of the Gestational Iodine Cohort. Pregnancy occurred during a period of mild ID in the population, with the children subsequently growing up in an iodine-replete environment. Participants were children whose mothers attended The Royal Hobart Hospital (Tasmania) antenatal clinics between 1999 and 2001. Australian national curriculum and Tasmanian state curriculum educational assessment data for children in year 3 were analyzed. Children whose mothers had UIC <150 µg/L had reductions of 10.0% in spelling (−41.1 points, 95% confidence interval [CI], −68.0 to −14.3, P = .003), 7.6% in grammar (−30.9 points, 95% CI, −60.2 to −1.7, P = .038), and 5.7% in English-literacy (−0.33 points, 95% CI, −0.63 to −0.03, P = .034) performance compared with children whose mothers' UICs were ≥150 µg/L. These associations remained significant after adjustment for a range of biological factors (maternal age at birth of child, gestational length at time of birth, gestational age at time of urinary iodine collection, birth weight, and sex). Differences in spelling remained significant after further adjustment for socioeconomic factors (maternal occupation and education). This study provides preliminary evidence that even mild iodine deficiency during pregnancy can have long-term adverse impacts on fetal neurocognition that are not ameliorated by iodine sufficiency during childhood.

The role of diet in the behavior of children has been controversial, but the association of several nutritional factors with childhood behavioral disorders has been continually suggested. In Chapter 8, Woo and colleagues conducted a case-control study to identify dietary patterns associated with attention deficit hyperactivity disorder (ADHD). The study included 192 elementary school students aged seven to 12 years. Three non-consecutive 24-h recall (HR) interviews were employed to assess dietary intake, and 32 predefined food groups were considered in a principal components analysis (PCA). PCA identified four major dietary patterns: the "traditional" pattern, the "seaweed-egg" pattern, the "traditional-healthy" pattern, and the "snack" pattern. The traditional-healthy pattern is characterized by a diet low in fat and high in carbohydrates as well as high intakes of fatty acids and minerals. The multivariate-adjusted odds ratio (OR) of ADHD for the highest tertile of the traditional-healthy pattern in comparison with the lowest tertile was 0.31 (95% CI: 0.12–0.79). The score of the snack pattern was positively associated with the risk of ADHD, but a significant association was observed only in the second tertile. A significant association between ADHD and the dietary pattern score was not found for the other two dietary patterns. In conclusion, the traditional-healthy dietary pattern was associated with lower odds having ADHD.

Abnormalities in folate-dependent one-carbon metabolism have been reported in many children with autism. Because inadequate choline and betaine can negatively affect folate metabolism and in turn downstream methylation and antioxidant capacity, Hamlin and colleauges sought in Chapter 9 to determine whether dietary intake of choline and betaine in children with autism was adequate to meet nutritional needs based on national recommendations. Three-day food records were analyzed for 288 children with autism (ASDs) who participated in the national Autism Intervention Research Network for Physical Health (AIR-P) Study on Diet and Nutrition in children with autism. Plasma concentrations of choline and betaine were measured in a subgroup of 35 children with ASDs and 32 age-matched control children. The results indicated that 60–93% of children with ASDs were consuming less than the recommended Adequate Intake (AI) for choline. Strong positive correlations were found between dietary intake and plasma concentrations of choline and betaine in autistic children as well as lower plasma concentrations compared to the control group. The authors conclude that choline and betaine intake is inadequate in a significant subgroup of children with ASDs and is reflected in lower plasma levels. Inadequate intake of choline and betaine may contribute to the metabolic abnormalities observed in many children with autism and warrants attention in nutritional counseling.

A great deal of evidence has shown that iron is an important component in cognitive, sensorimotor, and social-emotional development and functioning, because the development of central nervous system processes is highly dependent on iron-containing enzymes and proteins. Deficiency of iron in early life may increase the risk of psychiatric morbidity. Utilizing the National Health Insurance Database from 1996 to 2008, Chen and colleagues identified children and adolescents with a diagnosis of IDA in Chapter 10 and compared with age and gender-matched controls (1:4) in an investigation of the increased risk of psychiatric disorders. A total of 2957 patients with IDA, with an increased risk of unipolar depressive disorder (OR=2.34, 95% CI=1.58~3.46), bipolar disorder (OR=5.78, 95% CI=2.23~15.05), anxiety disorder (OR=2.17, 95% CI=1.49~3.16), autism spectrum disorder (OR=3.08, 95% CI=1.79~5.28), attention deficit hyperactivity disorder (OR=1.67, 95% CI=1.29~2.17), tic disorder (OR=1.70, 95% CI=1.03~2.78), developmental delay (OR=2.45, 95% CI=2.00~3.00), and mental retardation (OR=2.70, 95% CI=2.00~3.65), were identified. A gender effect was noted, in that only female patients with IDA had an increased OR of bipolar disorder (OR=5.56, 95% CI=1.98~15.70) and tic disorder (OR=2.95, 95% CI=1.27~6.86). Iron deficiency increased the risk of psychiatric disorders, including mood disorders, autism spectrum disorder, attention deficit hyperactivity disorder, and developmental disorders. Further study is required to clarify the mechanism in the association between IDA and psychiatric disorder.

Vitamin D deficiency is a re-emerging epidemic, especially in minority populations. Vitamin D is crucial not only for bone health but for proper brain development and functioning. Low levels of vitamin D are associated with depression, seasonal affective disorder, and schizophrenia in adults, but little is known about vitamin D and mental health in the pediatric population. In Chapter 11, Gracious and colleagues assessed one hundred four adolescents presenting for acute mental health treatment over a 16-month period for vitamin D status and the relationship of 25-OH vitamin D levels to severity of illness, defined by presence of psychotic features. Vitamin D deficiency (25-OH D levels <20 ng/ml) was present in 34%; vitamin D insufficiency (25-OH D levels 20–30 ng/ml) was present in 38%, with a remaining 28% in the normal range. Adolescents with psychotic features had lower vitamin D levels (20.4 ng/ml vs. 24.7 ng/ml; p=0.04, 1 df). The association for vitamin D deficiency and psychotic features was substantial (OR 3.5; 95% CI 1.4-8.9; p <0.009). Race was independently associated with vitamin D deficiency and independently associated with psychosis for those who were Asian or biracial vs. white

(OR=3.8; 95% CI 1.1–13.4; p<0.04). Race was no longer associated with psychosis when the results were adjusted for vitamin D level. Vitamin D deficiency and insufficiency are both highly prevalent in adolescents with severe mental illness. The preliminary associations between vitamin D deficiency and presence of psychotic features warrant further investigation as to whether vitamin D deficiency is a mediator of illness severity, result of illness severity, or both. Higher prevalence of vitamin D deficiency but no greater risk of psychosis in African Americans, if confirmed, may have special implications for health disparity and treatment outcome research.

Breakfast consumption is associated with positive outcomes for diet quality, micronutrient intake, weight status and lifestyle factors. Breakfast has been suggested to positively affect learning in children in terms of behavior, cognitive, and school performance. However, these assertions are largely based on evidence which demonstrates acute effects of breakfast on cognitive performance. Less research which examines the effects of breakfast on the ecologically valid outcomes of academic performance or in-class behavior is available. In Chapter 12, Adolphus and colleagues searched the literature for articles published between 1950–2013 indexed in Ovid MEDLINE, Pubmed, Web of Science, the Cochrane Library, EMBASE databases, and PsychINFO. Thirty-six articles examining the effects of breakfast on in-class behavior and academic performance in children and adolescents were included. The effects of breakfast in different populations were considered, including undernourished or well-nourished children and adolescents from differing socio-economic status (SES) backgrounds. The habitual and acute effects of breakfast and the effects of school breakfast programs (SBPs) were considered. The evidence indicated a mainly positive effect of breakfast on on-task behavior in the classroom. There was suggestive evidence that habitual breakfast (frequency and quality) and SBPs have a positive effect on children's academic performance with clearest effects on mathematic and arithmetic grades in undernourished children. Increased frequency of habitual breakfast was consistently positively associated with academic performance. Some evidence suggested that quality of habitual breakfast, in terms of providing a greater variety of food groups and adequate energy, was positively related to school performance. However, these associations can be attributed, in part, to confounders such as SES and to methodological weaknesses such as the subjective nature of the observations of behavior in class.

Evidence suggests that flavonoid-rich foods are capable of inducing improvements in memory and cognition in animals and humans. However, there is a lack of clarity concerning whether flavonoids are the causal agents in inducing such behavioral responses. In Chapter 13, Rendeiro and colleagues show that supplementation with pure anthocyanins or pure flavanols for 6 weeks, at levels similar to that found in blueberry (2% w/w), results in an enhancement of spatial memory in 18 month old rats. Pure flavanols and pure anthocyanins were observed to induce significant improvements in spatial working memory ($p = 0.002$ and $p = 0.006$ respectively), to a similar extent to that following blueberry supplementation ($p = 0.002$). These behavioral changes were paralleled by increases in hippocampal brain-derived neurotrophic factor ($R = 0.46$, $p<0.01$), suggesting a common mechanism for the enhancement of memory. However, unlike protein levels of BDNF, the regional enhancement of BDNF mRNA expression in the hippocampus appeared to be predominantly enhanced by anthocyanins. The data support the claim that flavonoids are likely causal agents in mediating the cognitive effects of flavonoid-rich foods.

Extensive studies have demonstrated that oxidative stress plays a vital role in the pathology of several neurological diseases, including autism spectrum disorder (ASD); those studies proposed that GSH and antioxidant enzymes have a pathophysiological role in autism. Furthermore, camel milk has emerged to have potential therapeutic effects in autism. The aim of Al-Ayadhi and Elamin in Chapter 14 was to evaluate the effect of camel milk consumption on oxidative stress biomarkers in autistic children, by measuring the plasma levels of glutathione, superoxide dismutase, and myeloperoxidase before and 2 weeks after camel milk consumption, using the ELISA technique. All measured parameters exhibited significant increase after camel milk consumption. These findings suggest that camel milk could play an important role in decreasing oxidative stress by alteration of antioxidant enzymes and nonenzymatic antioxidant molecules levels, as well as the improvement of autistic behaviour as demonstrated by the improved Childhood Autism Rating Scale (CARS).

A central issue when designing multidimensional biological and psychosocial interventions for children who are exposed to multiple developmental risks is identification of the age period(s) in which such interventions will have the strongest and longest lasting effects (sensitive periods). In Chapter 15, Wachs and colleagues review nutritional, neuroscientific, and psychological evidence on this issue. Nutritional evidence is used to identify nutrient-sensitive periods of age-linked dimensions of brain development, with specific reference to iron deficiency. Neuroscience evidence is used to assess the importance of timing of exposures to environmental stressors for maintaining neural, neuroendocrine, and immune systems integrity. Psychological evidence illustrates the sensitivity of cognitive and social–emotional development to contextual risk and protective influences encountered at different ages. Evidence reviewed documents that the early years of life are a sensitive period when biological or psychosocial interventions or exposure to risk or protective contextual influences can produce unique long-term influences upon human brain, neuroendocrine, and cognitive or psychosocial development. However, the evidence does not identify the early years as the sole sensitive time period within which to have a significant influence upon development. Choice of age(s) to initiate interventions should be based on what outcomes are targeted and what interventions are used.

PART I

NUTRITION AND NEUROCOGNITIVE DEVELOPMENT

CHAPTER 1

NUTRITIONAL INFLUENCES ON HUMAN NEUROCOGNITIVE FUNCTIONING

MICHAEL A. SMITH AND ANDREW B. SCHOLEY

The notion that good nutrition is essential for adequate growth and sound physical wellbeing is very well established. Further, in recent years, there has been an overwhelming increase in research dedicated to better understanding how nutritional factors influence cognition and behavior (Riby et al., 2012). An aim of this Research Topic was to bring together Review, Opinion and Original Research articles reflecting the current science in this discipline. These include the effects of a range of foods and nutritional substrates on acute and chronic human neurocognitive functioning. The 13 accepted papers which form this Research Topic cover a diverse range of topics relating nutritional factors to neurocognitive functioning and performance. The articles demonstrate that neurocognitive performance is influenced by nutritional factors ranging from the dietary level (e.g., whole diet and meal composition) through to effects of macronutrients (such as glucose and omega-3 fatty acids) and micronutrients (vitamins, iron) on neurocognitive performance.

Nutritional Influences on Human Neurocognitive Functioning. © *Smith MA and Scholey AB.* Frontiers in Human Neuroscience, **8**,*358 (2014). doi:10.3389/fnhum.2014.00358. Licensed under Creative Commons Attribution 3.0 Unported License, http://creativecommons.org/licenses/by/3.0/.*

An objective of this research topic was to consider how various nutritional factors impact upon neurocognitive functioning at different stages of the lifespan. A number of the submissions focused on effects of nutrition in childhood, during which time nutrition plays an important role in growth and development, including via influences on constituents of the human central nervous system. A review by Nyaradi et al. (2013) considered the role of nutrition from a very broad perspective on neurocognitive development from the prenatal period through to childhood. This suggested that while observational studies have supported an important role for several individual nutrients (such as omega-3 fatty acids, B vitamins, iron) in the neurocognitive development of children, intervention studies aimed at supplementing intake of these individual nutrients have demonstrated inconclusive benefits. The authors of this review also highlighted the beneficial neurocognitive effects of breastfeeding and regular breakfast consumption as well as the impairing neurocognitive effects of childhood malnutrition. Kitsao-Wekulo et al. (2013) aimed to extend current understanding of this link between childhood malnutrition and poor cognitive outcomes, by investigating nutritional status as a mediator of the relationship between several socio-demographic variables and cognitive function in a sample of predominantly rural-dwelling Kenyan children. Nutritional status was found to mediate the relationship between socio-demographic factors and (i) language, (ii) motor function, and (iii) executive functioning in this study. With respect to specific micronutrient deficiencies that translate to adverse neurocognitive outcomes, Radlowski and Johnson (2013) reviewed the literature relating to the most common global nutrient deficiency, namely iron deficiency. They report that maternal anemia during the perinatal period increases the risk of delayed neurocognitive development. A further nutrient for which intake is typically below recommended levels in Western individuals is the omega-3 docosahexaenoic acid (DHA). Low dietary levels of this essential fatty acid are potentially problematic given (i) the involvement of this nutrient in mediating several critical brain functions, and (ii) DHA is derived from the diet alone. Similarly to the review of Nyaradi et al. (2013), Heaton et al. (2013) review concludes that dietary and plasma DHA levels in infancy appear to be associated with enhanced cognitive development, but that RCTs investigating infant DHA supplementation have been inconclusive with respect to beneficial effects on cognitive development. However, these authors note substantial methodological issues with RCTs of infant DHA supplementation studies, which could in part explain the equivocal findings (see also Meldrum et al., 2011). In a further review by Whiteley et al. (2013), it was argued that several dietary interventions have been effective in attenuating the neurocognitive and other adverse psychological outcomes in developmental disorders. The authors focused specifically on an intervention involving dietary elimination of gluten (the major protein in wheat, barley and rye) and casein (found in mammalian dairy products), and reported that this gluten and casein free dietary intervention was effective in enhancing such functions as language, attention and motor control in individuals with autism spectrum disorders.

Caroline Edmonds has conducted several studies investigating the influence of hydration status on cognitive functioning, with previous studies observing that access to water improves cognitive performance in children (Edmonds and Jeffes, 2009). In the paper included in this Research Topic, Edmonds et al. (2013) observed that beneficial effects of water consumption may be limited to individuals with relatively higher levels of subjective thirst, with thirsty individuals who were not provided with water exhibiting slower simple reaction times compared with (i) those who were administered water and (ii) those who were not administered water but reported lower levels of subjective thirst. In a further empirical study, Gibson et al. (2013) found that younger women with a higher dietary intake of saturated fat showed deficits in learning and memory.

Three papers accepted into our Research Topic considered the role of breakfast, which has been argued by many nutritionists to be the "most important meal of the day," in neurocognitive performance. A review by Adolphus et al. (2013) reported that (i) the quality and frequency of the habitual breakfast meal and (ii) engagement with school breakfast programmes in children and adolescents influences academic attainment. In addition Defeyter and Russo (2013) investigated the acute effect of breakfast consumption (compared to fasting) in adolescent non-habitual breakfast consumers, and observed that breakfast consumption enhanced verbal memory (under conditions of greater cognitive load) and backwards counting performance. However, no effects were observed in a range of other cognitive domains. Conversely, Zilberter and Zilberter (2013) highlight the equivocal findings of previous studies investigating the relationship between breakfast consumption and neurocognitive performance. These authors report that several different breakfast effects which have been investigated previously (e.g., glycemic load of the breakfast meal, nutritional composition, breakfast vs. no breakfast) have yielded positive, negative, and null effects on neurocognitive performance across a range of different populations under investigation. Thus it appears that more studies are needed to ascertain the specific benefits of breakfast on neurocognitive performance.

Finally, in recent years neuroimaging studies have made a substantial contribution to our understanding of the neurocognitive mechanisms underpinning nutritional influences on human cognitive performance. Three papers within this Research Topic specifically discuss the role of neuroimaging in investigating the link between nutrition and cognitive functioning. With respect to carbohydrate intake and neurocognitive performance, it is well established that glucose ingestion enhances memory performance, but no such beneficial memory effect of glucose is typically observed for emotionally laden stimuli (Smith et al., 2011). Schopf et al. (2013) report that following glucose ingestion, the hypothalamus becomes inactive in response to emotional material, providing a mechanistic explanation for the previously observed behavioral observations. Further, Jackson and Kennedy (2013) discuss the ways in which near-infrared spectroscopy has proven useful in detecting changes in cerebral blood flow following ingestion of dietary constituents including caffeine, polyphenols and omega-3 fatty acids. A paper which reviewed the literature relating to neuroimaging studies that have investigated the mechanisms underpinning the influence of early diet on cognitive and brain development by Isaacs (2013) provides a sound overview of the work which has been conducted on this topic.

In summary, it is clear that nutritional status, diet and the ingestion of a range of nutrients impacts upon neurocognitive development, function, and performance. The papers within this Research Topic consider a range of these effects. However, equivocal findings have emerged from many studies which have investigated the relationship between nutrition and cognition. Neuroimaging studies are informative with respect to the precise mechanisms which mediate these effects, and future studies in this area will contribute greatly to our understanding of the relationship between nutrition, diet and human neurocognitive functioning.

REFERENCES

1. Adolphus K., Lawton C. L., Dye L. (2013). The effects of breakfast on behavior and academic performance in children and adolescents. Front. Hum. Neurosci. 7:425 10.3389/fnhum.2013.00425

2. Defeyter M. A., Russo R. (2013). The effect of breakfast cereal consumption on adolescents' cognitive performance and mood. Front. Hum. Neurosci. 7:789 10.3389/fnhum.2013.00789

3. Edmonds C. J., Crombie R., Gardner M. R. (2013). Subjective thirst moderates changes in speed of responding associated with water consumption. Front. Hum. Neurosci. 7:363 10.3389/fnhum.2013.00363

4. Edmonds C. J., Jeffes B. (2009). Does having a drink help you think? 6-7-Year-old children show improvements in cognitive performance from baseline to test after having a drink of water. Appetite 53, 469–472 10.1016/j.appet.2009.10.002

5. Gibson E. L., Barr S., Jeanes Y. M. (2013). Habitual fat intake predicts memory function in younger women. Front. Hum. Neurosci. 7:838 10.3389/fnhum.2013.00838

6. Heaton A. E., Meldrum S. J., Foster J. K., Prescott S. L., Simmer K. (2013). Does docosahexaenoic acid supplementation in term infants enhance neurocognitive functioning in infancy? Front. Hum. Neurosci. 7:774 10.3389/fnhum.2013.00774

7. Isaacs E. B. (2013). Neuroimaging, a new tool for investigating the effects of early diet on cognitive and brain development. Front. Hum. Neurosci. 7:445 10.3389/fnhum.2013.00445

8. Jackson P. A., Kennedy D. O. (2013). The application of near infrared spectroscopy in nutritional intervention studies. Front. Hum. Neurosci. 7:473 10.3389/fnhum.2013.00473

9. Kitsao-Wekulo P., Holding P., Taylor H. G., Abubakar A., Kvalsvig J., Connolly K. (2013). Nutrition as an important mediator of the impact of background variables on outcome in middle childhood. Front. Hum. Neurosci. 7:713 10.3389/fnhum.2013.00713

10. Meldrum S. J., Smith M. A., Prescott S. L., Hird K., Simmer K. (2011). Achieving definitive results in long-chain polyunsaturated fatty acid supplementation trials of term infants: factors for consideration. Nutr. Rev. 69, 205–214 10.1111/j.1753-4887.2011.00381.x

11. Nyaradi A., Li J., Hickling S., Foster J., Oddy W. H. (2013). The role of nutrition in children's neurocognitive development, from pregnancy through childhood. Front. Hum. Neurosci. 7:97 10.3389/fnhum.2013.00097

12. Radlowski E. C., Johnson R. W. (2013). Perinatal iron deficiency and neurocognitive development. Front. Hum. Neurosci. 7:585 10.3389/fnhum.2013.00585

13. Riby L. M., Smith M. A., Foster J. K., editors. (eds.). (2012). Nutrition and Mental Performance: A Lifespan Perspective. London: Palgrave MacMillan

14. Schopf V., Fischmeister F. P., Windischberger C., Gerstl F., Wolzt M., Karlsson K. A. E., et al. (2013). Effects of individual glucose levels on the neuronal correlates of emotions. Front. Hum. Neurosci. 7:212 10.3389/fnhum.2013.00212
15. Smith M. A., Riby L. M., Eekelen J. A., Foster J. K. (2011). Glucose enhancement of human memory: a comprehensive research review of the glucose memory facilitation effect. Neurosci. Biobehav. Rev. 35, 770–783 10.1016/j.neubiorev.2010.09.008
16. Whiteley P., Shattock P., Knivsberg A. M., Seim A., Reichelt K. L., Todd L., et al. (2013). Gluten- and casein-free dietary intervention for autism spectrum conditions. Front. Hum. Neurosci. 6:344 10.3389/fnhum.2012.00344
17. Zilberter T., Zilberter E. Y. (2013). Breakfast and cognition: sixteen effects in nine populations, no single recipe. Front. Hum. Neurosci. 7:631 10.3389/fnhum.2013.00631

CHAPTER 2

DIETARY PATTERNS IN PREGNANCY AND EFFECTS ON NUTRIENT INTAKE IN THE MID-SOUTH: THE CONDITIONS AFFECTING NEUROCOGNITIVE DEVELOPMENT AND LEARNING IN EARLY CHILDHOOD (CANDLE) STUDY

ESZTER VÖLGYI, KECIA N. CARROLL, MARION E. HARE, KAREN RINGWALD-SMITH, CHANDRIKA PIYATHILAKE, WONSUK YOO, AND FRANCES A. TYLAVSKY

2.1 INTRODUCTION

Pregnancy is a time when in utero exposures may impact the long term programming for onset of diseases in offspring [1,2,3]. Dietary intake during pregnancy has the potential to influence birth outcomes [4,5] and cognitive development via gene expression [6]. As dietary habits are often cultural and influenced by the food available for consumption, under-

Dietary Patterns in Pregnancy and Effects on Nutrient Intake in the Mid-South: The Conditions Affecting Neurocognitive Development and Learning in Early Childhood (CANDLE) Study. © Völgyi E, Carroll KN, Hare ME, Ringwald-Smith K, Piyathilake C, Yoo W and Tylavsky FA. Nutrients, **5**,5 (2013). doi:10.3390/nu5051511. Licensed under Creative Commons Attribution 3.0 Unported License, http://creativecommons.org/licenses/by/3.0/.

standing the characteristics of diet within a study population may provide a basis for future interventions to improve lifelong health.

Multivariate statistical methods such as factor analysis has become a well-accepted and popular method [7] to describe dietary patterns in nutritional research. Much of the work has investigated the effects of diet on the risk of adverse outcomes such as colorectal cancer [8,9,10], diabetes and obesity [11,12], and stroke [13]. More recently this approach has been used to characterize diet during pregnancy and relate patterns to nutrient intake, lifestyle and socio-demographic characteristics [14,15,16]. These efforts have provided evidence that dietary patterns may reflect differences in nutrient intake and are sensitive to differences across socio-economic strata or cultural habits.

The Conditions Affecting Neurocognitive Development and Learning in Early Childhood (CANDLE) study is a prospective study that includes a cohort of mother-child dyads. Enrollment for this cohort occurs during the second trimester of pregnancy. The study's primary aim is to identify factors from in utero through early childhood that contribute to cognitive development by age 3. Consistent with life course theory [17] capturing dietary exposure during gestation may be critical in untangling the role of nutrition in the trajectory of early childhood cognitive development. The objectives of this study are to describe a unique process to determine dietary patterns from a food frequency questionnaire (FFQ) that are region specific for the Mid-South, and to examine how these patterns relate to socio-demographic status of the study population, and nutrients (omega 3 fatty acids, folate, pyridoxine, iron, zinc, cobalamin, choline) [18] plausibly linked to neurocognitive development.

2.2 EXPERIMENTAL SECTION

2.2.1 STUDY POPULATION

Data from pregnant women who enrolled in the CANDLE study between December 2006 and July 2011 were included in this study. Inclusion criteria included being: a resident of Shelby County Tennessee, able to speak and understand English, aged between 16 and 40 years old, and 16–28 weeks of gestation with a singleton pregnancy.

Exclusion criteria included: an existing chronic disease requiring medication (hypertension, insulin dependent or Type II diabetes mellitus, sickle cell disease or trait, renal disease, hepatitis, lupus erythematous, scleroderma, pulmonary disease, heart disease, human immunodeficiency virus); pregnancy complications including maternal red cell alloimmunization (Rh factor incompatibility permitted); prolapsed or ruptured membranes; oligohydraminios; complete placenta previa; and not intending to deliver at one of four participating hospitals. The study was conducted in accordance with the Helsinki Declaration and was approved and reviewed by the Institutional Review Board of the University of Tennessee Health Science Center. Informed consent was given by all subjects 18 years or older and assent was given by those aged 16–17.9 years with consent provided by their legally authorized representative prior to the assessments.

2.2.2 DEMOGRAPHIC, LIFESTYLE AND SOCIOECONOMIC ASSESSMENT

Research assistants collected information on family income, participant race, ethnicity, marital status, and parity and household composition through self-administered questionnaires. Pre-pregnancy body height and weight were recorded based on self report of the women. We calculated pre-pregnancy body mass index (BMI) as weight (kg) per height (m²).

2.2.3 DIETARY ASSESSMENT

The Block (2005) food frequency questionnaire (FFQ) was administered during the second trimester by trained research assistants to elicit usual intake of 111 food and beverage groups from the previous three months. Interviewers were trained by registered dietitians and re-certified by a registered dietician based on a taped interview every six months to obtain the frequency of intake and quantity consumed with the aid of standardized food pictures. The FFQ was processed by Nutrition Quest (Berkley, CA, USA) to yield macro and micronutrients, serving size and frequency of intake of the food items. The full Block FFQ has been shown to be a valid and reliable method to describe nutrient intake from diet for groups and rank individuals according to nutrients [19,20,21,22,23].

Of 1503 women who completed the enrollment visit, we excluded respondents who reported implausibly low (<1000) or high (>5000) kcal/day of total energy intake (n = 152). Willett [24] reports using an allowable energy range of 500–3500 for non-pregnant, non-lactating women which we adapted for the increased energy needs of pregnancy. Due to technical issues, 196 participants' FFQ data was unable to be retrieved for determining nutrient intake. The final sample size for this study was 1155.

2.2.4 FOOD PATTERN DETERMINATION

Exploratory factor analysis with principal component extraction and varimax rotation method was performed on the frequency of the 111 food and beverage groups to extract the factors that make up distinct dietary patterns. To decide the number of factors to retain, we used the scree plot and the eigenvalues of the principal components, and subjective criteria. We tested solutions for number of models with two to five factors in order to evaluate the interpretability of the dietary patterns. Food groups with a factor loading above 0.30 were considered as the most important contributors to each factor, and were used to identify the dietary patterns. Three factors were identified in our population. These single dietary patterns were termed "Healthy", "Processed", and "US-Southern" based on the food groups that loaded for each of the three factors. For each participant, a factor score in the respective single dietary pattern was estimated as a sum of the daily frequency of intake of each food group multiplied by the loading score for the food group. Theoretically the food groups with high daily intake and high factor loading contributed most to the individual's score in the respective single dietary pattern.

Because the total explained variance of the three single dietary patterns was 15.4%, we explored the use of rank percentiles in order to combine the three major dietary factors, as done elsewhere [16]. After carefully evaluating the factor scores, combined food patterns were created based on the individuals' rank order in each single factor. Five quintiles were created in each factor based on the individual's factor scores. (1) Single food patterns (Healthy, Processed, and US Southern dietary patterns) were created if the woman was at least two quintiles higher in one factor than in the other two single dietary factors. (2) A combined dietary pattern was assigned if the individual was at least two quintiles higher in two single dietary patterns than in the third factor. In this way, combined dietary patterns were created as Healthy-Processed (H-P), Healthy-US Southern (H-S), and Processed-US Southern (P-S). (3) If the study participant had less than two quintiles difference between all three single dietary patterns, she was classified with the overall Mixed dietary pattern. As a result, women were grouped into seven mutually exclusive dietary patterns (Healthy, Processed, US Southern, H-P, H-S, P-S, and Mixed), reflecting their primary food choices. Initially, we separated dairy products, salad dressing, and some meat products into low fat and high fat groups. Differential consumption of these foods did not seem to have effect on factor loadings; therefore, we kept low and high fat items in one group.

2.2.5 STATISTICAL ANALYSIS

All continuous data were checked for normality by Shapiro-Wilk's W test and for homogeneity by Levene's test before each analysis. Descriptive results are reported as mean ± SE. Body mass index for adults was classified as underweight (<18.5 kg/m^2), normal (18.5–24.9 kg/m^2), overweight (25–29.9 kg/m^2), and obese (>30.0 kg/m^2). Median test and Kruskal-Wallis ANOVA were used to describe the differences in the demographics and food items among the dietary patterns. Analysis of covariance (ANCOVA) with daily energy intake (kcal/day) as a covariate was used to describe the differences in the macro- and micronutrients among the dietary patterns. The post-hoc group differences were evaluated using a Tukey adjustment for multiple comparisons. Multiple regression analysis was performed to describe the explained variance in the macro- and micronutrients by the energy adjusted dietary patterns. All analyses were performed using Statistica v10 (StatSoft Inc., Tulsa, OK, USA) and JMP v9.0 (SAS Institute,

Cary, NC, USA). A p-value of less than 0.05 was considered statistically significant.

2.3 RESULTS

2.3.1 DESCRIPTION OF THE STUDY PARTICIPANTS

Overall, the mean age of the study population was 26.5 ± 5.4 years (range 16 to 40 years). One third of the women in the study population were obese (30%) and one quarter were overweight (24%) before their pregnancies. The women were predominantly African-American (AA) (62%) and 54% of the total sample had a high school degree or less. The number of individuals living in the household ranged from 2 to 11 with the average household size of 4.3 persons, and 37% were single (data not shown).

2.3.2 DIETARY PATTERNS

Factor loadings of the food items for each of the single dietary patterns that had a minimum of 0.30 factor loading are presented in Table 1. The Healthy dietary pattern was characterized by high factor loadings of vegetables, fruits, non-fried fish and chicken, and water. The Processed dietary pattern represents those who consume primarily processed meat, fast food items (items typically obtained from Western-style fast food restaurants), snacks, sweets, and soft drinks. The US Southern pattern was characterized by the typical US Southern foods such as eggs, cooked cereals, peaches, corn, fried fish, beans, greens, cabbage, sweet potatoes, liver, pig's feet, neck bones oxtails, and tongue, pork, and real fruit juices.

Our statistical approach resulted in 135 (12%) women categorized as Healthy; 98 (8%) as Processed; 120 (10%) as US Southern; 136 (12%) as P-S; 123 (11%) as H-P; 98 (8%) as H-S; and 445 (39%) as Mixed (Table 2). The seven dietary patterns reflect differences in the daily frequency of intakes for the 62 food and beverage groups that loaded from factor analyses from ($p < 0.001$). There were no differences in foods that were commonly consumed by all participants such as cold cereal and milk on cereal and for foods consumed relatively infrequently by only a few participants (menudo, oysters and diet shakes). Overall the daily frequency of the food and beverage items/groups reflects the influence of the respective single pattern when combining the single diet pattern scores. The overall Mixed dietary pattern obtained from the Healthy, Processed and US Southern reflect foods from all of the single, i.e., H-P pattern represents primarily healthy foods but contains some pertinent processed foods. The largest group of mixed patterns contained pertinent food items from all single diet patterns. There were no food items that distinguished it from the three single and three combined dietary patterns. The contribution of the food items from the single diet patterns' (Healthy, US Southern, Processed) to the mixed groups (H-S, H-P, S-P) could be considered as positive influences (fruits, nuts, seeds, vegetables) or negative influences (salty snacks, higher fat items) on the nutrient density of the diets. For example, in the H-S group there was a slightly higher intake of yogurt than those who reported a "pure US Southern diet", which has positive influences on calcium and the B complex nutrients. On the other hand, in the H-S group, there was a mildly negative influence of salty snacks that could increase a lower nutrient dense diet. Of the 62 food groups that loaded on the three main groups, there were increases in daily frequency for 39 "healthy" foods that would boost the nutrient density of the diet (62%) and a negative influence on nutrient density from 6 (10%) "less healthy foods" for those in the H-S pattern (Table 2). In contrast the mixed groups that had combined with the Processed group, showed a 25% increase in "negative nutrient dense foods" and 32% increase in nutrient dense foods for the H-P pattern and only a 20% increase in positive nutrient dense foods for those consuming a P-S pattern. From regression analyses the energy adjusted dietary patterns explained 90% of the variance in total fat intake, 84% for protein, 89% for carbohydrate. Regression analyses also showed the energy adjusted dietary patterns explained 62% of the variance for omega3, 65% for sugar, 62% for fiber, 75% for iron, 76% for zinc, 65% for B_6, 51% for B_{12}, 59% for folate, 78% for thiamine, 76% for niacin, 74% for riboflavin, 73% for total choline and 78% for free choline. The explained variances are based on the R^2 of the regression model.

TABLE 1: Factor loadings of food and beverage items/groups in the three main factors.

Food Item (Variance Explained)	Healthy (5.8%)	Processed (5.1%)	US Southern (4.4%)
BREAKFAST ITEMS			
Eggs			0.344
Breakfast sausage including in sandwiches/biscuits		0.301	0.311
Bacon			0.367
Cooked cereals (oatmeal, grits, cream of wheat)			0.320
Breakfast or cereal bars	0.308		
DAIRY			
Yogurt, including frozen	0.434		
Cheese, sliced or spreads		0.332	
Milk as a beverage	0.303		
FRUITS			
Banana	0.334		
Apples or pears	0.355		
Peaches or nectarines, fresh			0.352
Canned fruit			0.374
Strawberries or other berries in season	0.383		
VEGETABLES			
Broccoli	0.331		0.312
Carrots or mixed vegetables with carrots	0.471		
Corn			0.316
Green beans or green peas			0.407
Spinach, cooked	0.370		
Greens (collards, turnip, or mustard)			0.517
Sweet potatoes, yams			0.360
Fried potatoes (French fries, home fries, hash browns)		0.563	
Cole slaw, cabbage, Chinese cabbage			0.444
Green salad, lettuce salad	0.600		
Tomatoes, raw	0.524		
Other vegetables (squash, cauliflower, okra, peppers)	0.547		
Pinto, black or baked beans, chili with beans	0.304		
Vegetable, vegetable-beef or tomato soup	0.337		

TABLE 1: *Cont.*

Food Item (Variance Explained)	Healthy (5.8%)	Processed (5.1%)	US Southern (4.4%)
BREADS			
Sandwich buns		0.469	
Bagels, English muffins, dinner rolls	0.339		
Cornbread, corn muffins, hush puppies			0.380
Sliced bread (white, dark, whole wheat)		0.310	
CONDIMENTS			
Salad dressing, regular or low fat	0.541		
Mayonnaise, sandwich breads		0.372	
Ketchup, salsa or chili peppers		0.450	
Mustard, barbecue sauce, soy sauce, gravy etc.		0.322	
SWEETS AND SNACKS			
Donuts		0.304	
Cake, snack cakes, cupcakes, Ho-Hos, pastries		0.437	
Cookies		0.407	
Chocolate candy		0.392	
Candy, hard, skittles, starburst etc.		0.358	
Snack chips like potato chips, tortilla chips, Fritos, Doritos, popcorn		0.552	
MEAT, FISH, POULTRY, MEAT SUBSTITUTES			
Pizza		0.328	
Meat substitutes (veggie burgers, chicken, hot dogs or lunch meats)	0.346		
Hamburgers or cheese burgers		0.504	
Hot dogs or sausage (Polish, Italian or chorizo)		0.342	
Lunch meats (turkey or regular)		0.393	
Tacos, burritos, enchiladas, tamales with meat or chicken		0.306	
Ribs, spareribs			0.373
Liver (chicken livers or liverwurst)			0.319
Pigs feet, neck bones, oxtails, tongue			0.419
Beef or pork dishes (beef stew, pot pie, hamburger helper)			0.319
Fried chicken (nuggets, wings or patties)		0.497	

TABLE 1: *Cont.*

Food Item (Variance Explained)	Healthy (5.8%)	Processed (5.1%)	US Southern (4.4%)
Roasted or broiled chicken or turkey	0.354		
Fried fish or fish sandwich			0.378
Fish not fried	0.435		
Peanut Butter	0.378		
Peanuts, sunflower seeds, or other nuts and seeds	0.348		
BEVERAGES			
100% orange or grapefruit juice			0.310
Hi-C, Cranberry Juice Cocktail, Hawaiian Punch, Tang		0.309	
Kool-aid, lemonade, sports drinks, or fruit flavored drinks		0.356	
Soft drinks (Coke, Sprite, Orange) regular or diet		0.377	
Water tap or bottled	0.320		

Only those food items are presented that had a minimum of 0.30 factor loading. In a supplementary table, all food and beverage items' factor loadings are available for each main factor (Supplementary Table S1).

2.3.3 CHARACTERISTICS OF PARTICIPANTS

The characteristics of the study participants according by dietary patterns appear in Table 3. Compared to the US Southern, Processed or Mixed dietary patterns women with the Healthy dietary pattern were more likely to be older ($p < 0.0001$), have a higher level of education ($p < 0.0001$), less likely to be single mothers ($p < 0.0001$), and less likely to be obese prior to pregnancy ($p = 0.0044$). The diet patterns aligned across race categories (Figure 1). Healthy and H-P patterns were consumed more by Caucasians and women in the "other" race category (Asians, American Indians, Alaska Native, Native Hawaiian, other Pacific Islander). In contrast, African Americans disproportionately were the highest consumers of the Processed, US Southern, P-S, and H-S dietary patterns. There were no significant differences in ethnicity, household size, and parity among the dietary patterns.

TABLE 2: Average monthly frequency of intake of food groups in the seven dietary patterns[1].

Food Groups	Healthy (n = 135)	Processed (n = 98)	Southern (n = 120)	H-P (n = 123)	H-S (n = 98)	P-S (n = 136)	Mixed (n = 445)
BREAKFAST ITEMS							
Eggs	4.4 ± 0.6	4.6 ± 0.7	7.2 ± 0.6	4.3 ± 0.6	10 ± 0.7	7.9 ± 0.6	5.7 ± 0.3
Breakfast sausage including in sandwiches/biscuits	0.8 ± 0.5	4.9 ± 0.6	5.8 ± 0.5	3.0 ± 0.5	3.3 ± 0.6	9.7 ± 0.5	4.0 ± 0.3
Bacon	1.7 ± 0.6	5.5 ± 0.6	7.4 ± 0.6	2.9 ± 0.6	5.2 ± 0.6	8.5 ± 0.5	4.5 ± 0.3
Cooked cereals (oatmeal, grits, cream of wheat)	5.2 ± 0.7	2.8 ± 0.8	7.5 ± 0.7	3.1 ± 0.7	11.0 ± 0.8	5.2 ± 0.7	5.1 ± 0.4
Breakfast or cereal bars	6.6 ± 0.6	2.4 ± 0.7	2.8 ± 0.6	7.0 ± 0.6	4.9 ± 0.7	1.8 ± 0.6	4.6 ± 0.3
DAIRY							
Yogurt, including frozen	11.1 ± 0.7	2.0 ± 0.8	3.5 ± 0.7	7.2 ± 0.7	9.6 ± 0.8	2.8 ± 0.7	5.6 ± 0.4
Cheese, sliced or spreads	16.3 ± 0.8	18.9 ± 1.0	10.7 ± 0.9	21.2 ± 0.9	13.9 ± 1.0	15.5 ± 0.8	15.5 ± 0.5
Milk as a beverage	16.7 ± 1.0	6.9 ± 1.2	8.7 ± 1.1	14.7 ± 1.1	14.7 ± 1.2	7.2 ± 1.0	12.0 ± 0.6
FRUITS							
Banana	9.7 ± 0.7	3.7 ± 0.8	6.2 ± 0.8	6.8 ± 0.7	11.2 ± 0.8	5.4 ± 0.7	6.6 ± 0.4
Apples or pears	11.1 ± 0.7	3.2 ± 0.8	7.4 ± 0.8	6.2 ± 0.7	13.7 ± 0.8	7.2 ± 0.7	7.3 ± 0.4
Canned fruit	2.5 ± 0.3	5.0 ± 0.8	7.9 ± 0.8	4.3 ± 0.6	8.8 ± 1.0	7.7 ± 0.8	6.1 ± 0.4
Peaches or nectarines, fresh	2.3 ± 0.5	1.3 ± 0.6	5.0 ± 0.5	1.9 ± 0.5	7.4 ± 0.6	3.5 ± 0.5	3.2 ± 0.3
Strawberries or other berries in season	9.2 ± 0.6	2.8 ± 0.7	4.7 ± 0.7	6.3 ± 0.7	9.8 ± 0.7	3.9 ± 0.6	5.9 ± 0.3
VEGETABLES							
Broccoli	4.3 ± 0.5	1.9 ± 0.6	4.2 ± 0.5	3.8 ± 0.5	8.6 ± 0.6	3.7 ± 0.5	4.1 ± 0.3
Carrots or mixed vegetables with carrots	6.6 ± 0.5	1.3 ± 0.6	2.4 ± 0.5	4.5 ± 0.5	7.5 ± 0.6	2.0 ± 0.5	3.7 ± 0.3
Corn	3.4 ± 0.5	3.2 ± 0.5	4.9 ± 0.5	5.0 ± 0.5	6.8 ± 0.5	4.9 ± 0.5	5.0 ± 0.3

TABLE 2: *Cont.*

Food Groups	Healthy (n = 135)	Processed (n = 98)	Southern (n = 120)	H-P (n = 123)	H-S (n = 98)	P-S (n = 136)	Mixed (n = 445)
Green beans or green peas	5.1 ± 0.5	3.6 ± 0.6	6.5 ± 0.5	5.5 ± 0.5	10.2 ± 0.6	5.6 ± 0.5	6.3 ± 0.3
Spinach, cooked	2.6 ± 0.3	0.6 ± 0.4	1.3 ± 0.3	1.9 ± 0.3	4.5 ± 0.4	0.6 ± 0.3	1.2 ± 0.2
Greens (collards, turnip, or mustard)	0.6 ± 0.3	1.0 ± 0.4	3.3 ± 0.4	0.9 ± 0.3	4.8 ± 0.4	3.1 ± 0.3	2.3 ± 0.2
Sweet potatoes, yams	1.4 ± 0.2	0.8 ± 0.3	1.8 ± 0.2	0.8 ± 0.2	3.3 ± 0.3	1.4 ± 0.2	1.3 ± 0.1
Fried potatoes (French fries, home fries, hash browns)	3.0 ± 0.6	13.1 ± 0.7	4.6 ± 0.6	8.9 ± 0.6	4.0 ± 0.7	11.7 ± 0.6	7.6 ± 0.3
Cole slaw, cabbage, Chinese cabbage	1.00 ± 0.2	0.7 ± 0.3	2.0 ± 0.3	0.8 ± 0.3	4.1 ± 0.3	1.7 ± 0.2	1.6 ± 0.1
Green salad, lettuce salad	13.20 ± 0.6	3.9 ± 0.7	5.0 ± 0.6	10.4 ± 0.6	12.1 ± 0.7	3.5 ± 0.6	7.6 ± 0.3
Tomatoes, raw	10.40 ± 0.6	2.6 ± 0.7	2.2 ± 0.6	9.7 ± 0.6	7.5 ± 0.7	2.2 ± 0.6	5.3 ± 0.3
Other vegetables (squash, cauliflower, okra, peppers)	7.00 ± 0.4	0.7 ± 0.5	1.4 ± 0.5	5.1 ± 0.5	8.4 ± 0.5	1.0 ± 0.4	2.7 ± 0.2
Pinto, black or baked beans, chili with beans	3.30 ± 0.3	1.6 ± 0.3	1.3 ± 0.3	2.9 ± 0.3	2.3 ± 0.3	1.6 ± 0.3	2.2 ± 0.1
Vegetable, vegetable-beef or tomato soup	2.1 ± 0.2	0.6 ± 0.3	1.2 ± 0.2	1.2 ± 0.2	2.3 ± 0.3	0.7 ± 0.2	1.5 ± 0.1
BREADS							
Sandwich buns	3.0 ± 0.5	9.4 ± 0.5	3.1 ± 0.5	7.1 ± 0.5	2.5 ± 0.5	6.6 ± 0.5	5.5 ± 0.3
Bagels, English muffins, dinner rolls	4.8 ± 0.4	2.2 ± 0.5	1.6 ± 0.5	6.1 ± 0.5	3.6 ± 0.5	1.9 ± 0.4	3.7 ± 0.2
Cornbread, corn muffins, hush puppies	0.6 ± 0.3	2.0 ± 0.4	2.1 ± 0.3	1.1 ± 0.3	2.3 ± 0.4	3.8 ± 0.3	2.5 ± 0.2
Sliced bread (white, dark, whole wheat)	12.6 ± 0.8	15.8 ± 1.0	8.3 ± 0.9	16.2 ± 0.9	11.1 ± 1	11.2 ± 0.8	12.2 ± 0.5
CONDIMENTS							
Salad dressing, regular or low fat	12.1 ± 0.6	4.9 ± 0.7	5.2 ± 0.7	10.7 ± 0.7	11.9 ± 0.7	4.4 ± 0.6	8.5 ± 0.3
Mayonnaise, sandwich breads	3.3 ± 0.6	9.8 ± 0.7	3.5 ± 0.7	6.9 ± 0.6	4 ± 0.7	8.7 ± 0.6	6.1 ± 0.3
Ketchup, salsa or chili peppers	6.3 ± 0.6	11.9 ± 0.7	3.4 ± 0.7	11 ± 0.6	3.7 ± 0.7	9 ± 0.6	6.7 ± 0.3

TABLE 2: *Cont.*

Food Groups	Healthy (n = 135)	Processed (n = 98)	Southern (n = 120)	H-P (n = 123)	H-S (n = 98)	P-S (n = 136)	Mixed (n = 445)
Mustard, barbecue sauce, soy sauce, gravy, etc.	6.3 ± 0.6	8.5 ± 0.7	3.3 ± 0.6	9.3 ± 0.6	5.5 ± 0.7	6.4 ± 0.6	6.0 ± 0.3
SWEETS AND SNACKS							
Donuts	0.7 ± 0.2	1.2 ± 0.2	0.4 ± 0.2	1.6 ± 0.2	0.4 ± 0.2	1.5 ± 0.2	1.1 ± 0.1
Cake, snack cakes, cupcakes, Ho-Hos, pastries	1.8 ± 0.5	8.2 ± 0.5	1.5 ± 0.5	4.6 ± 0.5	1.3 ± 0.5	5.3 ± 0.5	2.9 ± 0.3
Cookies	3.6 ± 0.5	5.5 ± 0.5	1.5 ± 0.5	7.1 ± 0.5	1.7 ± 0.5	4.0 ± 0.5	3.7 ± 0.3
Chocolate candy	4.2 ± 0.6	9.6 ± 0.7	1.3 ± 0.6	8.2 ± 0.6	1.9 ± 0.7	5.5 ± 0.6	4.3 ± 0.3
Candy, hard, skittles, starburst, etc.	2.3 ± 0.6	6.6 ± 0.6	2.4 ± 0.6	4.8 ± 0.6	2.4 ± 0.6	6.1 ± 0.6	4.3 ± 0.3
Snack chips like potato chips, tortilla chips, Fritos, Doritos, popcorn	6.3 ± 0.7	17.9 ± 0.8	4.5 ± 0.7	12.1 ± 0.7	5.2 ± 0.8	14.6 ± 0.7	8.7 ± 0.4
MEAT, FISH, POULTRY, MEAT SUBSTITUTES							
Pizza	2.7 ± 0.4	5.2 ± 0.4	2.7 ± 0.4	4.6 ± 0.4	2.4 ± 0.4	5.5 ± 0.4	3.7 ± 0.2
Meat substitutes (veggie burgers, chicken, hot dogs or lunch meats)	1.7 ± 0.2	0.0 ± 0.2	0 ± 0.2	0.8 ± 0.2	0.5 ± 0.2	0.0 ± 0.2	0.2 ± 0.1
Hamburgers or cheese burgers	1.7 ± 0.4	9.0 ± 0.5	3.2 ± 0.4	4.6 ± 0.4	2 ± 0.5	7.9 ± 0.4	4.2 ± 0.2
Hot dogs or sausage (Polish, Italian or chorizo)	0.8 ± 0.3	3.9 ± 0.4	2.6 ± 0.4	2.0 ± 0.4	1.9 ± 0.4	5.8 ± 0.3	2.6 ± 0.2
Lunch meats (turkey or regular)	4.8 ± 0.6	9.5 ± 0.7	4.1 ± 0.6	7.8 ± 0.6	4.6 ± 0.7	9.0 ± 0.6	6.2 ± 0.3
Tacos, burritos, enchiladas, tamales with meat or chicken	2.2 ± 0.3	3.8 ± 0.3	1.8 ± 0.3	3.8 ± 0.3	1.8 ± 0.3	3.4 ± 0.3	2.7 ± 0.2
Ribs, spareribs	0.2 ± 0.1	0.5 ± 0.1	0.6 ± 0.1	0.2 ± 0.1	0.5 ± 0.1	1.2 ± 0.1	0.6 ± 0.1
Liver (chicken livers or liverwurst)	0.1 ± 0.1	0.1 ± 0.1	0.2 ± 0.1	0.0 ± 0.1	0.7 ± 0.1	0.3 ± 0.1	0.2 ± 0.1
Pig's feet, neck bones, oxtails, tongue	0.0 ± 0.1	0.2 ± 0.1	0.4 ± 0.1	0.0 ± 0.1	0.2 ± 0.1	0.8 ± 0.1	0.2 ± 0.1

TABLE 2: *Cont.*

Food Groups	Healthy (n = 135)	Processed (n = 98)	Southern (n = 120)	H-P (n = 123)	H-S (n = 98)	P-S (n = 136)	Mixed (n = 445)
Beef or pork dishes (beef stew, pot pie, hamburger helper)	0.6 ± 0.1	1.5 ± 0.2	1.8 ± 0.2	0.8 ± 0.2	1 ± 0.2	2.7 ± 0.2	1.3 ± 0.1
Fried chicken (nuggets, wings or patties)	1.2 ± 0.5	8.2 ± 0.6	4.4 ± 0.5	3.9 ± 0.5	3.0 ± 0.6	9.5 ± 0.5	5.1 ± 0.3
Roasted or broiled chicken or turkey	5.2 ± 0.4	2.6 ± 0.5	2.1 ± 0.4	4.5 ± 0.4	5.9 ± 0.5	2.4 ± 0.4	3.9 ± 0.2
Fried fish or fish sandwich	0.3 ± 0.2	1.1 ± 0.2	1.6 ± 0.2	0.6 ± 0.2	1.2 ± 0.2	2.4 ± 0.2	1.4 ± 0.1
Fish not fried	2.5 ± 0.2	0.3 ± 0.2	0.4 ± 0.2	1.6 ± 0.2	1.7 ± 0.2	0.3 ± 0.2	0.8 ± 0.1
Peanut Butter	6.7 ± 0.5	2.4 ± 0.6	1.9 ± 0.6	8.6 ± 0.6	4.8 ± 0.6	2.0 ± 0.5	4.1 ± 0.3
Peanuts, sunflower seeds, or other nuts and seeds	5.5 ± 0.4	0.9 ± 0.5	1.5 ± 0.5	3.7 ± 0.4	4.3 ± 0.5	1.3 ± 0.4	2.3 ± 0.2
BEVERAGES							
100% orange or grapefruit juice	5.4 ± 0.8	8.3 ± 0.9	9.4 ± 0.8	8.3 ± 0.8	12.5 ± 0.9	10.5 ± 0.8	9.4 ± 0.4
Hi-C, Cranberry Juice Cocktail, Hawaiian Punch, Tang	0.8 ± 0.6	6.6 ± 0.8	5.5 ± 0.7	2.6 ± 0.7	3.3 ± 0.8	9.2 ± 0.6	4.7 ± 0.4
Kool-aid, lemonade, sports drinks, or fruit flavored drinks	3.4 ± 0.7	10.9 ± 0.9	5.8 ± 0.8	5.6 ± 0.8	3.5 ± 0.9	12.8 ± 0.7	6.7 ± 0.4
Soft drinks (Coke, Sprite, Orange) regular or diet	5.9 ± 0.8	17.4 ± 0.9	2.7 ± 0.8	12.6 ± 0.8	2.5 ± 0.9	11.0 ± 0.8	7.5 ± 0.4
Water tap or bottled	29.9 ± 0.6	23 ± 0.7	25.3 ± 0.7	28.8 ± 0.7	29 ± 0.7	21.6 ± 0.6	26.9 ± 0.3
Coffee, regular or decaffeinated	9.7 ± 0.6	1.7 ± 0.7	0.4 ± 0.7	7.4 ± 0.7	1.2 ± 0.7	0.7 ± 0.6	2.0 ± 0.3

H-P, Healthy-Processed pattern; H-S, Healthy-US Southern pattern; P-S, Processed-US Southern pattern.1 All values represent means ± SE; ANOVA conducted to examine differences across the seven dietary patterns for each food item showed differences at $p < 0.001$.

TABLE 3: Basic characteristics of the study participants by dietary patterns.

Variable	Healthy	Processed	US Southern	H-P	H-S	P-S	Mixed	p 1
N	135	98	120	123	98	136	445	
Age, y (mean ± SE)	30.3 ± 0.38	24.1 ± 0.49	25.2 ± 0.52	28.5 ± 4.95	27.7 ± 0.74	23.4 ± 0.40	26.2 ± 0.24	<0.0001
Height, cm (mean ± SE)	166 ± 0.64	163 ± 0.79	163 ± 0.65	164 ± 0.67	166 ± 0.74	163 ± 0.59	164 ± 0.24	0.0009
Pre-pregnancy weight, kg (mean ± SE)	68.3 ± 1.40	75.1 ± 2.35	78.1 ± 2.45	72.4 ± 1.69	77.5 ± 2.10	71.9 ± 1.82	76.2 ± 0.99	0.0005
Race, n (%)								
Caucasian	121 (90)	19 (19)	8 (7)	97 (79)	13 (13)	3 (2)	140 (32)	<0.001
African American	7 (5)	79 (81)	110 (92)	24 (20)	74 (76)	131 (98)	294 (66)	
Other	7 (5)	0 (0)	2 (2)	2 (2)	11 (11)	0 (0)	9 (2)	
Ethnicity, n (%)								
Hispanic	3 (2)	0 (0)	1 (1)	4 (3)	2 (2)	1 (1)	15 (3)	0.2424
Non-Hispanic	132 (98)	97 (100)	119 (99)	117 (97)	95 (98)	133 (99)	425 (97)	
Pre-pregnancy BMI 2, n (%)								
Underweight	7 (5)	3 (3)	5 (4)	1 (1)	3 (3)	9 (7)	19 (4)	0.0044
Normal	83 (61)	38 (39)	48 (40)	64 (52)	37 (38)	55 (40)	146 (33)	
Overweight	19 (14)	25 (25)	17 (14)	28 (23)	23 (23)	36 (26)	134 (30)	
Obese	26 (19)	32 (33)	47 (39)	30 (24)	35 (36)	36 (26)	145 (33)	
Parity, n (%)								
Primipara	66 (49)	44 (45)	57 (48)	49 (40)	37 (38)	47 (65)	189 (42)	0.2051
Multipara	69 (51)	54 (55)	63 (53)	74 (60)	61 (62)	89 (35)	256 (58)	
Education, n (%)								

TABLE 3: *Cont.*

Variable	Healthy	Processed	US Southern	H-P	H-S	P-S	Mixed	p 1
Less than high school	0 (0)	16 (16)	16 (13)	3 (2)	7 (7)	29 (21)	37 (8)	<0.0001
High school or GED	23 (17)	55 (56)	62 (52)	37 (30)	41 (42)	80 (59)	216 (49)	
Technical school	8 (6)	10 (10)	12 (10)	9 (7)	11 (11)	17 (13)	49 (11)	
College or professional	102 (77)	17 (17)	30 (25)	74 (60)	39 (40)	9 (7)	143 (32)	
Marital Status, n (%)								
Single	5 (4)	53 (54)	71 (59)	12 (10)	39 (40)	84 (62)	160 (36)	<0.0001
Co-habitation	127 (95)	43 (44)	45 (38)	110 (90)	54 (54)	48 (35)	272 (61)	
Do not know	2 (1)	2 (2)	4 (3)	0 (0)	4 (4)	4 (3)	12 (3)	
Household size, (mean ± SE)	3.9 ± 0.1	4.7 ± 0.2	4.4 ± 1.2	4.1 ± 0.1	4.2 ± 0.2	4.6 ± 0.2	4.3 ± 0.1	0.0188
Insurance, n (%)								
Medicaid (Tenncare)	17 (13)	69 (70)	78 (65)	31 (25)	50 (51)	118 (87)	246 (55)	<0.0001
Other	117 (87)	28 (29)	39 (33)	92 (75)	44 (45)	17 (13)	188 (42)	
Missing	1 (0)	1 (1)	3 (2)	0 (0)	4 (4)	1 (0)	11 (3)	

H-P, Healthy-Processed pattern; H-S, Healthy-US Southern pattern; P-S, Processed-US Southern pattern. The numbers do not always add up because of rounding errors.1 To test the significant differences, Kruskal-Wallis ANOVA and median test were performed.2 Based on the categories established by the Institute of Medicine [25] for adults and based on age specific cut offs between age 16 and 18 years [26,27].

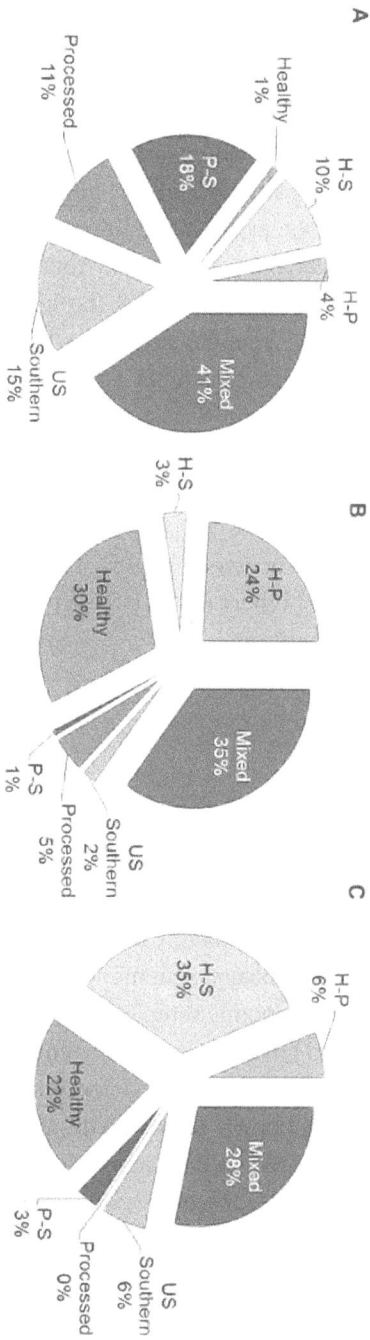

FIGURE 1: Distribution of dietary patterns during pregnancy in the Conditions Affecting Neurocognitive Development and Learning in Early Childhood (CANDLE) Cohort by race. (a) African American; (b) Caucasian; (c) Other.

The differences in mean daily macronutrient and energy adjusted mean daily micronutrient intakes among the dietary patterns appear in Table 4. Energy intake and all macro- and micronutrient intake differed among the dietary patterns ($p < 0.001$). The lowest consumption of energy adjusted nutrients was mirrored by low consumption of fruits and vegetables. The Processed and the P-S patterns had the highest energy intakes, and the Healthy and the US Southern had the lowest. The Healthy, US Southern and H-S patterns had the lowest fat and total sugar intake and highest protein intake while Processed and P-S the highest fat and sugar intake and the lowest protein intake. Regarding carbohydrate intake, there was little difference between patterns, with a significant difference found only between the Healthy and the P-S patterns ($p = 0.011$), where the Healthy group had the highest, and P-S had the lowest intake. The Healthy, H-P and H-S diets were the highest in fiber, while the Processed and P-S were the lowest. Cholesterol intake was high in the US Southern patterns and low in the Healthy and Processed patterns. The vitamin, mineral, and trace element intake was the highest in the US Southern and H-S and lowest in the Processed dietary patterns.

2.4 DISCUSSION

Three major dietary patterns, namely Healthy, Processed and US Southern were identified among pregnant women from the Mid-South using factor analysis. Combining the factor scores with quintile rankings of the factors we developed seven distinct mutually exclusive dietary patterns. This is the first study that examined dietary patterns within a geographical region that includes a diverse socioeconomic sample from the US. These dietary patterns were different ($p < 0.001$) from each other in almost all the food items, macro- and micro nutrients and aligned across socioeconomic and racial groups.

Dietary patterns are known to vary with age, gender, economics, and cultural habits [28]. Residents of Shelby County Tennessee reflect a diverse population that includes a preponderance of African-Americans across a wide range of incomes. The CANDLE study has enrolled participants reflective of the birth mothers of Shelby County Tennessee, thus diet characterization must be sensitive to the different segments of the population. Our approach to identifying dietary patterns appears to have been successful in identifying various segments of our study population based on race, income, and education. While this report is not unique with regard to dietary patterns [15] as they relate to segments of the population, it did identify types and combinations of foods that have distinct differences in nutrient composition with regard to nutrients linked to neurocognitive development [18,29].

Our findings that healthy eating patterns are reflective of older and more educated individuals are in concert with other reports [14]. Our Southern diet pattern is reflective of foods traditionally ascribed to the southeastern US [30]. The identified patterns in this paper are comparable and representative of the Southern US regions that differ from the national patterns [31,32,33]. Substantial segments of our sample retained core southern foods while also incorporating items from the healthy and from the processed foods patterns, reflecting a wider variety of food selection that translated into different nutrient intakes. Those with the H-S dietary pattern had higher levels of omega-3 fatty acids, iron, vitamin B6, folate, thiamine, niacin, riboflavin, total choline, and free choline than those with the pure Southern diet pattern, implying that individuals in this category capitalized on the foods with the highest nutrient density of both eating patterns. The Processed dietary pattern was characterized by a lower nutrient density and high energy content, yielding a decreased energy adjusted nutrient intake when combined with other dietary patterns. This is consistent with diets associated with food globalization, urbanization, and lower economic status [34]. The diversity of food selection among the African-American and Caucasian participants in our study underscores cultural sensitivity at the local level is important when collecting dietary information [30].

One limitation of our study was the significant amount of missing data due to technical problems and too low or high energy intake. The excluded sample consisted mainly of African American women due to the study design at recruitment. Therefore the missing sample is not representative of the overall study population presented in this paper, but after stratification, it is representative of the African American study population. Since our results show racial difference in the distribution of study participants across the dietary patterns, we think that this limitation has no significant effect on our analysis.

TABLE 4: Daily intake of total energy, macro- and energy adjusted micronutrients in the seven dietary patterns.

Nutrient	Healthy (n = 135)	Processed (n = 98)	Southern (n = 120)	H-P (n = 123)	H-S (n = 98)	P-S (n = 136)	Mixed (n = 445)	ANCOVA[1] p
Energy (kcal/day)	1801 ± 73.4[a]	2958 ± 86.2[b]	1887 ± 77.9[a]	2579 ± 76.9[c]	2347 ± 86.2[c]	3081 ± 73.2[b]	2360 ± 40.5[c]	<0.0001
Fat (% of E)	34.3 ± 0.43	37.6 ± 0.50	36.3 ± 0.46	36.6 ± 0.45	35.8 ± 0.50	37.9 ± 0.43	36.3 ± 0.24	<0.0001
Protein (% of E)	16.5 ± 0.20	13.5 ± 0.24	14.8 ± 0.21	14.9 ± 0.21	15.9 ± 0.24	14.2 ± 0.20	14.9 ± 0.11	<0.0001
Carbohydrate (% of E)	52.0 ± 0.56	50.4 ± 0.66	50.9 ± 0.59	50.5 ± 0.59	50.7 ± 0.66	49.2 ± 0.56	50.7 ± 0.31	0.0351
Saturated fat (g)	30.1 ± 0.50	33.6 ± 0.59	32.5 ± 0.53	32.2 ± 0.51	29.9 ± 0.58	34.0 ± 0.51	32.0 ± 0.27	<0.0001
Omega 3 fatty acids (g)	2.17 ± 0.05[b]	1.75 ± 0.06[c]	2.09 ± 0.06[b]	2.08 ± 0.05[b]	2.44 ± 0.06[a]	1.82 ± 0.05[c]	2.10 ± 0.03[b]	<0.0001
Total Sugar (g)	10.6 ± 0.64	21.7 ± 0.75	13.2 ± 0.68	16.5 ± 0.67	8.60 ± 0.75	19.4 ± 0.64	15.2 ± 0.35	<0.0001
Fiber (g)	27.4 ± 0.48	15.4 ± 0.55	20.8 ± 0.50	22.3 ± 0.49	26.0 ± 0.54	15.2 ± 0.48	20.5 ± 0.26	<0.0001
Fe (mg)	19.2 ± 0.32[a,b]	15.6 ± 0.37[d]	17.6 ± 0.34[c]	17.9 ± 0.33[b,c]	19.5 ± 0.37[a]	16.1 ± 0.32[d]	17.7 ± 0.17[c]	<0.0001
Zn (mg)	14.3 ± 0.23	12.2 ± 0.26	12.9 ± 0.24	13.3 ± 0.23	13.5 ± 0.26	12.5 ± 0.23	13.2 ± 0.12	<0.0001
Vit B6 (mg)	2.69 ± 0.05[a]	1.93 ± 0.06[c]	2.37 ± 0.05[b]	2.40 ± 0.05[b]	2.72 ± 0.06[a]	2.03 ± 0.05[c]	2.33 ± 0.03[b]	<0.0001
Vit B12 (µg)	6.54 ± 0.20[a,b]	5.00 ± 0.23[d]	6.01 ± 0.20[a,b,c]	5.64 ± 0.20[c,d]	6.69 ± 0.22[a]	5.76 ± 0.20[b,c,d]	6.03 ± 0.10[a,b,c]	<0.0001
Folate (µg)	777 ± 17.0	544 ± 19.7	656 ± 17.9	715 ± 17.4	775 ± 19.4	559 ± 17.1	671 ± 9.11	<0.0001
Thiamine (mg)	2.09 ± 0.03[a]	1.62 ± 0.04[d]	1.95 ± 0.03[b]	1.89 ± 0.03[b,c]	2.10 ± 0.04[a]	1.76 ± 0.03[c,d]	1.91 ± 0.02[b]	<0.0001
Niacin (mg)	27.4 ± 0.45[a]	23.0 ± 0.53[d]	24.7 ± 0.48[c,d]	25.8 ± 0.46[a,b,c]	27.1 ± 0.52[a,b]	24.0 ± 0.46[c,d]	25.5 ± 0.24[b,c]	<0.0001
Riboflavin (mg)	2.77 ± 0.04[a]	2.00 ± 0.05[d]	2.40 ± 0.05[c]	2.46 ± 0.04[b,c]	2.65 ± 0.05[a,b]	2.11 ± 0.04[d]	2.42 ± 0.02[c]	<0.0001
Total Choline (mg)	386 ± 7.08[b]	272 ± 8.22[f]	377 ± 7.44[b,c]	334 ± 7.23[d,e]	435 ± 8.08[a]	328 ± 7.11[e]	354 ± 3.79[c,d]	<0.0001
Free Choline (mg)	98.3 ± 1.33[a]	63.8 ± 1.54[d]	79.5 ± 1.39[c]	88.2 ± 1.35[b]	94.0 ± 1.51[a,b]	65.9 ± 1.33[d]	81.9 ± 0.71[c]	<0.0001

H-P, Healthy-Processed pattern; H-S, Healthy-US Southern pattern; P-S, Processed-US Southern pattern. Results are given as mean ± SE. [1] Covariate: Energy intake (kcal/day). [a,b,c,d,e,f] Means that do not share the same superscript are significantly different from each other

Statistical approaches have been well documented in establishing dietary patterns. Depicting dietary patterns using factor analyses can account for 15%–32% of the variance in dietary intake [7,15,35,36]. Explained variance in factor analysis is influenced by the amount of variables that are used in the analysis. Our result of the 15.4% is comparable with previously published literature in Mexican Americans [37], however they used 63 food items to identify dietary patterns which means potentially less variance, as the 111 items in our analysis. Most approaches are based on a 1 or 2 step process that may or may not allow for accurate calculation of total variance. However, the dietary patterns in our study accounted for 89%–90% of the variance in energy adjusted macronutrients and 50%–78% of the variance in the energy adjusted micronutrients. Thus, our patterns may be more robust in examining associations with cognitive development than single nutrients alone.

The complexity of a two-step process in assigning dietary patterns allowed us to capture mixed patterns. An individual with a high score on one factor may have another high score on another factor; therefore, the person's dietary pattern is a mixed pattern and not a pure dietary pattern of the highest score. The interpretation of these cases is analytically challenging because there are no cutoffs for these cases. Investigators using factor analysis should be cautious about this problem. To overcome this problem, we created mixed dietary patterns based on the individuals' rank orders in each factor. In this way H-P, H-S, P-S, and overall Mixed patterns were identified. The analysis of the individual food items and energy, macronutrient, and micronutrient intake of these patterns confirm that they are significantly distinct from the other main food patterns. Knudsen and colleagues [16] have used this method of analysis where they identified two factors, i.e., healthy and unhealthy patterns, and then created a third, mixed dietary pattern based on quintiles of the factor scores. Two thirds of their study population belonged to this intermediate group, which is consistent with our results. We found that 70% of the participants in our study ate foods consistent with the mixed dietary pattern.

Our statistical approach was to use all 111 food groups compared to condensing the food items into smaller groups. While decreasing the number of groups may increase the variance explained by the factor analysis, it decreases the ability to identify unique dietary patterns within sub groups of the population perspective [38]. For example condensing food items to 46 groups may yield two-three factors and thus limits the description of the dietary patterns. We also examined if incorporating the fat content of food item yielded additional information pertinent to dietary patterns. In our sample, this did not yield any additional information.

The goal of determining diet patterns is often to identify combinations of foods and beverages that reflect a specific type of diet that may be beneficial or harmful to a health outcome. The strengths and limitations of classifying individuals into specific patterns are that they may reflect an overall pattern of intake that may be targeted for community interventions; however, this may not be useful in examining a specific nutrient/disease relationship. Use of the seven patterns may not be readily translated into individual diet counseling, but it does identify key foods that could be targeted for community-based interventions to improve nutrient intake. Selectively over or under reporting by individuals of various socio-demographic groups, may bias the results of a study using nutrients as the exposure [39]. Diet patterns appear to be unaffected by under reporting or the report of consuming a food item [40]. Our approach in classifying diets, clearly links consumption of more processed foods (low nutrient density) with a higher percentages of overweight and obesity, thereby suggesting that under reporting may not be a large factor in this study.

2.5 CONCLUSIONS

Our study is the first to provide unique dietary patterns consumed by a cohort of women living in the mid-southern US. The diet patterns reflect a gamut of food stuffs that describe the traditional southern diet in the US, a highly processed diet, a primarily healthy food and dietary pattern combinations that reflect nutrition transition. The goal of creating diet patterns for this prospective study is to use examine the association of maternal nutritional factors during pregnancy to brain and cognitive development by age 3. How the dietary patterns during pregnancy relate to the child's cognitive development or help explain epigenetic expression of disease or health condition remains to be determined. In our longitudinal study, we will investigate whether maternal nutrient intake and diet patterns during pregnancy are somewhat stable and examine the influence on early child-hood development as part of the life course history.

REFERENCES

1. Barker, D.J. The fetal origins of adult hypertension. J. Hypertens. 1992, 10, S39–S44.
2. Barker, D.J. The fetal origins of diseases of old age. Eur. J. Clin. Nutr. 1992, 46, S3–S9.
3. Barker, D.J.; Martyn, C.N. The maternal and fetal origins of cardiovascular disease. J. Epidemiol. Community Health 1992, 46, 8–11.
4. Christian, P. Micronutrients, birth weight, and survival. Annu. Rev. Nutr. 2010, 30, 83–104.
5. Haider, B.A.; Yakoob, M.Y.; Bhutta, Z.A. Effect of multiple micronutrient supple-mentation during pregnancy on maternal and birth outcomes. BMC Public Health 2011, 11, doi:10.1186/1471-2458-11-S3-S19.
6. Gecz, J.; Mulley, J. Genes for cognitive function: Developments on the X. Genome Res. 2000, 10, 157–163.
7. Newby, P.K.; Tucker, K.L. Empirically derived eating patterns using factor or cluster analysis: A review. Nutr. Rev. 2004, 62, 177–203.
8. Dixon, L.B.; Balder, H.F.; Virtanen, M.J.; Rashidkhani, B.; Mannisto, S.; Krogh, V.; van Den Brandt, P.A.; Hartman, A.M.; Pietinen, P.; Tan, F.; et al. Dietary patterns as-sociated with colon and rectal cancer: Results from the Dietary Patterns and Cancer (DIETSCAN) Project. Am. J. Clin. Nutr. 2004, 80, 1003–1011.
9. Fung, T.; Hu, F.B.; Fuchs, C.; Giovannucci, E.; Hunter, D.J.; Stampfer, M.J.; Cold-itz, G.A.; Willett, W.C. Major dietary patterns and the risk of colorectal cancer in women. Arch. Intern. Med. 2003, 163, 309–314.
10. Slattery, M.L.; Boucher, K.M.; Caan, B.J.; Potter, J.D.; Ma, K.N. Eating patterns and risk of colon cancer. Am. J. Epidemiol. 1998, 148, 4–16.
11. Gittelsohn, J.; Wolever, T.M.; Harris, S.B.; Harris-Giraldo, R.; Hanley, A.J.; Zin-man, B. Specific patterns of food consumption and preparation are associated with diabetes and obesity in a Native Canadian community. J. Nutr. 1998, 128, 541–547.
12. Van Dam, R.M.; Rimm, E.B.; Willett, W.C.; Stampfer, M.J.; Hu, F.B. Dietary pat-terns and risk for type 2 diabetes mellitus in U.S. men. Ann. Intern. Med. 2002, 136, 201–209.
13. Fung, T.T.; Stampfer, M.J.; Manson, J.E.; Rexrode, K.M.; Willett, W.C.; Hu, F.B. Prospective study of major dietary patterns and stroke risk in women. Stroke 2004, 35, 2014–2019.
14. Northstone, K.; Emmett, P.; Rogers, I. Dietary patterns in pregnancy and associations with socio-demographic and lifestyle factors. Eur. J. Clin. Nutr. 2008, 62, 471–479.
15. Northstone, K.; Emmett, P.M.; Rogers, I. Dietary patterns in pregnancy and associa-tions with nutrient intakes. Br. J. Nutr. 2008, 99, 406–415.

16. Knudsen, V.K.; Orozova-Bekkevold, I.M.; Mikkelsen, T.B.; Wolff, S.; Olsen, S.F. Major dietary patterns in pregnancy and fetal growth. Eur. J. Clin. Nutr. 2008, 62, 463–470.

17. Elder, G.H., Jr. The life course as developmental theory. Child Dev. 1998, 69, 1–12.

18. Bourre, J.M. Effects of nutrients (in food) on the structure and function of the nervous system: Update on dietary requirements for brain. Part 1: Micronutrients. J. Nutr. Health Aging 2006, 10, 377–385.

19. Block, G.; Coyle, L.M.; Hartman, A.M.; Scoppa, S.M. Revision of dietary analysis software for the Health Habits and History Questionnaire. Am. J. Epidemiol. 1994, 139, 1190–1196.

20. Mares-Perlman, J.A.; Klein, B.E.; Klein, R.; Ritter, L.L.; Fisher, M.R.; Freudenheim, J.L. A diet history questionnaire ranks nutrient intakes in middle-aged and older men and women similarly to multiple food records. J. Nutr. 1993, 123, 489–501.

21. Johnson, B.A.; Herring, A.H.; Ibrahim, J.G.; Siega-Riz, A.M. Structured measurement error in nutritional epidemiology: Applications in the Pregnancy, Infection, and Nutrition (PIN) Study. J. Am. Stat. Assoc. 2007, 102, 856–866.

22. Subar, A.F.; Thompson, F.E.; Kipnis, V.; Midthune, D.; Hurwitz, P.; McNutt, S.; McIntosh, A.; Rosenfeld, S. Comparative validation of the Block, Willett, and National Cancer Institute food frequency questionnaires: The Eating at America's Table Study. Am. J. Epidemiol. 2001, 154, 1089–1099.

23. Block, G.; Hartman, A.M.; Dresser, C.M.; Carroll, M.D.; Gannon, J.; Gardner, L. A data-based approach to diet questionnaire design and testing. Am. J. Epidemiol. 1986, 124, 453–469.

24. Willet, W. Nutritional Epidemiology, 2nd ed.; Oxford University Press: New York, NY, USA, 1998.

25. IOM. Weight Gain During Pregnancy: Reexamining the Guidelines; The National Academies Press: Washington, DC, USA, 2009.

26. Cole, T.J.; Bellizzi, M.C.; Flegal, K.M.; Dietz, W.H. Establishing a standard definition for child overweight and obesity worldwide: International survey. BMJ 2000, 320, 1240–1243.

27. Cole, T.J.; Flegal, K.M.; Nicholls, D.; Jackson, A.A. Body mass index cut offs to define thinness in children and adolescents: International survey. BMJ. 2007, 335.

28. Satia, J.A. Dietary acculturation and the nutrition transition: An overview. Appl. Physiol. Nutr. Metab. 2010, 35, 219–223.

29. Bourre, J.M. Effects of nutrients (in food) on the structure and function of the nervous system: Update on dietary requirements for brain. Part 2: Macronutrients. J. Nutr. Health Aging 2006, 10, 386–399.

30. Bovell-Benjamin, A.C.; Dawkin, N.; Pace, R.D.; Shikany, J.M. Use of focus groups to understand African-Americans' dietary practices: Implications for modifying a food frequency questionnaire. Prev. Med. 2009, 48, 549–554.

31. Smith, S.L.; Quandt, S.A.; Arcury, T.A.; Wetmore, L.K.; Bell, R.A.; Vitolins, M.Z. Aging and eating in the rural, southern United States: Beliefs about salt and its effect on health. Soc. Sci. Med. 2006, 62, 189–198.

32. Tucker, K.L.; Maras, J.; Champagne, C.; Connell, C.; Goolsby, S.; Weber, J.; Zaghloul, S.; Carithers, T.; Bogle, M.L. A regional food-frequency questionnaire for the US Mississippi Delta. Public Health Nutr. 2005, 8, 87–96.

33. Jefferson, W.K.; Zunker, C.; Feucht, J.C.; Fitzpatrick, S.L.; Greene, L.F.; Shewchuk, R.M.; Baskin, M.L.; Walton, N.W.; Phillips, B.; Ard, J.D. Use of the Nominal Group Technique (NGT) to understand the perceptions of the healthiness of foods associated with African Americans. Eval. Program Plann. 2010, 33, 343–348.

34. Popkin, B.M. Global nutrition dynamics: the world is shifting rapidly toward a diet linked with noncommunicable diseases. Am. J. Clin. Nutr. 2006, 84, 289–298.

35. Smith, A.D.; Emmett, P.M.; Newby, P.K.; Northstone, K. A comparison of dietary patterns derived by cluster and principal components analysis in a UK cohort of children. Eur. J. Clin. Nutr. 2011, 65, 1102–1109.

36. Sotres-Alvarez, D.; Herring, A.H.; Siega-Riz, A.M. Latent class analysis is useful to classify pregnant women into dietary patterns. J. Nutr. 2010, 140, 2253–2259.

37. Tseng, M.; DeVellis, R.F.; Maurer, K.R.; Khare, M.; Kohlmeier, L.; Everhart, J.E.; Sandler, R.S. Food intake patterns and gallbladder disease in Mexican Americans. Public Health Nutr. 2000, 3, 233–243.

38. Tucker, K.L. Dietary patterns, approaches, and multicultural perspective. Appl. Physiol. Nutr. Metab. 2010, 35, 211–218.

39. Bailey, R.L.; Mitchell, D.C.; Miller, C.; Smiciklas-Wright, H. Assessing the effect of underreporting energy intake on dietary patterns and weight status. J. Am. Diet. Assoc. 2007, 107, 64–71.

40. Millen, A.E.; Tooze, J.A.; Subar, A.F.; Kahle, L.L.; Schatzkin, A.; Krebs-Smith, S.M. Differences between food group reports of low-energy reporters and non-low-energy reporters on a food frequency questionnaire. J. Am. Diet. Assoc. 2009, 109, 1194–1203.

CHAPTER 3

THE ROLE OF NUTRITION IN CHILDREN'S NEUROCOGNITIVE DEVELOPMENT, FROM PREGNANCY THROUGH CHILDHOOD

ANETT NYARADI, JIANGHONG LI, SIOBHAN HICKLING, JONATHAN FOSTER, AND WENDY H. ODDY

3.1 INTRODUCTION

Cognition represents a complex set of higher mental functions subserved by the brain, and includes attention, memory, thinking, learning, and perception (Bhatnagar and Taneja, 2001). Cognitive development in preschoolers is predictive of later school achievement (Tramontana et al., 1988; Clark et al., 2010; Engle, 2010). As Ross and Mirowsky (1999) state: "Schooling builds human capital—skills, abilities, and resources—which ultimately shapes health and well-being." Indeed, more education has been linked to better jobs, higher income, higher socio-economic status, better health care access and housing, better lifestyle, nutrition, and physical activity (Florence et al., 2008), which are all well-known health determinants. Education increases an individual's sense of personal control and self-esteem; these factors have also been shown to influence bet-

The Role of Nutrition in Children's Neurocognitive Development, from Pregnancy Through Child-hood. © *Nyaradi A, Li J, Hickling S, Foster J, and Oddy WH.* Frontiers in Human Neuroscience, *7,97 (2013). doi:10.3389/fnhum.2013.00097. Licensed under Creative Commons Attribution 3.0 Unported License, http://creativecommons.org/licenses/by/3.0/.*

ter health behavior (Ross and Mirowsky, 1999; Logi Kristjánsson et al., 2010). Academic achievement is important for future personal health, and is therefore a significant concern for public health.

Cognitive development is influenced by many factors, including nutrition. There is an increasing body of literature that suggests a connection between improved nutrition and optimal brain function. Nutrients provide building blocks that play a critical role in cell proliferation, DNA synthesis, neurotransmitter and hormone metabolism, and are important constituents of enzyme systems in the brain (Bhatnagar and Taneja, 2001; Lozoff and Georgieff, 2006; Zeisel, 2009; De Souza et al., 2011; Zimmermann, 2011). Brain development is faster in the early years of life compared to the rest of the body (Benton, 2010a), which may make it more vulnerable to dietary deficiencies.

In this literature review, we assess the current research evidence for a link between nutritional intake in pregnancy and childhood and children's cognitive development. We first discuss individual micronutrients and single aspects of diet, which represents earlier research in this area. We next consider the more encompassing aspects of diet, which have emerged as researchers became more interested in diet as a comprehensive measurement. The most recent research trend in this area suggests a broader analysis of the role of nutrition in neurocognitive development, which we offer here in comparison to previous reviews (Black, 2003b; Bellisle, 2004; Stevenson, 2006; Georgieff, 2007; Benton, 2010a).

3.2 BRAIN DEVELOPMENT IN HUMANS

The understanding of the functional and structural development of the human brain has emerged from a range of methodologies (including clinical lesion and experimental animal studies) and lately as a result of greatly improved neuroimaging methods, in particular Positron Emission Tomography and Magnetic Resonance Imaging (MRI) (Levitt, 2003; Uddin et al., 2010). Brain development is a temporally extended and complex process, with different parts and functions of the brain developing at different times (Grossman et al., 2003). By 5 weeks after conception in humans, the anterior-posterior and dorsal-ventral axes of the neural tube have already developed (Levitt, 2003). The cortical plate (which is the forerunner of the cerebral cortex) and some inter-neuronal connections form from 8 to 16 weeks of gestation (Kostović et al., 2002; Levitt, 2003). From 24 weeks of gestation until the perinatal period, the neurons in the cortical plate die and are replaced by more mature cortical neurons. During this time, significant refinement in neural connections take place (Levitt, 2003). From 34 weeks post-conception until 2 years of age, peak synapse development, and significant brain growth occurs (Huttenlocher and Dabholkar, 1997; Levitt, 2003). By preschool age, synaptic density has reached the adult level. The myelination of some parts of the brain (particularly those that control higher cognitive functions, such as the frontal lobes) continues well into adolescence, whilst myelination occurs earlier in other parts of the brain that coordinate more primary functions (Toga et al., 2006). Although the gray matter (which contains the bodies of nerve cells) reaches asymptote by the age of 7–11 in different regions of the brain, it is thought that the growth of the white matter (which represents axonal nerve tracts) continues beyond 20 years of age. Studies have shown that the maturation of specific brain areas during childhood is associated with development of specific cognitive functions such as language, reading, and memory (Nagy et al., 2004; Deutsch et al., 2005; Giedd et al., 2010). The development of the frontal lobes, which are believed to control higher cognitive functions (including planning, sequencing and self-regulation), appears to occur in growth spurts during the first 2 years of life, and then again between 7 and 9 years of age and also around 15 years of age (Thatcher, 1991; Bryan et al., 2004). The development of some subcortical structures including the basal ganglia, amygdala, and hippocampus (which are also centrally involved in some mediating higher cognitive functions, including memory, executive functions, and emotion) also continues until late adolescence. In addition, a meta-analysis has confirmed a connection between the size of the hippocampus and memory performance during brain development in children and young adults (Van Petten, 2004). Overall, the research evidence suggests that cognitive development is strongly connected with micro and macro-anatomical changes which take place throughout childhood (Levitt, 2003; Herlenius and Lagercrantz, 2004; Ghosh et al., 2010).

Individual brain development follows a genetic program which is influenced by environmental factors including nutrition (Bryan et al., 2004;

Toga et al., 2006; Giedd et al., 2010). Environmental influences may modify gene expression through epigenetic mechanisms, whereby gene function is altered through the processes of DNA methylation, histone modification and the modulating effect of non-coding RNAs, without the alteration of the gene sequence per se. These epigenetic factors can cause long lasting or even heritable changes in biological programs (Levi and Sanderson, 2004; Rosales et al., 2009; Murgatroyd and Spengler, 2011; Lillycrop and Burdge, 2012). It has been shown in animal and more recently in human studies that nutrition is one of the most salient environmental factors, and that nutrition can have a direct effect on gene expression (Levi and Sanderson, 2004; Rosales et al., 2009; Attig et al., 2010; Lillycrop and Burdge, 2011; Jiménez-Chillarón et al., 2012). One of the first and best known human studies in the rapidly growing field of "Nutritional Epigenomics" relates to the Dutch Hunger Winter during the 1940's in which the offspring of mothers exposed to famine during pregnancy had an increased risk of cardiovascular, kidney, lung, and metabolic disorders and reduced cognitive functions (Roseboom et al., 2006; De Rooij et al., 2010). More specifically, evidence has been obtained of hypo- and hypermethylated DNA segments from the blood cells of the affected individuals (Heijmans et al., 2008).

Evidence suggests that the timing of nutritional deficiencies can significantly affect brain development. For example, it is well known that folic acid deficiency between 21 and 28 days after conception (when the neural tube closes) predisposes the foetus to a congenital malformation, called a neural tube defect. Hence, this is a critical period, because during that time an irreversible change in the brain structure and function occurs if there is inadequate folic acid present (Blencowe et al., 2010). A critical period is a specific period within a sensitive timeframe (Knudsen, 2004). A sensitive period tends to reflect a broader timeframe; during such a developmental period the brain is more sensitive to specific interventions. However, skills and abilities can still be acquired outside this time period, albeit with less proficiency (Knudsen, 2004). An example is that deaf children who receive cochlear implants within a sensitive period for brain development (i.e., before the age of 3–5 years) show better language development than those who receive a cochlear implant after this period (Penhune, 2011).

Since rapid brain growth occurs during the first 2 years of life (and by the age of 2 the brain reaches 80% of its adult weight), this period of life may be particularly sensitive to deficiencies in diet (Bryan et al., 2004; Lenroot and Giedd, 2006). Adolescence is also a significant and sensitive developmental period, with research indicating that structural reorganization, brain and cognitive maturation and—in particular—major developments in the prefrontal cortex take place during puberty (Luna and Sweeney, 2001; Sisk, 2004; Peper et al., 2009; Asato et al., 2010; Blakemore et al., 2010).

3.3 DIETARY INFLUENCES ON COGNITIVE DEVELOPMENT

3.3.1 MICRONUTRIENTS AND COGNITIVE DEVELOPMENT

3.3.1.1 OMEGA-3 FATTY ACIDS

In recent years, there has been an increasing interest in the effect of essential fatty acids, particularly long chain polyunsaturated fatty acids (LCPUFA), on cognitive brain development. Of the human brain's dry weight 60% is comprised of lipids, of which 20% are docosahexaenoic acid (DHA; which is an omega-3 fatty acid) and arachidonic acid (AA; an omega-6 fatty acid). These represent the two core fatty acids found in gray matter (Benton, 2010b; De Souza et al., 2011). Furthermore, the supply of LCPUFAs from food, especially the omega-3 fatty acids, including DHA and eicosapentaenoic acid (EPA), is frequently inadequate for children as well as for adults (Schuchardt et al., 2010).

Essential fatty acids play a central functional role in brain tissue. They are not only the basic components of neuronal membranes, but they modulate membrane fluidity and volume and thereby influence receptor and enzyme activities in addition to affecting ion channels. Essential fatty acids are also precursors for active mediators that play a key role in inflammation and immune reaction. They promote neuronal and dendritic spine growth and synaptic membrane synthesis, and hence influence signal processing, and neural transmission. In addition, essential fatty acids regulate gene expression in the brain (McCann and Ames, 2005; Eilander et al., 2007; Innis, 2007; Cetina, 2008; Wurtman, 2008; Ramakrishnan et al., 2009; Ryan et al., 2010; Schuchardt et al., 2010; De Souza et al., 2011). Therefore, the existing literature strongly suggests that essential fatty acids are critical for brain development and function.

It has been suggested that the fast growth of the human cerebral cortex during the last two million years was strongly related to the balanced dietary intake of LCPUFAs (Broadhurst et al., 1998), specifically with an equal ratio of omega-6 and omega-3 fatty acids in the diet (Simopoulos, 1999). Evidence proposes that the modern *Homo sapiens*, whose brain developed significantly relative to its ancestors, lived near rivers and oceans, where seafood and fish were abundant (Crawford et al., 1999). The rise in intellectual and brain development in Homo Sapiens also coincided with tool making and language development (Crawford et al., 1999; Broadhurst et al., 2002). During the last 150 years, it is believed that the balance of omega-6 to omega-3 fatty acids has shifted in favor of omega-6 fatty acids in the diet, resulting in a ratio of 20–25:1 and a dietary deficiency in omega-3 fatty acids (Simopoulos, 1999). A diet that is deficient in omega-3 fatty acids may have health and developmental implications (Simopoulos, 2008).

A number of epidemiological studies have shown a positive association between maternal fish intake (which is a rich source of omega-3 fatty acids) during pregnancy and cognitive development in children (Daniels et al., 2004; Hibbeln et al., 2007; Jacobson et al., 2008; Oken et al., 2008a,b; Boucher et al., 2011). Data from the Avon Longitudinal Study of Parents and Children (ALSPAC) in the UK regarding fish consumption and child cognitive development were analyzed in two studies (Daniels et al., 2004; Hibbeln et al., 2007). The earlier study found evidence that higher maternal fish consumption was associated with higher language and social skills (after appropriate adjustments) in 7421 British children assessed at 15 months, using the MacArthur Communicative Development Inventory (MCDI), and at 18 months using the Denver Developmental Screening test (Daniels et al., 2004). The later ALSPAC study demonstrated that those children whose mothers consumed lower levels of seafood during pregnancy had lower IQ, measured by the Wechsler Intelligence Scale for

Children III (WISC-III) at the age of 8 (after adjusting for a wide range of relevant covariates). Lower maternal seafood consumption was also linked to suboptimal behavior at age seven (measured using the Child Behavior Checklist) and to lower levels of social, fine motor and language development (measured using the Denver Developmental Screening test) at six, 18, 30, and 42 months of age in the same study (Hibbeln et al., 2007). Although higher fish intake may result in higher erythrocyte mercury concentration (which has been shown to alter neurodevelopment adversely), research in American schoolchildren (Project Viva, a prospective pre-birth cohort study) demonstrated that higher maternal fish intake was still positively associated with improved language scores on the Peabody Picture Vocabulary Test (PPVT), after adjustment for many potential confounders and covariates (Oken et al., 2008a). The Danish National Birth Cohort study investigated the developmental milestones of 25,446 six- and 18-month old children on a developmental scale created by the researchers, and found that higher maternal fish intake was beneficial for cognitive development even after adjusting for breastfeeding and many sociodemographic factors (Oken et al., 2008b). Two other studies of Inuit children in Arctic Quebec, Canada, showed that higher umbilical cord DHA concentration was associated with: (1) improved infant cognitive development, measured on the Fagan Test of Infant Intelligence at 6 months, (2) on the Bayley Scales of Infant Development test used at 11 months (Jacobson et al., 2008), and (3) better memory performance of school children on both the Digit Span Forward subtest of the WISC-IV and the California Verbal Learning Test-Children Version (Boucher et al., 2011). These results were independent of mercury contamination in seafood. Both studies adjusted for a wide range of socioeconomic and demographic factors. However, these investigations used smaller samples, specifically 109 infants (Jacobson et al., 2008) and 154 schoolchildren (Boucher et al., 2011), compared to the previously described studies. In conclusion, the positive association between maternal fish intake and cognitive development is supported by evidence from the studies cited above.

However, intervention studies of LCPUFA supplementation during pregnancy have produced conflicting results so far. Some studies have reported positive associations between DHA supplementation and cognitive developmental parameters (Helland et al., 2003, 2008; Colombo et al.,

2004; Judge et al., 2007; Dunstan et al., 2008). A randomized placebo-controlled double- blind study undertaken by Helland et al. (2003) in Norway
used a design which supplemented women from 18 weeks of pregnancy
until 3 months postpartum with cod liver oil containing 1183 mg DHA.
Children's cognitive status was assessed at 6 and 9 months on the Fagan
Test of Infant Intelligence (Helland et al., 2001), and at 4 years of age by
the Kaufman Assessment Battery for Children (K-ABC), specifically the
Mental Processing Composite comprising the Sequential Processing, Si-
multaneous Processing, and Non-verbal Scales (which reflects children's
problem solving and information processing skills; Helland et al., 2003).
The results indicated that maternal DHA supplementation improved children's mental processing skills at 4 years of age (Helland et al., 2003), but
not recognition memory at 6 and 9 months of age (Helland et al., 2001).
However, in a follow-up study conducted at the age of 7, there was no
difference in overall IQ between supplemented versus non-supplemented
children, but a positive correlation was observed between the concentration of α-linolenic acid (ALA) and DHA in maternal plasma phospholipid
and performance on the Sequential Processing scale (Helland et al., 2008).
A possible explanation of these findings is that by 7 years of age cognitive
development is influenced by many other intervening factors, and the test
battery used in the research may not have been sensitive enough to detect
the association between diet and cognition at this later age (Helland et
al., 2008). The results of a study reported by Judge et al. (2007) also supported the findings of the previous study, providing evidence that maternal
DHA supplementation results in better problem solving ability (speed of
processing) in 9 month old infants on the Infant Planning Test, but not on
recognition memory evaluated using the Fagan Test of Infant Intelligence.
These findings may indicate that DHA is more important in the development of problem solving and processing ability than other cognitive functions such as memory. Visual attention or look duration declines during the
first year of life, giving place to more complex mental processing (Frick
et al., 1999; Colombo et al., 2004; Judge et al., 2007). Colombo et al.
(2004) reported an association between maternal DHA supplementation
and faster decline in visual attention during infancy, and better resistance
to distractibility during the second year of life. Researchers in Western
Australia supplemented a small sample of women (n = 98) from 20 weeks

of gestation until delivery with high dose (2200 mg) DHA or olive oil and showed significant improvements in hand and eye coordination in the supplemented group at 2½ years of age, after adjusting for maternal age, maternal education, and breastfeeding (Dunstan et al., 2008). These researchers also demonstrated better performance in other elements of cognitive development (locomotor, social, speech and hearing performance, and practical reasoning), evaluated using the Griffiths Mental Development Scales, and on language development, evaluated using the PPVT (Dunstan et al., 2008). However, these latter differences were not statistically significant, perhaps due to the relatively small sample size in the study.

Contrary to expectations, some studies did not find a relationship between LCPUFA supplementation during pregnancy and cognitive development in children (Tofail, 2006; Makrides et al., 2010; Campoy et al., 2011). One of these studies was conducted in a developing country, Bangladesh, where a high proportion of mothers suffer from undernutrition, and possibly from multiple micronutrient deficiencies important for brain development. The pregnant mothers in this study were randomized into fish-oil or soy-oil supplemented groups, and their infants' cognitive development was measured on the Bayley Scales of Infant Development at ten months of age. In this study, the mothers were only given supplements during the third trimester, which may not have represented a sufficient timeframe for supplement administration (Tofail, 2006). In a recent study conducted in Europe on 270 women from three countries, cognitive development was measured on the K-ABC at 6½ years of age after 500 mg DHA prenatal supplementation. In this study, the co-authors did not find significant differences in intelligence between the intervention and control groups (Campoy et al., 2011). The explanation offered was that the positive effect of prenatal supplementation may have been overshadowed by other important factors (not all of which it is possible to control for) including social stimulation, other nutrients taken, diet as a whole, illnesses, and drugs prescribed by the age of 6–7 years (Helland et al., 2008). Makrides et al. (2010) conducted a well-designed multicenter double-blind randomized controlled trial in Australia on 2399 women between 2005 and 2009 from 21 weeks of gestation until birth and did not find any difference on the Bayley Scales of Infant and Toddler Development at the age of 18 months between intervention (supplemented with 800 mg DHA) and control groups (supplemented with vegetable oil capsules), after adjustment for potential confounders. Given the size of this study, the Makrides et al. (2010) investigation was certainly adequately powered to detect a statistically significant difference; yet, no such difference was observed.

Some published studies have also considered supplementation in lactating mothers in order to examine the effect of increased omega fats in breast milk on the cognitive development of children. Reviews of these studies have concluded that there are indications that supplementing lactating mothers with fish oil may positively influence cognitive development in children (Eilander et al., 2007; Hoffman et al., 2009).

In conclusion, the current findings show inconsistencies in the efficacy of maternal supplementation with omega-3 fatty acid. In seeking to account for the contrasting findings, it seems that the following considerations may be relevant: the interventions were applied in different groups of women, using a wide range of DHA dosage, with different durations of supplementation, and the outcomes were measured on different cognitive instruments and at different ages. The more consistent results obtained in epidemiological studies (compared with supplementation trials using only omega-3 fatty acid) may be explained by the possibility that fish is a whole food, and it contains other nutrients important to cognitive development. Furthermore, by eating fish rather than taking fish supplements, other possibly unhealthy or potentially inflammatory foods may also be displaced—i.e., red meat and processed meats. Epidemiological studies may also be better powered but they may also potentially have less control for confounding.

Postnatal studies have considered the effect of omega-3 fatty acid supplementations on term and preterm infants. Epidemiological studies and supplementation trials have also been undertaken in older children in relation to cognitive development. The DHA component is believed to be one of the main reasons why breast milk may improve the cognitive performance of children. Humans are able endogenously to synthesize DHA from precursor α-linolenic acid. However, the conversion rate varies according to genetically determined polymorphisms in two genes, namely FADS1 and FADS2. Moreover, in infants the conversion to DHA seems to be very limited (Hoffman et al., 2009; Guesnet and Alessandri, 2011). Research consistently shows that the blood levels of DHA in formula-fed infants are lower than in breastfed infants, irrespective of the level of precursors in formulas (Hoffman et al., 2009). Therefore, this topic has generated a great deal of scientific interest, especially with respect to the results of clinical trials that have supplemented infant formulas with LCPUFA and investigated the relationship with cognitive development in either term or preterm infants.

A Cochrane review undertaken by Simmer et al. (2008) included 11 studies and concluded that there is currently not enough evidence to support the supplementation of infant formulas with LCPUFA to benefit cognitive development in children born at term. Another review by McCann and Ames (2005) considered animal as well as human supplementation studies. These authors found that, although animal studies provided convincing evidence for DHA supplementation and improved cognitive performance, these studies were undertaken under extreme dietary conditions in which (in most cases) animals were severely deficient in essential fatty acids. By contrast, in formula and breastfed infants the differences in brain DHA concentrations are small, such that the positive effects of LCPUFA on cognitive development may be difficult to detect. Eilander et al. (2007) also concluded that there is no evidence that formula supplementation in term infants is beneficial for cognitive development. On the other hand, Hoffman et al. (2009) reviewed 20 studies and suggested that those trials which supplemented formula milk with a similar level of DHA to breast milk (i.e., to an average of 0.32%) found beneficial outcomes. A major intake of DHA in the brain happens in the last trimester of pregnancy; therefore, preterm infants are disadvantaged and have decreased brain concentration of this vital LCPUFA. Eilander et al. (2007) indicated that supplementing formula milk with LCPUFA may be beneficial for the cognitive development of preterm infants. However, a recent Cochrane review undertaken on preterm infants reported no significant outcome of supplementation with LCPUFA on their cognitive development (Schulzke et al., 2011).

Since brain development continues through childhood, there have been much interest in the association between cognitive development and omega-3 fat levels through diet and/or supplementation in children. Ryan et al. (2010) reviewed the available epidemiological studies and supplementation trials to date and concluded that, although the results were inconsistent,

it appears that those studies that supplemented with higher doses and longer durations of DHA achieved a favorable positive outcome in cognitive
development in childhood.

3.3.1.2 VITAMIN B12, FOLIC ACID, AND CHOLINE

B12 and folate deficiency resulting in anaemia is rare around the world.
However, it can occur in both developing and developed countries especially in older people, in those with absorption problems and in vegetar-
ians (De Benoist, 2008). Folate fortification of bread products has been
made mandatory in Australia and in many other countries, which has reduced this deficiency significantly (Brown et al., 2011). In recent years,
there has been an increasing interest in the association between vitamin
B12, folic acid, choline metabolism, and cognitive development. Folate
affects neural stem cell proliferation and differentiation, decreases apoptosis, alters DNA biosynthesis, and has an important role in homocysteine and S-adenosylmethionine biosynthesis (Zeisel, 2009; Zhang et al.,
2009). It is believed that choline has similar roles in brain development as
folate (Meck and Williams, 2003; McCann et al., 2006; Zeisel, 2006a,b,
2009; Signore et al., 2008). Furthermore, folate, choline and vitamin B12
metabolism are interconnected at the homocysteine-methionine-S-ade-
nosylmethionine pathway (Zeisel, 2009). S-adenosylmethionine is one
of the main methyl donors in different metabolic methylation reactions,
including DNA methylation. Therefore, choline and folate deficiency
may result in DNA hypomethylation, thereby altering gene transcription
(Zeisel, 2009). In addition, choline is a component of phospholipids in cell
membranes and a precursor for the neurotransmitter acetylcholine (Zeisel,
2006b). Vitamin B12 has a role in axon myelination that is important for
impulse conduction from cell to cell, and it also protects neurons from
degeneration. Vitamin B12 may also alter the synthesis of different cytokines, growth factors and oxidative energy metabolites such as lactic acid
(Dror and Allen, 2008).

   In children, the association between vitamin B12 and cognitive development has been mainly observed in infants born of vegetarian/vegan
mothers or mothers on a macrobiotic diet. These diets can result in vitamin

B12 deficiency, as vitamin B12 is largely found in animal products. A pooled analysis that included 48 case studies of infants with vitamin B12 deficiencies reported a variety of abnormal clinical and radiological signs, including: hypotonic muscles, involuntary muscle movements, apathy, cerebral atrophy, and demyelination of nerve cells (Dror and Allen, 2008). After vitamin B12 treatment, a rapid improvement in neurological symptoms is reported in deficient infants, but many of these infants remained seriously delayed in cognitive and language development in the longer term (Dror and Allen, 2008). The long-lasting effect of vitamin B12 deficiency is supported by the findings of Louwman et al. (2000). These researchers investigated the cognitive functioning of adolescents who consumed a macrobiotic diet until the age of 6 years, compared to children with an omnivorous diet. Those adolescents who consumed a macrobiotic diet until 6 years of age had lower levels of fluid intelligence, spatial ability and short term memory (even with currently normal vitamin B12 status) than the control subjects. Although vitamin B12 deficiency is not likely to occur in non-vegetarian people in western countries, Pepper and Black (2011) raised concern about the more frequent gastric bypass surgeries in obese women and the increased incidence of coeliac disease and inflammatory bowel diseases (such as Crohn's and ulcerative colitis). In these conditions, the absorption of vitamin B12 is substantially decreased in the intestine, thereby potentially adversely affecting the development of future children born to these women.

The association between maternal blood folate status and cognitive development has been investigated in several studies (Tamura et al., 2005; Veena et al., 2010). Tamura et al. (2005) did not find any relationship between maternal blood folate status ("low" vs. "normal") during the second half of the pregnancy and cognitive development of their children at the age of 5–6 years on different cognitive tests including Differential Ability Scales, Visual and Auditory Sequential Memory, Knox Cube, the Gross Motor Scale and the Grooved Pegboard. These researchers conducted their study among African-American women of low socioeconomic status and their disadvantaged children. These children nevertheless did not present with signs or symptoms of any overt clinical deficiency (such as megaloblastic anaemia). On the other hand, Veena et al. (2010) reported that higher maternal blood folate concentration—but not folate status ("low" vs. "normal", similar to the previous study)—was associated with better cognitive performance on a wide range of tests (Atlantis, Word Order, Pattern Reasoning, Verbal Fluency, Koh's Block Design and WISC-III) in 9–10-year-old Indian children. Interestingly, most of the women (96%) in this study manifested blood folate levels within the normal range. However, the only positive association found between maternal vitamin B12 status and cognitive performance in these children was on verbal fluency, although almost half of the mothers (42.5%) manifested moderately low vitamin B12 level. It is possible that vitamin B12 affects some cognitive functions only if the person is severely deficient, as can be seen in vegetarian mothers and their children. Another reason for the limited findings may be that the tests conducted were not sensitive enough to detect small changes in different functions. Another research group in India showed that lower vitamin B12 levels during pregnancy impaired short term memory (Digit Span Test) and sustained attention (Color Trail Test) in 9 years old children after adjusting for covariates (Bhate, 2008) while non-verbal intelligence on Raven's Cultured Progressive Matrices and visual perception on a Visual Recognition Test were unaffected in this study.

Although there is no sufficient data about the requirements of choline in humans, choline does not seem to be deficient in the general population, with the exception of experimental conditions (Commonwealth of Australia, 2006). Evidence from numerous animal studies indicates that dietary choline has an important impact on the cognitive development of offspring (Meck and Williams, 2003; McCann et al., 2006). Choline in animal models alters the development of the hippocampus, which has a central role in memory and learning (Zeisel, 2006a). Like folate, choline also has a role in the closure of the foetal neural tube. A study among Californian mothers found an increased risk of neural tube defects of their children with lower maternal dietary choline intake, as identified from a food frequency questionnaire (Shaw et al., 2004). There is only one study to date that has evaluated the impact of maternal blood choline (represented across a wide range of concentrations) on intelligence (measured on the Wechsler Preschool and Primary Scale of Intelligence-Revised) in 5 year old children. However, the authors did not find a significant correlation between the two (Signore et al., 2008). In summary, the impact of vitamin B12, folate and choline on children's cognitive development has not been adequately researched to date in humans.

3.3.1.3 ZINC

Zinc deficiency appears to be a major problem worldwide, affecting 40% of the global population (Maret and Sandstead, 2006). Recent research suggests that toddlers, adolescents, older people and individuals with diabetes are possibly at a higher risk of zinc deficiency in Australia (Gibson and Heath, 2011). Animal studies have established a relationship between zinc and neurodevelopment (Shah and Sachdev, 2006; Summers et al., 2008; Coyle et al., 2009). It is believed that zinc is a vital nutrient for the brain, with important structural and functional roles (Bhatnagar and Taneja, 2001; Black, 2003a; Bryan et al., 2004; Shah and Sachdev, 2006; Georgieff, 2007). More specifically, zinc is a cofactor for more than 200 enzymes that regulate diverse metabolic activities in the body including protein, DNA and RNA synthesis. In addition, zinc plays a role in neurogenesis, maturation, and migration of neurons and in synapse formation (Bhatnagar and Taneja, 2001; Black, 2003a; Bryan et al., 2004; Shah and Sachdev, 2006; Georgieff, 2007). Zinc is also found in high concentrations in synaptic vesicles of hippocampal neurons (which are centrally involved in learning and memory), and seems to modulate some neurotransmitters including glutamate and gamma- aminobutyric acid (GABA) receptors (Bhatnagar and Taneja, 2001; Levenson, 2006).

Zinc supplementation has a positive effect on the immune status of infants and may prevent congenital malformations (Shah and Sachdev, 2006). However, the relationship between maternal zinc status and the child's cognitive development has not been fully investigated. In an observational study, low maternal zinc intake in Egyptian mothers was associated with lower levels of focused attention in newborns, measured with the Brazelton Neonatal Behavior Assessment Scale (Kirksey et al., 1994). Surprisingly, a placebo controlled randomized trial undertaken on poor Bangladeshi mothers found that 13 months old infants of zinc supplemented mothers scored less on the Bayley scales of infant development than infants born to mothers who received a placebo (Hamadani et al., 2002). In trying to explain their findings, these researchers argued that zinc supplementation alone may cause imbalances or even deficiencies of other micronutrients that are important for brain development, as micronutrients interact with one another (Hamadani et al., 2002)—a point which we will return to later in this review. Another double-blind randomized controlled trial of maternal zinc supplementation among African-American mothers showed no difference in the cognitive development of 5 years old children between the intervention and control groups, measured on the Differential Ability Scales, Visual and Auditory Sequential Memory, Knox Cube, Gross Motor Scale, and Grooved Pegboard (Tamura et al., 2003). In both studies, the mothers were supplemented only in the second half of their pregnancy. Overall, there are only a limited number of studies on this topic. Taken together, the findings do not consistently show a positive relationship between maternal zinc status and cognitive development of children.

Two articles that reviewed earlier observational and randomized control trials in children on zinc and cognitive development concluded that zinc deficiency can negatively influence cognitive development. Conversely, more recent randomized control trials from India (Taneja et al., 2005) and Bangladesh (Black et al., 2004), where malnutrition is common among children, did not find that zinc supplementation alone affects infants' cognitive development on the Bayley Scales of Infant Development test. Nevertheless, in the Bangladeshi trial, when zinc was combined with iron supplementation, it showed an improvement in cognition (Black et al., 2004). Additional studies are therefore needed to examine the long term benefit of zinc on brain development.

3.3.1.4 IRON

One of the most common nutritional deficiencies in both developing and developed countries is iron deficiency. In some parts of the world, such as in Sub-Saharan Africa and South-East Asia, the prevalence is more than 40%. In developed countries—including Australia—it could be as high as 20%, particularly in pregnant women and in children (World Health

Organization, 2008). Over the past decades, a considerable literature has been published on the association between iron status/anaemia and cognitive development in children, as well as in animal models (Grantham-McGregor and Ani, 2001). It is believed that iron is involved with different enzyme systems in the brain, including: the cytochrome c oxidase enzyme system in energy production, tyrosine hydroxylase for dopamine receptor synthesis, delta-9- desaturase for myelination, and fatty acid synthesis, and ribonucleotide reductase for brain growth regulation (Deungria, 2000; Lozoff and Georgieff, 2006; Georgieff, 2007; Rioux et al., 2011). In addition, iron appears to modify developmental processes in hippocampal neurons by altering dendritic growth (Jorgenson et al., 2003; Lozoff and Georgieff, 2006).

There are a limited number of studies that have examined the connection between maternal iron status or maternal iron supplementation and cognitive development. (In the below, treatment refers to anaemic individuals, and supplementation to non-anaemic children.) Tamura et al. (2002) found significantly inferior performance in language skills, fine motor skills and attention (and lower but not significant scores in every other test) in 5 years old children whose cord ferritin levels lay in the lowest quartile. Cognitive performance in this study was measured on the WISC-R, the Test for Auditory Comprehension of Language, fine and gross-motor scales of the Peabody Developmental Motor Scales and the Yale Children's Inventory for attention and tractability. The mothers who took part in the study were of African-American descent and low socioeconomic status, and a high proportion of the children were born small-for-gestational-age. However, a randomized placebo controlled iron supplementation trial in a representative sample of Australian pregnant women failed to find any difference between an iron supplemented vs. placebo group in the IQ of children at 4 years of age on the Stanford–Binet Intelligence Scale, despite maternal iron status having improved due to supplementation (Zhou et al., 2006). The authors suggested that supplementing pregnant women who are generally well-nourished with iron may not confer any additional health benefits, while Tamura's study was undertaken in disadvantaged mothers and small-for-gestational-age infants (Tamura et al., 2002; Zhou et al., 2006). A recent trial in Canada by Rioux et al. (2011) also found no evidence that better maternal iron and DHA status enhanced cognitive development in six months old infants, measured on the Brunet-Lezine Scale of Psychomotor Development of Early Childhood and the Bayley Scales of Infant Development. These researchers recruited a small sample size of mothers from a higher socioeconomic background and with better feeding practices, consistent with the methodology and findings of the Australian study cited above.

In children, the relationship between iron and cognitive development has been well researched. In addition, these investigations have been reviewed many times during the last decade. Grantham-McGregor and Ani (2001) reviewed a range of longitudinal studies and reported that anaemic infants had poorer cognitive and school performance in the long term, and that short-term iron treatment trials in anaemic children did not show benefits in cognitive development. A Cochrane review based on seven randomized controlled trials reached a similar conclusion, i.e., that short term iron treatment for anaemia in children less than 3 years old did not improve cognitive development (Logan et al., 2001). Sachdev et al. (2005) included 17 randomized controlled trials in their meta-analysis, and did not find convincing evidence of an association between iron supplementation and treatment for anaemic and cognitive development. However, treating older children with iron deficiency increased IQ significantly. A more recent review and meta-analysis on children (aged 6 years and older), adolescents and adults found that iron treatment increased IQ in anaemic individuals, but iron supplementation did not improve IQ in non-anaemic children (Falkingham et al., 2010).

In summary, there is a lack of epidemiological evidence or data from well-designed intervention trials demonstrating the impact of maternal iron supplementation on the cognitive development of healthy children. There is evidence that older anaemic children benefit from iron treatments. However, cognitive performance tests including the Bayley Scales of Infant Development and the Denver Developmental Screening Test may not be sensitive enough to detect small changes in short-term supplementation or treatment in young children (Armstrong, 2002). Furthermore, if iron deficiency occurs in very early life, the damage may be irreversible, and it may not be possible to reverse this damage with iron treatment (Beard, 2008).

3.3.1.5 IODINE

Iodine deficiency is a significant worldwide public health issue, especially in children and during pregnancy (World Health Organization, 2004). In Australia, the majority of children and pregnant women are mildly deficient in iodine, with some groups reaching moderate to severe deficiency (Gallego, 2010). Iodine deficiency in the soils in many countries has led to food fortification, most commonly the use of iodized salt (World Health Organization, 2004). The relationship between iodine and cognitive development is extensively researched. It is well known today that severe iodine deficiency during pregnancy may cause "cretinism" in children (Forrest, 2004; Zimmermann, 2007, 2009, 2011; Melse-Boonstra and Jaiswal, 2010). The clinical manifestation of cretinism depends on the severity of iodine deficiency; the features may include mental retardation, speech and hearing impairment, upper motor neuron and extrapyramidal lesions (Delong et al., 1985). Iodine is necessary for the production of thyroid hormones in the body; 70–80% of it is found in the thyroid gland (Melse-Boonstra and Jaiswal, 2010). Iodine deficiency manifests in hypothyroidism, causing underproduction of thyroid hormones including triiodothyronin (T3) and thyroxin (T4). Thyroid hormones play an important role in neurodevelopment and numerous neurological processes including neuronal cell differentiation, maturation and migration, myelination, neurotransmission, and synaptic plasticity (Zimmermann, 2009, 2011; Melse-Boonstra and Jaiswal, 2010). In addition, in animal models hypothyroidism alters neurogenesis and the development and functions of synapses in the hippocampus (Desouza et al., 2005; Gong et al., 2010).

Qian et al. (Qian, 2005) conducted a meta-analysis on studies from different locations in China where the soil is severely iodine deficient, and found a 12.3 point decrease in the IQ of those children whose mothers lived in iodine deficient areas compared to those living in iodine sufficient locations. The association between mild-moderate maternal iodine deficiency and cognitive development is not as clear as it is when iodine deficiency is severe (Forrest, 2004; Zimmermann, 2007, 2009, 2011; Melse-Boonstra and Jaiswal, 2010). In mild-moderate iodine deficiency, maternal thyroid stimulating hormone (TSH) and the thyroid hormone T3 level are unaffected, such that hypothyroidism is not clinically or even sub-clinically diagnosed. In such situations the level of maternal T4 may not be sufficient for the appropriate neurological development of the foetus (Melse-Boonstra and Jaiswal, 2010).

A number of observational studies from iodine sufficient or mildly iodine deficient areas of USA, Russia, The Netherlands, Italy and Spain have shown a significant association between mild maternal thyroid deficiency and cognitive impairment in children. The tests that were reviewed in these studies included the WISC, Neonatal Behavioral Assessment Scale, Bayley Scale of Infant Development, McCarthy Scales of Children's Abilities and the Gnome Mental Development Scale (Haddow et al., 1999; Pop, 2001; Pop et al., 2003; Vermiglio et al., 2004; Riano Galan et al., 2005; Kasatkina et al., 2006; Kooistra et al., 2006). By contrast, one study did not find any relationship between maternal T4 levels and cognitive development in children at 6 months (visual recognition memory) and 3 years of age (PPVT and Wide Range of Visual Motor Ability). However, this study included only a very small number of women with abnormal thyroid function (Oken et al., 2009). Berbel et al. (2009) carried out a trial in Spain that showed better gross and fine motor coordination and socialization (Brunet-Lezine Scale) in 18-month-old children whose mothers were supplemented with iodine from early pregnancy, compared to those who took the supplement from late pregnancy. Velasco et al. (2009) also found that those infants whose mothers took daily iodine supplements from the first trimester of pregnancy exhibited better psychomotor development (measured on the Bayley Scales of Infant Development), compared to those whose mothers were not supplemented with groups evaluated at different ages (5.5 and 12.4 months, respectively). Contrary to expectation, another study from Spain reported lower psychomotor development (measured on the Bayley Scale of Infant Development) in infants (especially in girls) born to mothers with maternal multivitamin supplementation that contained high amounts of iodine (100–149 µg/day), when compared to those infants with lesser amounts of maternal iodine supplementation (<100 µg/day) (Murcia et al., 2011). It is possible that the optimum dose of iodine for those mothers who are manifesting only mild iodine deficiency is less;

further research is needed to determine the safe level of iodine intake for mildly deficient pregnant women.

The vast number of studies on the iodine status and supplementation in children and its relationship to cognitive development in mild-moderate iodine deficient areas of the world has been reviewed several times. An earlier review and meta- analysis of 18 studies found a 13.5 point difference in IQ between iodine sufficient and iodine deficient children (Bleichrodt and Born, 1994). Other reviews reported that most observational studies on iodine deficient children found some degree of cognitive impairment (when compared to children from iodine sufficient areas), and iodine supplementation trials in school age children have provided some promising results with respect to improvement of some cognitive processes (Zimmermann, 2007, 2011; Melse-Boonstra and Jaiswal, 2010). More recent iodine supplementation trials from Albania and New Zealand found that supplementation of mildly iodine deficient 10–13 years old children improved matrix reasoning in both studies. In addition, fine motor skills and visual problem solving were improved in the Albanian trial (Zimmermann, 2006; Gordon et al., 2009). Relatively few studies have been conducted in very young children to support the significance of iodine in cognitive development (Melse-Boonstra and Jaiswal, 2010).

In conclusion, the above literature suggests that iodine is important for the cognitive development of older children. Furthermore, although iodine supplementation is critical for severely iodine deficient pregnant women, there is no general consensus about the effectiveness of iodine supplementation during pregnancy in countries with mild iodine deficiency.

3.3.2 MULTIVITAMIN AND MINERAL SUPPLEMENTATION

Although it is important to investigate nutrients individually, deficiencies of nutrients rarely occur in isolation, and an inadequate diet typically causes multiple micronutrient deficiencies. In addition, nutrients interact with each other and do not work separately (Benton, 2010a). Thus, it is important to investigate the association between multiple mineral and vitamins supplementation or deficiencies and cognitive development.

A recent systematic review of prenatal maternal micronutrient supplementation and children's cognitive and psychomotor development considered 18 studies, including six multiple-micronutrient supplementation trials. This review found some evidence that multivitamin and mineral supplementation might positively influence certain aspects of brain development in children (Leung et al., 2011). The review included six trials on multiple-micronutrient supplementations conducted in Peru, rural Taiwan, Tanzania (on HIV infected mothers), and in rural China, Indonesia and Bangladesh, where mothers were poorly nourished (Joos et al., 1983; Schmidt et al., 2004; McGrath et al., 2006; Tofail et al., 2008; Li et al., 2009; Caulfield et al., 2010). A very recent randomized controlled trial in Indonesia found that multiple micronutrient supplementation in undernourished pregnant mothers resulted in improved motor development, visual attention and spatial ability in pre-schoolers (Prado et al., 2012). All the above-mentioned trials are from low income countries, it is currently unknown whether the cognitive development of children of well-nourished mothers from higher income countries would benefit from multiple-micronutrient supplementation.

More consistent results from trials supplementing children with multiple-micronutrients have been shown. A meta-analysis investigated 20 randomized controlled trials published from 1970 to 2008 in developed as well as developing countries, and found that multiple-micronutrient supplementation may result in higher fluid intelligence (Eilander et al., 2010). However, this increase was only marginal, and no association was observed with crystallized intelligence in children. The finding of this review (i.e., that fluid intelligence, but not crystallized intelligence, may be influenced by multiple-micronutrient supplementation) is consistent with conclusions drawn from other studies (Benton, 2001, 2012). Fluid intelligence refers to reasoning ability that reflects the individual's current neurological potential (indexed by measures such as speed of processing) rather than their level of past attainment and acquired, crystallized knowledge (which is measured by abilities such as depth of vocabulary). Fluid ability is typically measured via non-verbal cognitive tests, while crystallized intelligence is more usually measured by administering verbal cognitive tests (Eilander et al., 2010; Benton, 2012).

3.3.3 OVERALL DIET, FOOD, AND COGNITIVE PERFORMANCE

3.3.3.1 BREASTFEEDING

A considerable amount of literature has been published on the possible connection between breastfeeding and cognitive development. Many of these studies demonstrate significantly positive associations between the two; however, the associations typically diminish or are no longer significant after controlling for confounders including maternal IQ, which is believed to be the strongest predictor of children's intelligence (Rey, 2003; McCann and Ames, 2005; Michaelsen et al., 2009). Furthermore, it remains unclear whether the remaining, diminished associations between breastfeeding and child cognitive development are further confounded by factors that have not been controlled for (Michaelsen et al., 2009). A meta-analysis of 20 studies undertaken in the late 1990's found that breastfeeding in normal birth weight infants increased IQ by 2.7 points and in low birth weight children by 5.2 points, but only six of the studies controlled for maternal IQ (Anderson et al., 1999). Three critical reviews conducted in the early 1990's concluded that the evidence linking breastfeeding and cognitive development has not yet been comprehensively demonstrated (Drane and Logemann, 2000; Jain et al., 2002; Rey, 2003). However, a more recent review by Michaelsen et al. (2009) concluded that the majority of studies found an association between breastfeeding and cognitive development, even after adjusting for confounders, and the difference in IQ related to breastfeeding is around 2–5 points at any age. This finding is supported by a large randomized control trial, where breastfeeding mothers were randomized into a breastfeeding promotion intervention trial that resulted in a higher breastfeeding rate up to 12 months after birth (43.3 vs. 6.4%). Intelligence tests were conducted at age 6½ years on the children in both groups (i.e., intervention vs. control) and associations between longer exclusive breastfeeding and improved cognitive development were found (Kramer et al., 2008). As noted earlier in this review, it has been suggested that one of the reasons behind the advantage of breastfeeding over formula feeding concerns the concentration of LCPUFA in breast milk, especially DHA (Michaelsen et al., 2009).

More recently, some studies have directly examined the effect of breastfeeding on brain development and structure. A study by Kafouri et al. (2012) reported that longer breastfeeding duration is positively associated with cortical thickness in the parietal lobe in adolescents, and in the same study they also found an association between intelligence (measured on WISC) and longer breastfeeding after adjusting for relevant confounders, which included maternal education. Herba et al. (2012) used cranial ultrasound in 2 months old infants; those infants who were breastfed exclusively had larger gangliothalamic diameter and head circumference, and smaller ventricular volume compared to bottle fed babies. Furthermore, breastfeeding has been associated previously with not only higher IQ (measured on the WISC) in adolescents but with increased white matter volume, especially in boys (Isaacs et al., 2010).

In summary, the debate concerning whether breastfeeding and cognitive development have a positive association appears to continue, but with more advanced neuroimaging technologies now available, future research may offer greater insights. Nevertheless, as Gökçay (2010) pointed out, breast milk provides the best nutritional intake for infants, regardless of its putative association with cognitive development.

3.3.3.2 MALNUTRITION

The number of malnourished (undernourished) children continues to rise in some regions, such as in Sub-Saharan Africa (De Onis, 2000). Every year, 20 million newborns (15.5% of all births) are low birth weight, most of them from developing countries (United Nations Children's Fund and World Health Organization, 2004). The effect of malnutrition on brain structures has been extensively researched in animal models. Malnutrition appears to alter cell numbers, cell migrations, myelinisation, synaptogenesis, hippocampal formation and neurotransmission in rats (Debassio et al., 1996; Mathangi and Namasivayam, 2001; Granados-Rojas et al., 2002; Alamy and Bengelloun, 2012). In a human study, researchers described fewer numbers of neurons with shorter dendrites and abnormal dendritic spines in individuals with malnutrition; however, this study was carried out just on 13 severely undernourished infants, compared to seven adequately fed babies (Benítez-Bribiesca et al., 1999). Because of small sample size, this study cannot provide definitive evidence of the effect of malnutrition on brain structure (although the fact that significant differences were observed even with a relatively small number of participants is potentially revealing, in terms of statistical power considerations). Moreover, malnourished children have less energy and interest for learning that negatively influences cognitive development (Engle, 2010).

Malnutrition can develop in utero, when the mother is malnourished (as often happens in low income countries). In Western countries, restricted foetal growth is often the result of a medical condition such as severe hypertension, or if the mother consumes higher levels of alcohol (Henriksen and Clausen, 2002; Feldman et al., 2012; Mustafa et al., 2012). For example, in uncontrolled severe hypertension during pregnancy the placental blood flow is restricted and there are placental abnormalities, which may prevent the foetus from obtaining the required oxygen and nutrients for development (Henriksen and Clausen, 2002). It has been shown that intrauterine growth retardation (IUGR) or small-for-gestational age (SGA) at birth is associated with cognitive developmental delays and a decrease of 4–8 points in IQ scores compared to infants with a birth weight that is appropriate-for-gestational-age (AGA; Pallotto and Kilbride, 2006). Apart from IUGR, stunting can be caused by a nutritional deficit (such as protein-energy malnutrition) during the rapid growth of young children. Most often intrauterine malnutrition is followed by poor postnatal nutrition, and the combined and persistent effect of malnutrition across both periods results in seriously stunted growth (Dewey and Begum, 2011). Indeed, evidence from developing countries shows that stunting in early childhood is associated with poorer cognitive development and academic performance in later childhood (Grantham-McGregor, 1995; Grantham-McGregor et al., 2007). A recent review concluded that even mild but persistent malnutrition in early life (i.e., during the first 2 years of life) negatively influences reasoning, visuospatial functions, IQ, language development, attention, learning, and academic achievement, while supplementation with food can improve cognitive performance (Laus, 2011). In an interesting study, researchers randomly assigned 425 preterm infants to a "standard nutrient" group (who received either breast milk or standard formula) and "high nutrient" group (who received a higher protein-energy and micronutrient diet). The cognitive development of the children was then measured at 7½–8 years of age, and it was found that IQ (measured on the WISC) was higher in the high nutrient group, especially with respect to verbal IQ in boys (Lucas et al., 1998). A subgroup of these children (n = 76) was assessed again at 16 years, and a persistent effect of the high nutrient diet on verbal IQ was demonstrated. At this stage, brain MRIs were also undertaken and showed a larger volume of the caudate (which was correlated with higher verbal IQ), but only in males (Isaacs et al., 2008, 2009).

Obesity is a special form of malnutrition (overnutrition, as opposed to undernutrition which has been previously considered here), because the diet is likely to have low nutrient-density in conjunction with a high fat and carbohydrate content (Tanumihardjo et al., 2007). Obesity is of growing concern worldwide, with the number of overweight and obese children dramatically increasing over the past two decades. It was estimated in 2010 that 43 million children worldwide (including 35 million from developing countries) were overweight or obese, and this number is expected to continue to grow to 60 million by 2020 (De Onis et al., 2010).

Animal studies suggest that there may be a biological link between obesity and impaired cognitive performance that is related to insulin resistance and altered glucose metabolism (Jurdak et al., 2008). Furthermore, when rats were fed a high fat diet, it decreased neurogenesis in the hippocampus (Lindqvist et al., 2006). In addition, a maternal high-fat diet in mice altered the development of hippocampus in the foetus (Niculescu and Lupu, 2009), which may mediated by a decrease in the level of brain-derived neurotrophic factor (Molteni et al., 2002). A recent literature review concluded that overweight and obesity may result in poorer academic performance (measured as literacy, numeracy, and school grades; Burkhalter and Hillman, 2011), but only a few studies have researched a possible connection between obesity/overweight and cognitive performance. Li et al. (2008) described an association in 8–16-year-old children and adolescents between increased body mass index (BMI) and reduced cognitive performance, specifically visuospatial functioning as measured on the block-design test (a subtest of the WISC), but not attention, working memory (digit-span subtest) and academic performance (Wide Range Achievement Test). This association remained after adjusting for a range of covariates and potential obesity mediating factors. Palermo and Dowd (2012) did not find a similar association between increased body weight and cognitive performance as measured by the Woodcock Johnson Revised Test of Achievement and the Memory for Digit Span test. Bisset et al. (2012) examined weight status trajectories in 4–7-year-old children; overweight was not associated with cognitive outcomes as measured on the Kaufman's Assessment Battery for Children. The inconsistent findings in humans between obesity and cognitive development may be the result of the complexity of factors underlying these outcomes (Li et al., 2008). Moreover, associations between obesity and cognition that have been reported may be mediated by sociodemographic factors that include discrimination and isolation rather than through biological mechanisms (Palermo and Dowd, 2012).

3.3.3.3 BREAKFAST

The level of glucose metabolism in children's brains increases from birth until 4 years of age, reaching twice that of the adults' metabolic rate. This rate of glucose metabolism in children remains elevated until 9–10 years of age, before it declines to the adult level by late adolescence (Chugani, 1998). Therefore, regular meals and continuous glucose supply (to provide the brain with the required glucose for its high metabolism) is more important in children than in adults (Bellisle, 2004). Accordingly, children are more prone to the adverse effect of overnight fasting, and breakfast is a very important meal to provide fuel to the brain in the morning (Bellisle, 2004). A systematic review concluded that having breakfast is beneficial for cognitive function and development, especially in malnourished children. A lack of studies conducted into the optimal breakfast including type, composition and portion size exists but (Hoyland, 2009) carbohydrate rich, low-glycaemic food for breakfast that provides a continuous supply of glucose is known to facilitate better cognitive performance (Bellisle, 2004; Ingwersen et al., 2007; Micha et al., 2011).

A recent study showed that the brain's gray and white matter volume differed in various parts of healthy children's brain, according to the type of breakfast they ate (Taki et al., 2010). The researchers suggested that the difference may be due to the different glycemic index of the different breakfast staple types. The authors also proposed that if different breakfast types affect gray and white matter volume in the brain, they may in turn influence cognitive function. Therefore, the type of breakfast children eat can potentially have a long-term influence on cognitive development (Taki et al., 2010).

3.3.3.4 DIETARY PATTERN AND DIET QUALITY

Since individuals consume combinations of foods (which may contain other bioactive compounds that could act synergistically or antagonistically within or between food groups; Tangney and Scarmeas, 2011), it is important to investigate diet as a broadly encompassing variable in association with cognitive outcomes. Furthermore, as Tangney and Scarmeas (2011) state, if research shows an association between diet (as comprehensively measured) and better health outcomes, it may be easier to implement changes in terms of dietary interventions.

Some researchers have investigated the influences of overall diet on neurocognitive development during childhood. Gale et al. (2009) considered dietary patterns in infancy in relation to cognitive development and found higher full-scale IQ (measured on the Wechsler Preschool and Primary Scale of Intelligence test) at 4 years of age in children who consumed higher amounts of fruit, vegetables and food prepared at home during infancy (i.e., between 6 and 12 months). The association remained significant after adjusting for a wide range of factors, including socioeconomic status, maternal IQ and education. A cross-sectional study reported by Theodore et al. (2009) examined the association between (i) the intake of specific food groups in 3½ years old children and in the same children again at 7 years of age and (ii) their cognitive development measuring on the Stanford–Binet Intelligence Scale (at 3 years) and on the WISC-III (at

7 years). These researchers found that a higher level of consumption of fish at 7 years of age and bread and cereals at 3½ years of age was associated with higher IQ scores, whereas those children at the age of 3½ who consumed margarine every day scored significantly lower on IQ. Northstone et al. (2011) reported that higher scores on the "health conscious" dietary pattern (which included more salad, rice, pasta, and fruits) at 3 years of age were associated with higher IQ score on the WISC-III when these same children were tested aged 8½ years, compared to those children on the "processed" dietary pattern (with high fat and sugar content), after adjusting for a wide variety of potential confounders. In the same study, Smithers et al. (2012) examined six different dietary patterns and found negative associations between (i) the "discretionary pattern" (which contains biscuits, sweets, soft drinks, and snacks) at 6, 15, and 24 months of age, and ready-prepared baby foods at 6 and 15 months of age and (ii) IQ scores at 8 years of age (measured on the WISC). Smithers et al. (2012) also reported positive associations between children's IQ at age 8 years and "breastfeeding pattern" (measured at 6 months), "home-made contemporary" (legumes, fruits, fruit juices, cheese, egg) at 15 and 24 months, "home-made traditional" (vegetables, meat, sauces) at 6 months (but not at 15 and 24 months), and "ready-to-eat" food pattern (biscuits, breads, cereals, yoghurt) at 24 months.

3.4 CONCLUSION AND RECOMMENDATIONS FOR FUTURE RESEARCH

The majority of studies, which have investigated the association between nutrition and cognitive development, have focused on individual micronutrients, including omega-3 fatty acids, vitamin B12, folic acid, zinc, iron, and iodine. The evidence is more consistent from observational studies, which suggest these micronutrients play an important role in the cognitive development of children. However, the results from intervention trials of single nutrients are inconsistent and inconclusive, prompting the need for better controlled and more adequately powered studies in the future. It is plausible that children living in poor countries may encounter more multiple micronutrient deficiencies, as opposed to children living in rich countries who are reasonably well nourished (and where a small deficiency in one nutrient may not result in measurable, long-term change in cognitive outcomes, due to compensation over time). These are important considerations, because nutrients do not act alone; rather, they have in some contexts synergistic and in other contexts antagonistic effects with each other.

Individuals consume combinations of food and poor overall diet can cause multiple macro-and micronutrient deficiencies and imbalances. If an overall healthy diet synergistically enhances cognitive development in children, then public health interventions should focus on the promotion of overall diet quality rather than isolated micronutrients or dietary components consumed by children and adolescents.

REFERENCES

1. Alamy M., Bengelloun W. A. (2012). Malnutrition and brain development: an analysis of the effects of inadequate diet during different stages of life in rat. Neurosci. Biobehav. Rev. 36, 1463–1480 10.1016/j.neubiorev.2012.03.009

2. Anderson J. W., Johnstone B. M., Remley D. T. (1999). Breast-feeding and cognitive development: a meta-analysis. Am. J. Clin. Nutr. 70, 525–535

3. Armstrong B. (2002). Review: iron treatment does not improve psychomotor development and cognitive function at 30 days in children with iron deficiency anaemia. Evid. Based. Ment. Health 5:17 10.1136/ebmh.5.1.17

4. Asato M. R., Terwilliger R., Woo J., Luna B. (2010). White matter development in adolescence: a DTI study. Cereb. Cortex 20, 2122–2131 10.1093/cercor/bhp282

5. Attig L., Gabory A., Junien C. (2010). Early nutrition and epigenetic programming: chasing shadows. Curr. Opin. Clin. Nutr. Metab. Care 13, 284–293 10.1097/MCO.0b013e328338aa61

6. Beard J. L. (2008). Why iron deficiency is important in infant development. J. Nutr. 138, 2534–2536

7. Bellisle F. (2004). Effects of diet on behaviour and cognition in children. Br. J. Nutr. 92, S227–S232 10.1079/BJN20041171

8. Benítez-Bribiesca L., De La Rosa-Alvarez I., Mansilla-Olivares A. (1999). Dendritic spine pathology in infants with severe protein-calorie malnutrition. Pediatrics 104, e21

9. Benton D. (2001). Micro-nutrient supplementation and the intelligence of children. Neurosci. Biobehav. Rev. 25, 297–309 10.1016/S0149-7634(01)00015-X

10. Benton D. (2010a). The influence of dietary status on the cognitive performance of children. Mol. Nutr. Food Res. 54, 457–470 10.1002/mnfr.200900158

11. Benton D. (2010b). Neurodevelopment and neurodegeneration: are there critical stages for nutritional intervention? Nutr. Rev. 68, S6–S10 10.1111/j.1753-4887.2010.00324.x

12. Benton D. (2012). Vitamins and neural and cognitive developmental outcomes in children. Proc. Nutr. Soc. 71, 14–26 10.1017/S0029665111003247

13. Berbel P., Mestre J. L., Santamaria A., Palazon I., Franco A., Graells M., et al. (2009). Delayed neurobehavioral development in children born to pregnant women with mild hypothyroxinemia during the first month of gestation: the importance of early iodine supplementation. Thyroid 19, 511–519 10.1089/thy.2008.0341

14. Bhate V. (2008). Vitamin B-12 status of pregnant Indian women and cognitive function in their 9-year-old children. Food Nutr. Bull. 29, 249–254

15. Bhatnagar S., Taneja S. (2001). Zinc and cognitive development. Br. J. Nutr. 85, S139–S145 10.1079/BJN2000306

16. Bisset S., Fournier M., Janosz M., Pagani L. (2012). Predicting academic and cognitive outcomes from weight status trajectories during childhood. Int. J. Obes. (Lond.). 37, 154–159 10.1038/ijo.2012.106

17. Black M. M. (2003a). The evidence linking zinc deficiency with children's cognitive and motor functioning. J. Nutr. 133, 1473S–1476S

18. Black M. M. (2003b). Micronutrient deficiencies and cognitive functioning. J. Nutr. 133, 3927S–3931S

19. Black M. M., Baqui A. H., Zaman K., Ake Persson L., El Arifeen S., Le K., et al. (2004). Iron and zinc supplementation promote motor development and exploratory behavior among Bangladeshi infants. Am. J. Clin. Nutr. 80, 903–910

20. Blakemore S.-J., Burnett S., Dahl R. E. (2010). The role of puberty in the developing adolescent brain. Hum. Brain Mapp. 31, 926–933 10.1002/hbm.21052

21. Bleichrodt N., Born M. (1994). A metaanalysis of research on iodine and its relationship to cognitive development, in The Damaged Brain of Iodine Deficiency, ed Stanbury J. B., editor. (New York, NY: Cognizant Communication;), 195–200

22. Blencowe H., Cousens S., Modell B., Lawn J. (2010). Folic acid to reduce neonatal mortality from neural tube disorders. Int. J. Epidemiol. 39, i110–i121 10.1093/ije/dyq028

23. Boucher O., Burden M. J., Muckle G., Saint-Amour D., Ayotte P., Dewailly E., et al. (2011). Neurophysiologic and neurobehavioral evidence of beneficial effects of prenatal omega-3 fatty acid intake on memory function at school age. Am. J. Clin. Nutr. 93, 1025–1037 10.3945/ajcn.110.000323

24. Broadhurst C. L., Cunnane S. C., Crawford M. A. (1998). Rift Valley lake fish and shellfish provided brain-specific nutrition for early Homo. Br. J. Nutr. 79, 3–21 10.1079/BJN19980004

25. Broadhurst C. L., Wang Y., Crawford M. A., Cunnane S. C., Parkington J. E., Schmidt W. F. (2002). Brain-specific lipids from marine, lacustrine, or terrestrial food resources: potential impact on early African Homo sapiens. Comp. Biochem. Physiol. B Biochem. Mol. Bio. 131, 653–673 10.1016/S1096-4959(02)00002-7

26. Brown R. D., Langshaw M. R., Uhr E. J., Gibson J. N., Joshua D. E. (2011). The impact of mandatory fortification of flour with folic acid on the blood folate levels of an Australian population. Med. J. Aust. 194, 65–67

27. Bryan J., Osendarp S., Hughes D., Calvaresi E., Baghurst K., Van Klinken J.-W. (2004). Nutrients for cognitive development in school-aged children. Nutr. Rev. 62, 295–306 10.1111/j.1753-4887.2004.tb00055.x

28. Burkhalter T. M., Hillman C. H. (2011). A narrative review of physical activity, nutrition, and obesity to cognition and scholastic performance across the human lifespan. Adv. Nutr. 2, 201S–206S 10.3945/an.111.000331

29. Campoy C., Escolano-Margarit M. V., Ramos R., Parrilla-Roure M., Csábi G., Beyer J., et al. (2011). Effects of prenatal fish-oil and 5-methyltetrahydrofolate supplementation on cognitive development of children at 6.5 y of age. Am. J. Clin. Nutr. 94, 1880S–1888S 10.3945/ajcn.110.001107

30. Caulfield L. E., Putnick D. L., Zavaleta N., Lazarte F., Albornoz C., Chen P., et al. (2010). Maternal gestational zinc supplementation does not influence multiple aspects of child development at 54 mo of age in Peru. Am. J. Clin. Nutr. 92, 130–136 10.3945/ajcn.2010.29407

31. Cetina I. (2008). Long-chain omega-3 fatty acid supply in pregnancy and lactation. Curr. Opin. Clin. Nutr. Metab. Care 11, 297–302 10.1097/MCO.0b013e3282f795e6

32. Chugani T. (1998). A critical period of brain development: studies of cerebral glucose utilization with PET. Prev. Med. 27, 184–188 10.1006/pmed.1998.0274

33. Clark C. A., Pritchard V. E., Woodward L. J. (2010). Preschool executive functioning abilities predict early mathematics achievement. Dev. Psychol. 46, 1176–1191 10.1037/a0019672

34. Colombo J., Kannass K. N., Jill Shaddy D., Kundurthi S., Maikranz J. M., Anderson C. J., et al. (2004). Maternal DHA and the development of attention in infancy and toddlerhood. Child Dev. 75, 1254–1267 10.1111/j.1467-8624.2004.00737.x

35. Commonwealth of Australia. (2006). Nutrient reference values for Australia and New Zealand. Canberra, ACT.

36. Coyle P., Tran N., Fung J. N. T., Summers B. L., Rofe A. M. (2009). Maternal dietary zinc supplementation prevents aberrant behaviour in an object recognition task in mice offspring exposed to LPS in early pregnancy. Behav. Brain Res. 197, 210–218 10.1016/j.bbr.2008.08.022

37. Crawford M., Bloom M., Broadhurst C., Schmidt W., Cunnane S., Galli C., et al. (1999). Evidence for the unique function of docosahexaenoic acid during the evolution of the modern hominid brain. Lipids 34, S39–S47

38. Daniels J. L., Longnecker M. P., Rowland A. S., Golding J. (2004). Fish intake during pregnancy and early cognitive development of offspring. Epidemiology 15, 394–402 10.1097/01.ede.0000129514.46451.ce

39. De Benoist B. (2008). Conclusions of a WHO Technical Consultation on folate and vitamin B12 deficiencies. Food Nutr. Bull. 29, S238–S244

40. De Onis M. (2000). Is malnutrition declining? An analysis of changes in levels of child malnutrition since 1980. Bull. World Health Organ. 78, 1222

41. De Onis M., Blössner M., Borghi E. (2010). Global prevalence and trends of overweight and obesity among preschool children. Am. J. Clin. Nutr. 92, 1257–1264 10.3945/ajcn.2010.29786

42. De Rooij S. R., Wouters H., Yonker J. E., Painter R. C., Roseboom T. J. (2010). Prenatal undernutrition and cognitive function in late adulthood. Proc. Natl. Acad. Sci. U.S.A. 107, 16881–16886 10.1073/pnas.1009459107

43. De Souza A. S., Fernandes F. S., Do Carmo M. G. (2011). Effects of maternal malnutrition and postnatal nutritional rehabilitation on brain fatty acids, learning, and memory. Nutr. Rev. 69, 132–144 10.1111/j.1753-4887.2011.00374.x

44. Debassio W. A., Kemper T. L., Tonkiss J., Galler J. R. (1996). Effect of prenatal protein deprivation on postnatal granule cell generation in the hippocampal dentate gyrus. Brain Res. Bull. 41, 379–383 10.1016/S0361-9230(96)00214-6

45. Delong G. R., Stanbury J. B., Fierro-Benitez R. (1985). Neurological signs in congenital iodine-deficiency disorder (endemic cretinism). Dev. Med. Child Neurol. 27, 317–324

46. Desouza L. A., Ladiwala U., Daniel S. M., Agashe S., Vaidya R. A., Vaidya V. A. (2005). Thyroid hormone regulates hippocampal neurogenesis in the adult rat brain. Mol. Cell. Neurosci. 29, 414–426 10.1016/j.mcn.2005.03.010

47. Deungria M. (2000). Perinatal iron deficiency decreases cytochrome c oxidase (CytOx) activity in selected regions of neonatal rat brain. Pediatr. Res. 48, 169–176 10.1203/00006450-200008000-00009

48. Deutsch G. K., Dougherty R. F., Bammer R., Siok W. T., Gabrieli J. D. E., Wandell B. (2005). Children's reading performance is correlated with white matter structure measured by diffusion tensor imaging. Cortex 41, 354–363

49. Dewey K. G., Begum K. (2011). Long-term consequences of stunting in early life. Matern. Child Nutr. 7, 5–18 10.1111/j.1740-8709.2011.00349.x

50. Drane D. L., Logemann J. A. (2000). A critical evaluation of the evidence on the association between type of infant feeding and cognitive development. Paediatr. Perinat. Epidemiol. 14, 349–356 10.1046/j.1365-3016.2000.00301.x

51. Dror D. K., Allen L. H. (2008). Effect of vitamin B12 deficiency on neurodevelopment in infants: current knowledge and possible mechanisms. Nutr. Rev. 66, 250–255 10.1111/j.1753-4887.2008.00031.x

52. Dunstan J. A., Simmer K., Dixon G., Prescott S. L. (2008). Cognitive assessment of children at age 2½ years after maternal fish oil supplementation in pregnancy: a randomised controlled trial. Arch. Dis. Child Fetal. Neonatal. Ed. 93, F45–F50 10.1136/adc.2006.099085

53. Eilander A., Gera T., Sachdev H. S., Transler C., Knaap H. V. D., Kok F. J., et al. (2010). Multiple micronutrient supplementation for improving cognitive performance in children: systematic review of randomized controlled trials. Am. J. Clin. Nutr. 91, 115–130 10.3945/ajcn.2009.28376

54. Eilander A., Hundscheid D. C., Osendarp S. J., Transler C., Zock P. L. (2007). Effects of n-3 long chain polyunsaturated fatty acid supplementation on visual and cognitive development throughout childhood: a review of human studies. Prostaglandins Leukot. Essent. Fatty Acids 76, 189–203 10.1016/j.plefa.2007.01.003

55. Engle P. L. (2010). INCAP studies of malnutrition and cognitive behavior. Food Nutr. Bull. 31, 83–94

56. Falkingham M., Abdelhamid A., Curtis P., Fairweather-Tait S., Dye L., Hooper L. (2010). The effects of oral iron supplementation on cognition in older children and adults: a systematic review and meta-analysis. Nutr. J. 9:4 10.1186/1475-2891-9-4

57. Feldman H. S., Jones K. L., Lindsay S., Slymen D., Klonoff-Cohen H., Kao K., et al. (2012). Prenatal alcohol exposure patterns and alcohol-related birth defects

and growth deficiencies: a prospective study. Alcohol. Clin. Exp. Res. 36, 670–676 10.1111/j.1530-0277.2011.01664.x

58. Florence M. D., Asbridge M., Veugelers P. J. (2008). Diet quality and academic performance. J. Sch. Health 78, 209–215 10.1111/j.1746-1561.2008.00288.x

59. Forrest D. (2004). The developing brain and maternal thyroid hormone: finding the links. Endocrinology 145, 4034–4036 10.1210/en.2004-0603

60. Frick J. E., Colombo J., Saxon T. F. (1999). Individual and developmental differences in disengagement of fixation in early infancy. Child Dev. 70, 537–548 10.1111/1467-8624.00039

61. Gale C. R., Martyn C. N., Marriott L. D., Limond J., Crozier S., Inskip H. M., et al. (2009). Dietary patterns in infancy and cognitive and neuropsychological function in childhood. J. Child Psychol. Psychiatry 50, 816–823 10.1111/j.1469-7610.2008.02029.x

62. Gallego G. (2010). Iodine deficiency in Australia: is iodine supplementation for pregnant and lactating women warranted? Med. J. Aust. 192, 461–463

63. Georgieff M. K. (2007). Nutrition and the developing brain: nutrient priorities and measurement. Am. J. Clin. Nutr. 85, 614S–620S

64. Ghosh S. S., Kakunoori S., Augustinack J., Nieto-Castanon A., Kovelman I., Gaab N., et al. (2010). Evaluating the validity of volume-based and surface-based brain image registration for developmental cognitive neuroscience studies in children 4 to 11 years of age. Neuroimage 53, 85–93 10.1016/j.neuroimage.2010.05.075

65. Gibson R., Heath A.-L. (2011). Population groups at risk of zinc deficiency in Australia and New Zealand. Nutr. Diet. 68, 97–108

66. Giedd J., Stockman M., Weddle C., Liverpool M., Alexander-Bloch A., Wallace G., et al. (2010). Anatomic magnetic resonance imaging of the developing child and adolescent brain and effects of genetic variation. Neuropsychol. Rev. 20, 349–361 10.1007/s11065-010-9151-9

67. Gökçay G. (2010). Breastfeeding and child cognitive development. Child. Care. Health Dev. 36, 591 10.1111/j.1365-2214.2009.01070.x

68. Gong J., Dong J., Wang Y., Xu H., Wei W., Zhong J., et al. (2010). Developmental iodine deficiency and hypothyroidism impair neural development, up-regulate caveolin-1 and down-regulate synaptophysin in rat hippocampus. J. Neuroendocrinol. 22, 129–139 10.1111/j.1365-2826.2009.01943.x

69. Gordon R. C., Rose M. C., Skeaff S. A., Gray A. R., Morgan K. M., Ruffman T. (2009). Iodine supplementation improves cognition in mildly iodine-deficient children. Am. J. Clin. Nutr. 90, 1264–1271 10.3945/ajcn.2009.28145

70. Granados-Rojas L., Larriva-Sahd J., Cintra L., Gutiérrez-Ospina G., Rondán A., DíAz-Cintra S. A. (2002). Prenatal protein malnutrition decreases mossy fibers-CA3 thorny excrescences asymmetrical synapses in adult rats. Brain Res. 933, 164–171 10.1016/S0006-8993(02)02314-4

71. Grantham-McGregor S. (1995). A review of studies of the effect of severe malnutrition on mental development. J. Nutr. 125, 2233–2238

72. Grantham-McGregor S., Ani C. (2001). A review of studies on the effect of iron deficiency on cognitive development in children. J. Nutr. 131, 649S–666S

73. Grantham-McGregor S., Cheung Y. B., Cueto S., Glewwe P., Richter L., Strupp B. (2007). Developmental potential in the first 5 years for children in developing countries. Lancet 369, 60–70 10.1016/S0140-6736(07)60032-4

74. Grossman A. W., Churchill J. D., McKinney B. C., Kodish I. M., Otte S. L., Greenough W. T. (2003). Experience effects on brain development: possible contributions to psychopathology. J. Child Psychol. Psychiatry 44, 33–63 10.1111/1469-7610.t01-1-00102

75. Guesnet P., Alessandri J.-M. (2011). Docosahexaenoic acid (DHA) and the developing central nervous system (CNS) - Implications for dietary recommendations. Biochimie 93, 7–12 10.1016/j.biochi.2010.05.005

76. Haddow J. E., Palomaki G. E., Allan W. C., Williams J. R., Knight G. J., Gagnon J., et al. (1999). Maternal thyroid deficiency during pregnancy and subsequent neuropsychological development of the child. New Eng. J. Med. 341, 549–555 10.1056/NEJM199908193410801

77. Hamadani J. D., Fuchs G. J., Osendarp S. J. M., Huda S. N., Grantham-McGregor S. M. (2002). Zinc supplementation during pregnancy and effects on mental development and behaviour of infants: a follow-up study. Lancet 360, 290–294 10.1016/S0140-6736(02)09551-X

78. Heijmans B. T., Tobi E. W., Stein A. D., Putter H., Blauw G. J., Susser E. S., et al. (2008). Persistent epigenetic differences associated with prenatal exposure to famine in humans. Proc. Natl. Acad. Sci. U.S.A. 105, 17046–17049 10.1073/pnas.0806560105

79. Helland I. B., Saugstad O. D., Smith L., Saarem K., Solvoll K., Ganes T., et al. (2001). Similar effects on infants of n-3 and n-6 fatty acids supplementation to pregnant and lactating women. Pediatrics 108, e82 10.1542/peds.108.5.e82

80. Helland I. B., Smith L., Blomén B., Saarem K., Saugstad O. D., Drevon C. A. (2008). Effect of supplementing pregnant and lactating mothers with n-3 very-long-chain fatty acids on children's IQ and body mass index at 7 years of age. Pediatrics 122, e472–e479 10.1542/peds.2007-2762

81. Helland I. B., Smith L., Saarem K., Saugstad O. D., Drevon C. A. (2003). Maternal supplementation with very-long-chain n-3 fatty acids during pregnancy and lactation augments children's IQ at 4 years of age. Pediatrics 111, e39–e44 10.1542/peds.111.1.e39

82. Henriksen T., Clausen T. (2002). The fetal origins hypothesis: placental insufficiency and inheritance versus maternal malnutrition in well-nourished populations. Acta Obstet. Gynecol. Scand. 81, 112–114 10.1034/j.1600-0412.2002.810204.x

83. Herba C. M., Roza S., Govaert P., Hofman A., Jaddoe V., Verhulst F. C., et al. (2012). Breastfeeding and early brain development: the Generation R study. Matern. Child Nutr. [Epub ahead of print]. 10.1111/mcn.12015

84. Herlenius E., Lagercrantz H. (2004). Development of neurotransmitter systems during critical periods. Exp. Neurol. 190, 8–21 10.1016/j.expneurol.2004.03.027

85. Hibbeln J. R., Davis J. M., Steer C., Emmett P., Rogers I., Williams C., et al. (2007). Maternal seafood consumption in pregnancy and neurodevelopmental outcomes in childhood (ALSPAC study): an observational cohort study. Lancet 369, 578–585 10.1016/S0140-6736(07)60277-3

86. Hoffman D. R., Boettcher J. A., Diersen-Schade D. A. (2009). Toward optimizing vision and cognition in term infants by dietary docosahexaenoic and arachidonic acid supplementation: a review of randomized controlled trials. Prostaglandins Leukot. Essent. Fatty Acids 81, 151–158 10.1016/j.plefa.2009.05.003

87. Hoyland A. (2009). A systematic review of the effect of breakfast on the cognitive performance of children and adolescents. Nut. Res. Rev. 22, 220–243 10.1017/S0954422409990175

88. Huttenlocher P. R., Dabholkar A. S. (1997). Regional differences in synaptogenesis in human cerebral cortex. J. Comp. Neurol. 387, 167–178 10.1002/(SICI)1096-9861(19971020)387:2<167::AID-CNE1>3.0.CO;2-Z

89. Ingwersen J., Defeyter M. A., Kennedy D. O., Wesnes K. A., Scholey A. B. (2007). A low glycaemic index breakfast cereal preferentially prevents children's cognitive performance from declining throughout the morning. Appetite 49, 240–244 10.1016/j.appet.2006.06.009

90. Innis S. M. (2007). Dietary (n-3) fatty acids and brain development. J. Nutr. 137, 855–859

91. Isaacs E. B., Fischl B. R., Quinn B. T., Chong W. K., Gadian D. G., Lucas A. (2010). Impact of breast milk on intelligence quotient, brain size, and white matter development. Pediatr. Res. 67, 357–362 10.1203/PDR.0b013e3181d026da

92. Isaacs E. B., Gadian D. G., Sabatini S., Chong W. K., Quinn B. T., Fischl B. R., et al. (2008). The effect of early human diet on caudate volumes and IQ. Pediatr. Res. 63, 308–314 10.1203/PDR.0b013e318163a271

93. Isaacs E. B., Morley R., Lucas A. (2009). Early diet and general cognitive outcome at adolescence in children born at or below 30 weeks gestation. J. Pediatr. 155, 229–234 10.1016/j.jpeds.2009.02.030

94. Jacobson J. L., Jacobson S. W., Muckle G., Kaplan-Estrin M., Ayotte P., Dewailly E. (2008). Beneficial effects of a polyunsaturated fatty acid on infant development: evidence from the Inuit of Arctic Quebec. J. Pediatr. 152, 356–364, e351. 10.1016/j.jpeds.2007.07.008

95. Jain A., Concato J., Leventhal J. M. (2002). How good is the evidence linking breast-feeding and intelligence? Pediatrics 109, 1044–1053 10.1542/peds.109.6.1044

96. Jiménez-Chillarón J. C., Díaz R., Martínez D., Pentinat T., Ramón-Krauel M., Ribó S., et al. (2012). The role of nutrition on epigenetic modifications and their implications on health. Biochimie 94, 2242–2263 10.1016/j.biochi.2012.06.012

97. Joos S. K., Pollitt E., Mueller W. H., Albright D. L. (1983). The Bacon Chow Study: maternal nutritional supplementation and infant behavioral development. Child Dev. 54, 669–676

98. Jorgenson L. A., Wobken J. D., Georgieff M. K. (2003). Perinatal iron deficiency alters apical dendritic growth in hippocampal CA1 pyramidal neurons. Dev. Neurosci. 25, 412–420

99. Judge M. P., Harel O., Lammi-Keefe C. J. (2007). Maternal consumption of a docosahexaenoic acid–containing functional food during pregnancy: benefit for infant performance on problem-solving but not on recognition memory tasks at age 9 mo. Am. J. Clin. Nutr. 85, 1572–1577

100. Jurdak N., Lichtenstein A. H., Kanarek R. B. (2008). Diet-induced obesity and spatial cognition in young male rats. Nutr. Neurosci. 11, 48–54 10.1179/147683008X301333

101. Kafouri S., Kramer M., Leonard G., Perron M., Pike B., Richer L., et al. (2012). Breastfeeding and brain structure in adolescence. Int. J. Epidemiol. [Epub ahead of print]. 10.1093/ije/dys172

102. Kasatkina É., Samsonova L., Ivakhnenko V., Ibragimova G., Ryabykh A., Naumenko L., et al. (2006). Gestational hypothyroxinemia and cognitive function in offspring. Neurosci. Behav. Physiol. 36, 619–624 10.1007/s11055-006-0066-0

103. Kirksey A., Wachs T. D., Yunis F., Srinath U., Rahmanifar A., McCabe G. P., et al. (1994). Relation of maternal zinc nutriture to pregnancy outcome and infant development in an Egyptian village. Am. J. Clin. Nutr. 60, 782–792

104. Knudsen E. I. (2004). Sensitive periods in the development of the brain and behavior. J. Cogn. Neurosci. 16, 1412–1425 10.1162/0898929042304796

105. Kooistra L., Crawford S., Van Baar A. L., Brouwers E. P., Pop V. J. (2006). Neonatal effects of maternal hypothyroxinemia during early pregnancy. Pediatrics 117, 161–167 10.1542/peds.2005-0227

106. Kostović I., Judaš M., Radoš M., Hrabač P. (2002). Laminar organization of the human fetal cerebrum revealed by histochemical markers and magnetic resonance imaging. Cereb. Cortex 12, 536–544 10.1093/cercor/12.5.536

107. Kramer M. S., Aboud F., Mironova E., Vanilovich I., Platt R. W., Matush L., et al. (2008). Breastfeeding and child cognitive development:new evidence from a large randomized trial. Arch. Gen. Psychiatry 65, 578–584 10.1001/archpsyc.65.5.578

108. Laus M. (2011). Early postnatal protein-calorie malnutrition and cognition: a review of human and animal studies. Int. J. Environ. Res. Public Health 8, 590–612 10.3390/ijerph8020590

109. Lenroot R. K., Giedd J. N. (2006). Brain development in children and adolescents: insights from anatomical magnetic resonance imaging. Neurosci. Biobehav. Rev. 30, 718–729 10.1016/j.neubiorev.2006.06.001

110. Leung B., Wiens K., Kaplan B. (2011). Does prenatal micronutrient supplementation improve children's mental development? A systematic review. BMC Pregnancy Childbirth 11:12 10.1186/1471-2393-11-12

111. Levenson C. W. (2006). Regulation of the NMDA receptor: implications for neuropsychological development. Nutr. Rev. 64, 428–432 10.1111/j.1753-4887.2006. tb00228.x

112. Levi R. S., Sanderson I. R. (2004). Dietary regulation of gene expression. Curr. Opin. Gastroenterol. 20, 139–142

113. Levitt P. (2003). Structural and functional maturation of the developing primate brain. J. Pediatr. 143, 35–45 10.1067/S0022-3476(03)00400-1

114. Li Q., Yan H., Zeng L., Cheng Y., Liang W., Dang S., et al. (2009). Effects of maternal multimicronutrient supplementation on the mental development of infants in rural Western China: follow-up evaluation of a double-blind, randomized, controlled trial. Pediatrics 123, e685–e692 10.1542/peds.2008-3007

115. Li Y., Dai Q., Jackson J. C., Zhang J. (2008). Overweight is associated with decreased cognitive functioning among school-age children and adolescents. Obesity 16, 1809–1815 10.1038/oby.2008.296

116. Lillycrop K. A., Burdge G. C. (2011). The Effect of nutrition during early life on the epigenetic regulation of transcription and implications for human diseases. J. Nutrigenet. Nutrigenomics 4, 248–260 10.1159/000334857

117. Lillycrop K. A., Burdge G. C. (2012). Epigenetic mechanisms linking early nutrition to long term health. Best Pract. Res. Clin. Endocrinol. Metab. 26, 667–676 10.1016/j.beem.2012.03.009

118. Lindqvist A., Mohapel P., Bouter B., Frielingsdorf H., Pizzo D., Brundin P., et al. (2006). High-fat diet impairs hippocampal neurogenesis in male rats. Eur. J. Neurol. 13, 1385–1388 10.1111/j.1468-1331.2006.01500.x

119. Logan S., Martins S., Gilbert R. (2001). Iron therapy for improving psychomotor development and cognitive function in children under the age of three with iron deficiency anaemia. Cochrane Database Syst. Rev. CD001444 10.1002/14651858. CD001444

120. Logi Kristjánsson Á., Dóra Sigfúsdóttir I., Allegrante J. P. (2010). Health behavior and academic achievement among adolescents: the relative contribution of dietary habits, physical activity, body mass index, and self-esteem. Health Educ. Behav. 37, 51–64 10.1177/1090198107313481

121. Louwman M. W., Van Dusseldorp M., Van De Vijver F. J., Thomas C. M., Schneede J., Ueland P. M., et al. (2000). Signs of impaired cognitive function in adolescents with marginal cobalamin status. Am. J. Clin. Nutr. 72, 762–769

122. Lozoff B., Georgieff M. K. (2006). Iron deficiency and brain development. Semin. Pediatr. Neurol. 13, 158–165 10.1016/j.spen.2006.08.004

123. Lucas A., Morley R., Cole T. J. (1998). Randomised trial of early diet in preterm babies and later intelligence quotient. Br. Med. J. 317, 1481–1487 10.1136/bmj.317.7171.1481

124. Luna B., Sweeney J. A. (2001). Studies of brain and cognitive maturation through childhood and adolescence: a strategy for testing neurodevelopmental hypotheses. Schizophr. Bull. 27, 443–455

125. Makrides M., Gibson R. A., McPhee A. J., Yelland L., Quinlivan J., Ryan P., et al. (2010). Effect of DHA Supplementation during pregnancy on maternal depression and neurodevelopment of young children. J. Am. Med. Assoc. 304, 1675–1683 10.1001/jama.2010.1507

126. Maret W., Sandstead H. H. (2006). Zinc requirements and the risks and benefits of zinc supplementation. J. Trace Elem. Med. Biol. 20, 3–18 10.1016/j.jtemb.2006.01.006

127. Mathangi D. C., Namasivayam A. (2001). Effect of chronic protein restriction on motor co-ordination and brain neurotransmitters in albino rats. Food Chem. Toxicol. 39, 1039–1043 10.1016/S0278-6915(01)00051-5

128. McCann J. C., Ames B. N. (2005). Is docosahexaenoic acid, an n–3 long-chain polyunsaturated fatty acid, required for development of normal brain function? An overview of evidence from cognitive and behavioral tests in humans and animals. Am. J. Clin. Nutr. 82, 281–295

129. McCann J. C., Hudes M., Ames B. N. (2006). An overview of evidence for a causal relationship between dietary availability of choline during development and cognitive function in offspring. Neurosci. Biobehav. Rev. 30, 696–712 10.1016/j.neubiorev.2005.12.003

130. McGrath N., Bellinger D., Robins J., Msamanga G. I., Tronick E., Fawzi W. W. (2006). Effect of maternal multivitamin supplementation on the mental and psychomotor development of children who are born to HIV-1–infected mothers in Tanzania. Pediatrics 117, e216–e225 10.1542/peds.2004-1668

131. Meck W. H., Williams C. L. (2003). Metabolic imprinting of choline by its availability during gestation: implications for memory and attentional processing across the lifespan. Neurosci. Biobehav. Rev. 27, 385–399 10.1016/S0149-7634(03)00069-1

132. Melse-Boonstra A., Jaiswal N. (2010). Iodine deficiency in pregnancy, infancy and childhood and its consequences for brain development. Best Pract. Res. Clin. Endocrinol. Metab. 24, 29–38 10.1016/j.beem.2009.09.002

133. Micha R., Rogers P. J., Nelson M. (2011). Glycaemic index and glycaemic load of breakfast predict cognitive function and mood in school children: a randomised controlled trial. Br. J. Nutr. 106, 1552–1561 10.1017/S0007114511002303

134. Michaelsen K. F., Lauritzen L., Mortensen E. L. (2009). Effects of breast-feeding on cognitive function, in Breast-feeding: early influences on later health, eds Goldberg G., Prentice A., Prentice A., Filteau S., Simondon K., editors. (Netherlands: Springer;), 199–215 10.1007/978-1-4020-8749-3_15

135. Molteni R., Barnard R. J., Ying Z., Roberts C. K., Gómez-Pinilla F. (2002). A high-fat, refined sugar diet reduces hippocampal brain-derived neurotrophic factor, neuronal plasticity, and learning. Neuroscience 112, 803–814 10.1016/S0306-4522(02)00123-9

136. Murcia M., Rebagliato M., Iñiguez C., Lopez-Espinosa M.-J., Estarlich M., Plaza B., et al. (2011). Effect of iodine supplementation during pregnancy on infant neurodevelopment at 1 year of age. Am. J. Epidemiol. 173, 804–812 10.1093/aje/kwq424

137. Murgatroyd C., Spengler D. (2011). Epigenetics of early child development. Front. Psychiatry 2:16 10.3389/fpsyt.2011.00016

138. Mustafa R., Ahmed S., Gupta A., Venuto R. C. (2012). A comprehensive review of hypertension in pregnancy. J. Pregnancy 2012:105918 10.1155/2012/105918

139. Nagy Z., Westerberg H., Klingberg T. (2004). Maturation of white matter is associated with the development of cognitive functions during childhood. J. Cogn. Neurosci. 16, 1227–1233 10.1162/0898929041920441

140. Niculescu M. D., Lupu D. S. (2009). High fat diet-induced maternal obesity alters fetal hippocampal development. Int. J. Dev. Neurosci. 27, 627–633 10.1016/j.ijdevneu.2009.08.005

141. Northstone K., Joinson C., Emmett P., Ness A., Paus T. (2011). Are dietary patterns in childhood associated with IQ at 8 years of age? A population-based cohort study. J. Epidemiol. Comm. Health. 66, 624–628 10.1136/jech.2010.111955

142. Oken E., Braverman L. E., Platek D., Mitchell M. L., Lee S. L., Pearce E. N. (2009). Neonatal thyroxine, maternal thyroid function, and child cognition. J. Clin. Endocrinol. Metab. 94, 497–503 10.1210/jc.2008-0936

143. Oken E., Radesky J. S., Wright R. O., Bellinger D. C., Amarasiriwardena C. J., Kleinman K. P., et al. (2008a). Maternal fish intake during pregnancy, blood mercury levels, and child cognition at age 3 years in a US cohort. Am. J. Epidemiol. 167, 1171–1181 10.1093/aje/kwn034

144. Oken E., Usterdal M. L., Gillman M. W., Knudsen V. K., Halldorsson T. I., Strøm M., et al. (2008b). Associations of maternal fish intake during pregnancy and breast-feeding duration with attainment of developmental milestones in early childhood: a study from the Danish National Birth Cohort. Am. J. Clin. Nutr. 88, 789–796

145. Palermo T. M., Dowd J. B. (2012). Childhood obesity and human capital accumulation. Soc. Sci. Med. 75, 1989–1998 10.1016/j.socscimed.2012.08.004

146. Pallotto E. K., Kilbride H. W. (2006). Perinatal outcome and later implications of intrauterine growth restriction. Clin. Obstet. Gynecol. 49, 257–269

147. Penhune V. B. (2011). Sensitive periods in human development: evidence from musical training. Cortex 47, 1126–1137 10.1016/j.cortex.2011.05.010

148. Peper J. S., Brouwer R. M., Schnack H. G., Van Baal G. C., Van Leeuwen M., Van Den Berg S. M., et al. (2009). Sex steroids and brain structure in pubertal boys and girls. Psychoneuroendocrinology 34, 332–342 10.1016/j.psyneuen.2008.09.012

149. Pepper M. R., Black M. M. (2011). B12 in fetal development. Semin. Cell Dev. Biol. 22, 619–623 10.1016/j.semcdb.2011.05.005

150. Pop V. J. (2001). Low maternal free thyroxine concentrations during early pregnancy are associated with impaired psychomotor development in infancy. Clin. Endocrinol. 50, 149

151. Pop V. J., Brouwers E. P., Vader H. L., Vulsma T., Van Baar A. L., De Vijlder J. J. (2003). Maternal hypothyroxinaemia during early pregnancy and subsequent child development: a 3-year follow-up study. Clin. Endocrinol. 59, 282–288 10.1046/j.1365-2265.2003.01822.x

152. Prado E. L., Alcock K. J., Muadz H., Ullman M. T., Shankar A. H. (2012). Maternal multiple micronutrient supplements and child cognition: a randomized trial in Indonesia. Pediatrics 130, e536–e546 10.1542/peds.2012-0412

153. Qian M. (2005). The effects of iodine on intelligence in children: a meta-analysis of studies conducted in China. Asia Pac. J. Clin. Nutr. 14, 32

154. Ramakrishnan U., Imhoff-Kunsch B., Digirolamo A. M. (2009). Role of docosahexaenoic acid in maternal and child mental health. Am. J. Clin. Nutr. 89, 958S–962S 10.3945/ajcn.2008.26692F

155. Rey J. (2003). Breastfeeding and cognitive development. Acta Paediatr. 92, 11–18

156. Riano Galan I., Sanchez Martinez P., Pilar Mosteiro Diaz M., Rivas Crespo M. F. (2005). Psycho-intellectual development of 3 year-old children with early gestational iodine deficiency. J. Pediatr. Endocrinol.Metab. 18Suppl. 1, 1265–1272

157. Rioux F. M., Bélanger-Plourde J., Leblanc C. P., Vigneau F. (2011). Relationship between maternal DHA and iron status and infants' cognitive performance. Can. J. Diet. Pract. Res. 72, 76

158. Rosales F., Reznick J. S., Zeisel S. (2009). Understanding the role of nutrition in the brain and behavioral development of toddlers and preschool children: identifying and addressing methodological barriers. Nutr. Neurosci. 12, 190–202 10.1179/147683009X423454

159. Roseboom T., De Rooij S., Painter R. (2006). The Dutch famine and its long-term consequences for adult health. Early Hum. Dev. 82, 485–491 10.1016/j.earlhumdev.2006.07.001

160. Ross C. E., Mirowsky J. (1999). Refining the association between education and health: the effects of quantity, credential, and selectivity. Demography 36, 445–460

161. Ryan A. S., Astwood J. D., Gautier S., Kuratko C. N., Nelson E. B., Salem N., Jr. (2010). Effects of long-chain polyunsaturated fatty acid supplementation on neurodevelopment in childhood: a review of human studies. Prostaglandins Leukot. Essent. Fatty Acids 82, 305–314 10.1016/j.plefa.2010.02.007

162. Sachdev H., Gera T., Nestel P. (2005). Effect of iron supplementation on mental and motor development in children: systematic review of randomised controlled trials. Public Health Nutr. 8, 117–132 10.1079/PHN2004677

163. Schmidt M. K., Muslimatun S., West C. E., Schultink W., Hautvast J. G. (2004). Mental and psychomotor development in Indonesian infants of mothers supplemented with vitamin A in addition to iron during pregnancy. Br. J. Nutr. 91, 279–285 10.1079/BJN20031043

164. Schuchardt J., Huss M., Stauss-Grabo M., Hahn A. (2010). Significance of long-chain polyunsaturated fatty acids (PUFAs) for the development and behaviour of children. Eur. J. Pediatr. 169, 149–164 10.1007/s00431-009-1035-8

165. Schulzke S. M., Patole S. K., Simmer K. (2011). Long-chain polyunsaturated fatty acid supplementation in preterm infants. Cochrane Database Syst. Rev. CD000375. 10.1002/14651858.CD000375.pub4

166. Shah D., Sachdev H. P. S. (2006). Zinc deficiency in pregnancy and fetal outcome. Nutr. Rev. 64, 15–30 10.1111/j.1753-4887.2006.tb00169.x

167. Shaw G. M., Carmichael S. L., Yang W., Selvin S., Schaffer D. M. (2004). Periconceptional dietary intake of choline and betaine and neural tube defects in offspring. Am. J. Epidemiol. 160, 102–109 10.1093/aje/kwh187

168. Signore C., Ueland P. M., Troendle J., Mills J. L. (2008). Choline concentrations in human maternal and cord blood and intelligence at 5 y of age. Am. J. Clin. Nutr. 87, 896–902

169. Simmer K., Patole S., Rao S. (2008). Long-chain polyunsaturated fatty acid supplementation in infants born at term. Cochrane Database Syst. Rev. CD000376. 10.1002/14651858.CD000376.pub2

170. Simopoulos A. P. (1999). Evolutionary aspects of omega-3 fatty acids in the food supply. Prostaglandins Leukot. Essen. Fatty Acids 60, 421–429

171. Simopoulos A. P. (2008). The importance of the omega-6/omega-3 fatty acid ratio in cardiovascular disease and other chronic diseases. Exp. Biol. Med. 233, 674–688 10.3181/0711-MR-311

172. Sisk C. (2004). The neural basis of puberty and adolescence. Nat. Neurosci. 7, 1040 10.1038/nn1326

173. Smithers L. G., Golley R. K., Mittinty M. N., Brazionis L., Northstone K., Emmett P., et al. (2012). Dietary patterns at 6, 15 and 24 months of age are associated with IQ at 8 years of age. Eur. J. Epidemiol. 27, 525–535 10.1007/s10654-012-9715-5

174. Stevenson J. (2006). Dietary influences on cognitive development and behaviour in children. Proc. Nutr. Soc. 65, 361–365

175. Summers B. L., Henry C. M. A., Rofe A. M., Coyle P. (2008). Dietary zinc supplementation during pregnancy prevents spatial and object recognition memory impairments caused by early prenatal ethanol exposure. Behav. Brain Res. 186, 230–238 10.1016/j.bbr.2007.08.011

176. Taki Y., Hashizume H., Sassa Y., Takeuchi H., Asano M., Asano K., et al. (2010). Breakfast staple types affect brain gray matter volume and cognitive function in healthy children. PLoS ONE 5:e15213 10.1371/journal.pone.0015213

177. Tamura T., Goldenberg R. L., Chapman V. R., Johnston K. E., Ramey S. L., Nelson K. G. (2005). Folate status of mothers during pregnancy and mental and psycho-

motor development of their children at five years of age. Pediatrics 116, 703–708 10.1542/peds.2004-2189

178. Tamura T., Goldenberg R. L., Hou J., Johnston K. E., Cliver S. P., Ramey S. L., et al. (2002). Cord serum ferritin concentrations and mental and psychomotor development of children at five years of age. Obstet. Gynecol. Survey 57, 493–494 10.1067/mpd.2002.120688

179. Tamura T., Goldenberg R. L., Ramey S. L., Nelson K. G., Chapman V. R. (2003). Effect of zinc supplementation of pregnant women on the mental and psychomotor development of their children at 5 y of age. Am. J. Clin. Nutr. 77, 1512–1516

180. Taneja S., Bhandari N., Bahl R., Bhan M. K. (2005). Impact of zinc supplementation on mental and psychomotor scores of children aged 12 to 18 months: a randomized, double-blind trial. J. Pediatr. 146, 506–511 10.1016/j.jpeds.2004.10.061

181. Tangney C. C., Scarmeas N. (2011). The good, bad, and ugly?: how blood nutrient concentrations may reflect cognitive performance. Neurology 78, 230–231 10.1212/WNL.0b013e31824367da

182. Tanumihardjo S. A., Anderson C., Kaufer-Horwitz M., Bode L., Emenaker N. J., Haqq A. M., et al. (2007). Poverty, obesity, and malnutrition: an international perspective recognizing the paradox. J. Am. Diet. Assoc. 107, 1966–1972 10.1016/j.jada.2007.08.007

183. Thatcher R. W. (1991). Maturation of the human frontal lobes: physiological evidence for staging. Dev. Neuropsychol. 7, 397–419

184. Theodore R. F., Thompson J. M. D., Waldie K. E., Wall C., Becroft D. M. O., Robinson E., et al. (2009). Dietary patterns and intelligence in early and middle childhood. Intelligence 37, 506–513

185. Tofail F. (2006). Supplementation of fish-oil and soy-oil during pregnancy and psychomotor development of infants. J. Health Popul. Nutr. 24, 48–56

186. Tofail F., Persson L. Å., El Arifeen S., Hamadani J. D., Mehrin F., Ridout D., et al. (2008). Effects of prenatal food and micronutrient supplementation on infant development: a randomized trial from the Maternal and Infant Nutrition Interventions, Matlab (MINIMat) study. Am. J. Clin. Nutr. 87, 704–711

187. Toga A. W., Thompson P. M., Sowell E. R. (2006). Mapping brain maturation. Trends Neurosci. 29, 148–159 10.1016/j.tins.2006.01.007

188. Tramontana M. G., Hooper S. R., Selzer S. C. (1988). Research on the preschool prediction of later academic achievement: a review. Dev. Rev. 8, 89–146

189. Uddin L. Q., Supekar K., Menon V. (2010). Typical and atypical development of functional human brain networks: insights from resting-state fMRI. Front. Syst. Neurosci. 4:21 10.3389/fnsys.2010.00021

190. United Nations Children's Fund and World Health Organization, (2004). Low Birthweight: Country, Regional and Global Estimates. New York, NY: UNICEF

191. Van Petten C. (2004). Relationship between hippocampal volume and memory ability in healthy individuals across the lifespan: review and meta-analysis. Neuropsychologia 42, 1394–1413 10.1016/j.neuropsychologia.2004.04.006

192. Veena S. R., Krishnaveni G. V., Srinivasan K., Wills A. K., Muthayya S., Kurpad A. V., et al. (2010). Higher maternal plasma folate but not vitamin b-12 concentrations during pregnancy are associated with better cognitive function scores in 9- to 10-year-old children in South India. J. Nutr. 140, 1014–1022 10.3945/jn.109.118075

193. Velasco I., Carreira M., Santiago P., Muela J. A., García-Fuentes E., Sánchez-Muñoz B., et al. (2009). Effect of iodine prophylaxis during pregnancy on neurocognitive development of children during the first two years of life. J. Clin. Endocrinol. Metab. 94, 3234–3241 10.1210/jc.2008-2652

194. Vermiglio F., Lo Presti V. P., Moleti M., Sidoti M., Tortorella G., Scaffidi G., et al. (2004). Attention deficit and hyperactivity disorders in the offspring of mothers exposed to mild-moderate iodine deficiency: a possible novel iodine deficiency disorder in developed countries. J. Clin. Endocrinol. Metab. 89, 6054–6060 10.1210/jc.2004-0571

195. World Health Organization. (2004). Iodine Status Worldwide, WHO Global Database on Iodine Deficiency, Geneva.

196. World Health Organization. (2008). Worldwide Prevalence of Anaemia 1993-2005: WHO Global Database on Anaemia, Geneva

197. Wurtman R. J. (2008). Synapse formation and cognitive brain development: effect of docosahexaenoic acid and other dietary constituents. Metabolism 57, S6–S10 10.1016/j.metabol.2008.07.007

198. Zeisel S. (2006a). The fetal origins of memory: the role of dietary choline in optimal brain development. J. Pediatr. 149, S131–S136 10.1016/j.jpeds.2006.06.065

199. Zeisel S. H. (2006b). Choline: critical role during fetal development and dietary requirements in adults. Annu. Rev. Nutr. 26, 229–250 10.1146/annurev.nutr.26.061505.111156

200. Zeisel S. H. (2009). Importance of methyl donors during reproduction. Am. J. Clin. Nutr. 89, 673S–677S 10.3945/ajcn.2008.26811D

201. Zhang X.-M., Huang G.-W., Tian Z.-H., Ren D.-L., Wilson J. (2009). Folate stimulates ERK1/2 phosphorylation and cell proliferation in fetal neural stem cells. Nutr. Neurosci. 12, 226–232 10.1179/147683009X423418

202. Zhou S. J., Gibson R. A., Crowther C. A., Baghurst P., Makrides M. (2006). Effect of iron supplementation during pregnancy on the intelligence quotient and behavior of children at 4 y of age: long-term follow-up of a randomized controlled trial. Am. J. Clin. Nutr. 83, 1112–1117

203. Zimmermann M. (2006). Iodine supplementation improves cognition in iodine-deficient schoolchildren in Albania: a randomized, controlled, double-blind study. Am. J. Clin. Nutr. 83, 108–114

204. Zimmermann M. B. (2007). The adverse effects of mild-to-moderate iodine deficiency during pregnancy and childhood: a review. Thyroid 17, 829–835 10.1089/thy.2007.0108

205. Zimmermann M. B. (2009). Iodine deficiency in pregnancy and the effects of maternal iodine supplementation on the offspring: a review. Am. J. Clin. Nutr. 89, 668S–672S 10.3945/ajcn.2008.26811C

206. Zimmermann M. B. (2011). The role of iodine in human growth and development. Semin. Cell Dev. Biol. 22, 645–652 10.1016/j.semcdb.2011.07.009

CHAPTER 4

NUTRITION AND BRAIN DEVELOPMENT IN EARLY LIFE

ELIZABETH L. PRADO AND KATHRYN G. DEWEY

4.1 INTRODUCTION

Adequate nutrition is necessary for normal brain development. Nutrition is especially important during pregnancy and infancy, which are crucial periods for the formation of the brain, laying the foundation for the development of cognitive, motor, and socio-emotional skills throughout childhood and adulthood. Thus, nutritional deficiencies during pregnancy and infancy are likely to affect cognition, behavior, and productivity throughout the school years and adulthood. Focusing on this early period for the prevention of nutrient deficiencies may have long-term and widespread benefits for individuals and societies.

This article presents an overview of the pathway from early nutritional deprivation to long-term brain function, cognition, behavior, and productivity. Although nutrition is important for brain function throughout the

Printed with permission from Elizabeth L. Prado et al. Nutrition and brain development in early life.
Nutrition Reviews *(2014), 72: 267–284. doi: 10.1111/nure.12102.*

lifespan, this article focuses on nutrition during pregnancy and the first few years after birth, which is the period of most rapid brain development. Presented first are the biological mechanisms through which nutrient deficiencies in pregnancy and infancy may affect brain development. Most of this evidence at the cellular and molecular level is from animal studies. Although these animal models have demonstrated the importance of adequate nutrition for the developing brain, many factors influence whether undernutrition during pregnancy and infancy leads to permanent cognitive deficits in human populations. The second part of this article discusses four of those factors: 1) the amount and quality of stimulation the child receives from the environment; 2) the timing of nutrient deprivation; 3) the degree of nutrient deficiency; and 4) the possibility of recovery. Finally, a brief review of human studies is presented, focusing on research from low- and middle-income countries, where multiple nutrient deficiencies are prevalent among pregnant women and children. [1] Also addressed in this review are the long-term consequences of undernutrition in early life, randomized trials of food and protein/energy supplementation, and studies of breastfeeding practices, essential fatty acids, and certain specific micronutrients, in addition to implications for policy, programs, and future research.

4.2 ROLE OF NUTRIENTS IN BRAIN DEVELOPMENT

Approximately 22 days after conception, the neural plate begins to fold inward, forming the neural tube, which eventually becomes the brain and spinal cord.[2] Adequate nutrition is necessary from the beginning, with the formation of the neural plate and neural tube affected by nutrients such as folic acid, copper, and vitamin A. Seven weeks after conception, cell division begins within the neural tube, creating nerve cells (neurons) and glial cells (cells that support neurons). After a neuron is created, it migrates to its place in the brain, where it then grows axons and dendrites projecting out from its cell body. These branching projections make connections with other cells, called synapses, through which nerve signals travel from one cell to another. These neurodevelopmental processes begin during gestation and continue throughout infancy (see Table 1). Groups of neurons form pathways, which are refined through the programmed elimination of cells and connections. About half of all the cells that are produced in the brain are subsequently eliminated throughout childhood and adolescence. Synapses are also overproduced and then selectively eliminated. Some of this refining of neural pathways depends on the child's experience, or in other words, input from the child's environment. Cells and connections that are activated are retained and strengthened while those that are not used are eliminated. This is thought to be one of the primary mechanisms of brain plasticity, allowing the brain to organize itself to adapt to the environment and reorganize itself to recover from injury during development.[2]

Evidence from animal models of nutrient deficiency, and some evidence from human studies, clearly shows that many nutrients are necessary for brain development. Table 1 presents evidence for the effect of specific nutrient deficiencies during early development on five key neurodevelopmental processes: 1) neuron proliferation, 2) axon and dendrite growth, 3) synapse formation, pruning, and function, 4) myelination, and 5) neuron apoptosis (programmed cell death). Table 1 focuses on nutrients that have been studied in human as well as animal studies. Other nutrients, such as copper, which is also important for some of these neurodevelopmental processes, are not included since rigorous studies in human populations and intervention studies have not yet been conducted.

Although the necessity of nutrients for brain development is evident, the extent to which nutrient deprivation during gestation and infancy results in long-term effects on brain function in free-living human populations is not yet clear. The actual impact depends on several factors, including 1) the child's experience and input from the environment, 2) the timing of nutrient deprivation, 3) the degree of nutrient deficiency, and 4) the possibility of recovery. Each of these factors is discussed in the following sections, followed by a brief discussion of methodological factors that can also influence the results of nutrition studies.

TABLE 1: Evidence for the role of selected nutrients and experience in five key neurodevelopmental processes

Influence	Neurodevelopmental processes				
	Neuron proliferation	Axon and dendrite growth	Synapse formation, pruning, and function	Myelination	Apoptosis
Definition and timing	Neuron proliferation is the creation of new cells through cell division. This begins in week 7 of gestation and continues to at least 4.5 months postpartum.[2] Neuron proliferation is mostly completed at birth, but neurons can be created in adulthood.[3]	Axons and dendrites are branching projections that grow out from cell bodies to make connections with other cells. This process begins during gestation and continues through at least 2 years after birth. In some brain areas, axons reach their final destinations at 15 weeks gestation, in others at 32 weeks gestation. Dendrite growth begins at 15 weeks gestation and continues through the second year after birth in some brain areas.[2]	Synapses are connections between axons, dendrites, and cell bodies. Synapse formation begins during gestation (around week 23) and continues throughout the lifespan. Synaptic density reaches a peak at different times in different brain areas (for example, in the visual cortex between 4 and 12 months postpartum, and in the prefrontal cortex after 15 months postpartum).[3] The decrease in synaptic density that follows this peak in each area reflects synaptic pruning. Synapse overproduction is completed in the second year after birth, while synaptic pruning begins in the first year after birth and continues through adolescence.[2]	Myelin is white, fatty matter that covers axons and accelerates the speed of nerve impulses traveling from one cell to another. Myelination begins as early as 12–14 weeks of gestation in the spinal cord and continues until adulthood. The most significant period of myelination occurs from mid-gestation to age 2 years.[4] Before birth, myelination occurs in brain areas involved in orientation and balance. After birth, the rate of myelination of areas involved in vision and hearing reaches a peak before myelination of areas underlying language, coinciding with the emergence of these abilities.[2]	Apoptosis is programmed cell death. Of all the cells that are produced in the brain, about half die through a variety of mechanisms. One of these mechanisms is programmed cell death, which is regulated primarily by neurotrophic factors, such as BDNF and IGF-1. When levels of neurotrophic factors are below a certain threshold, molecules within the cell trigger degeneration. Neuron apoptosis coincides with the period of synaptogenesis, beginning during gestation and continuing through adolescence.[5] Small head size or brain volume may be caused by decreased neuron proliferation or increased apoptosis.

TABLE 1: *Cont.*

Influence	Neurodevelopmental processes				
	Neuron proliferation growth	Axon and dendrite growth	Synapse formation, pruning, and function	Myelination	Apoptosis
Protein-energy malnutrition	Human autopsy studies and magnetic resonance imaging studies have shown that infants with IUGR had fewer brain cells and cerebral cortical grey matter volume than normal-birth-weight infants.[6, 7] Human autopsy studies have also shown that infants with severe acute malnutrition have fewer brain cells than well-nourished infants.[8] IUGR in animals results in similar effects.[6]	A human autopsy study showed that undernutrition in 3–4-month-old infants with moderate malnutrition (low weight for age) had decreased dendritic span and arborization (complexity of branching projections) compared to well-nourished infants.[9] Rodent models have found similar effects of early postnatal undernutrition on dendrite growth.[10]	Both prenatal and postnatal undernutrition in rodents results in fewer synapses as well as synaptic structural changes.a[11, 12]	Adults who had been exposed to famine in utero during World War II showed increased white matter hyperintensities, shown by MRI.[13] Reduced myelination has been found in animal models of IUGR[6] and maternal nutrient restriction without resulting in IUGR.[14] IUGR decreases IGF-1 levels and IGF-1-binding protein expression, which influence myelin production.[6]	BDNF and IGF-1 levels decreased and cell death increased in the offspring of baboon mothers fed a nutrient-restricted diet during pregnancy (without IUGR).[14] Other animal models have also shown that IUGR decreases IGF-1 and IGF-1-binding protein expression.[6]

TABLE 1: *Cont.*

Influence	Neurodevelopmental processes				
	Neuron proliferation	Axon and dendrite growth	Synapse formation, pruning, and function	Myelination	Apoptosis
Fatty acids	Neurogenesis requires the synthesis of large amounts of membrane phospholipid from fatty acids. Reduced neuron proliferation has been shown in animals with gestational DHA deficiency.[15]		Arachidonic acid and docosahexaenoic acid (DHA) in membranes at synaptic sites play a role in the maturation of synapses and in neurotransmission.[16]	Fatty acids are structural components of myelin. Both prenatal and postnatal fatty acid deficiency in rodents reduces the amount and alters the composition of myelin.[17, 18]	
Iron	Iron is required for the enzyme ribonucleotide reductase that regulates central nervous system cell division.[6] While gestational and neonatal iron deficiency in rodents does not affect overall brain size, a decrease in the size of the hippocampus (a subcortical structure that underlies learning and memory) has been shown.[19]	Gestational and neonatal iron deficiency in rodents results in truncated dendritic branching in the hippocampus, which persists into adulthood despite iron repletion.[20]	Gestational and early postnatal iron deficiency in rodents results in decreased synaptic maturity and efficacy in the hippocampus, which persists despite iron repletion.[21] In adult rodents, iron deficiency decreases the number of dopamine D2 receptors and the density of dopamine transporter in the striatum and nucleus accumbens. [22] In both animal models and cell culture experiments, dopamine and norepinephrine metabolism are altered by iron deficiency.[23]	Iron plays a role in myelin synthesis. In animal models, even marginal iron deficiency during prenatal and early postnatal development decreases myelin synthesis and alters myelin composition, which is not corrected with iron repletion.[24]	

TABLE 1: *Cont.*

Influence	Neurodevelopmental processes				
	Neuron proliferation	Axon and dendrite growth	Synapse formation, pruning, and function	Myelination	Apoptosis
Iodine and thyroid hormones	Some fetuses aborted in months 6 and 8 of gestation in an iodine-deficient area of China had lower brain weight than fetuses in an iodine-sufficient area, while some showed increased cell density. Gestational iodine deficiency in sheep and marmosets resulted in reduced brain weight and cell number, which was not corrected with iodine repletion. No effect on brain weight or cell number was found in rodents with gestational iodine deficiency, but cell migration was impaired.[25]	Gestational iodine deficiency results in reduced dendritic branching in the cerebral cortex in rodents[26] and in the cerebellum in sheep and marmosets.[25] Early postnatal hypothyroidism in rodents results in decreased dendritic branching in the visual and auditory cortex and cerebellum.[27]	Gestational iodine deficiency in sheep resulted in decreased synaptic density, which was not corrected with iodine repletion.[25] Gestational and early postnatal hypothyroidism in rodents decreases the number and density of synapses in the cerebellum, and alters neurotransmitter levels.[27]	No myelination was detected in the cerebral cortex of fetuses aborted at month 8 of gestation in an iodine-deficient area of China.[28] Gestational iodine deficiency in sheep and rodents reduces myelination.[25] Gestational and early postnatal hypothyroidism in rodents leads to reduced myelination.[27]	

TABLE 1: *Cont.*

Influence	Neurodevelopmental processes				
	Neuron proliferation	Axon and dendrite growth	Synapse formation, pruning, and function	Myelination	Apoptosis
Zinc	Zinc is necessary for cell division due to its role in DNA synthesis. Gestational zinc deficiency in rodents results in decreased number of cells, as reflected by total brain DNA[29] and reduced regional brain mass in the cerebellum, limbic system, and cerebral cortex.[6]	Gestational zinc deficiency in rodents results in reduced dendritic arborization.[6]	Zinc released into synapses in the hippocampus and cerebral cortex modulates synapse function. Specifically, zinc modulates postsynaptic NMDA receptors for glutamate and inhibits GABAB receptor activation.[30]		In rodent pups, zinc deficiency decreased expression of IGF-1 and growth hormone receptor genes.[31]
Choline	Choline is essential for stem cell proliferation and is involved in transmembrane signaling during neurogenesis.[6] In rodents, gestational choline supplementation stimulates cell division.[32]		The neurotransmitter acetylcholine is synthesized from choline. Gestational choline deficiency in rodents has long-term effects on cholinergic neurotransmission despite repletion.[32]		Gestational choline deficiency increases the rate of apoptosis in the hippocampus in rodents.[32]

TABLE 1: *Cont.*

Influence	Neurodevelopmental processes				
	Neuron proliferation	Axon and dendrite growth	Synapse formation, pruning, and function	Myelination	Apoptosis
B-vitamins	Before neuron proliferation begins, during weeks 2–4 of gestation, the neural tube forms, which is comprised of progenitor (stem) cells that give rise to neurons and glial cells (cells that support neurons).[2] Maternal deficiency in folic acid and vitamin B12 is associated with neural tube defects, such as anencephaly and spina bifida.[33]	Gestational and early postnatal vitamin B6 deficiency in rodents results in reduced dendritic branching in the neocortex and cerebellum.[34, 35]	Gestational and early postnatal vitamin B6 deficiency in rodents results in decreased synaptic density in the neocortex,[35] reduced synaptic efficiency, particularly in NMDA receptors,[36] and lowered dopamine levels and dopamine D2 receptor binding in the striatum.[37]	Gestational and early postnatal vitamin B6 deficiency in rodents results in reduced myelination.[38]	

TABLE 1: *Cont.*

Influence	Neurodevelopmental processes				
	Neuron proliferation	Axon and dendrite growth	Synapse formation, pruning, and function	Myelination	Apoptosis
Experience	Rodents raised in enriched environments (large enclosures with objects that allow visual and tactile stimulation) show greater brain weight and cortical thickness than rodents raised in impoverished environments (standard lab cages).[39]	A human autopsy study showed that individuals with higher levels of education had more dendritic branching than those with lower education in Wernicke's area, a brain area underlying language processing. [40] Rodents raised in enriched environments (filled with toys and other rodents) have more dendritic spines than those raised in less complex environments. [41]	Rodents raised in enriched environments (large enclosures with objects that allow visual and tactile stimulation) show more synapses per neuron in visual and motor cortices than rodents raised in impoverished environments (standard lab cages). [39]	Children raised in Romanian orphanages and then adopted into US families, thus having experienced a degree of early socioemotional deprivation, showed structural changes in white matter tracts compared to control children who had not spent any time in an orphanage. [42] Practicing the piano in childhood correlated with myelination in areas underlying finger movements, as measured by fractional anistropy.[43] An enriched rearing environment affects myelination of the corpus callosum in rodents and monkeys. [44, 45]	

a The gestational period in rodents corresponds to the first half of pregnancy in humans, while the first 3 weeks after birth in rodents corresponds to the second half of pregnancy in humans.[46] Abbreviations: BDNF, brain-derived neurotrophic factor; GABAB, gamma-aminobutyric acid B; IGF-1, insulin-like growth factor-1; IUGR, intrauterine growth restriction; NMDA, N-methyl-D-aspartate.

Evidence from animal models of nutrient deficiency, and some evidence from human studies, clearly shows that many nutrients are necessary for brain development. Table 1 presents evidence for the effect of specific nutrient deficiencies during early development on five key neurodevelopmental processes: 1) neuron proliferation, 2) axon and dendrite growth, 3) synapse formation, pruning, and function, 4) myelination, and 5) neuron apoptosis (programmed cell death). Table 1 focuses on nutrients that have been studied in human as well as animal studies. Other nutrients, such as copper, which is also important for some of these neurodevelopmental processes, are not included since rigorous studies in human populations and intervention studies have not yet been conducted.

Although the necessity of nutrients for brain development is evident, the extent to which nutrient deprivation during gestation and infancy results in long-term effects on brain function in free-living human populations is not yet clear. The actual impact depends on several factors, including 1) the child's experience and input from the environment, 2) the timing of nutrient deprivation, 3) the degree of nutrient deficiency, and 4) the possibility of recovery. Each of these factors is discussed in the following sections, followed by a brief discussion of methodological factors that can also influence the results of nutrition studies.

4.3 FACTORS INFLUENCING THE IMPACT OF UNDERNUTRITION

4.3.1 EXPERIENCE AND INPUT FROM THE ENVIRONMENT

Brain development is affected by experience. Two types of processes are described as "experience-expectant" and "experience-dependent."[41] In experience-expectant processes, the brain relies on specific input for normal development. For example, the brain expects visual input through the optic nerve for normal development of the visual cortex.[41] The absence of these expected experiences impairs the neurodevelopmental processes that depend on them. These experience-expectant processes also depend on other types of sensory stimulation (e.g., auditory and tactile) and occur early in life. In contrast, "experience-dependent" processes refer to the way the brain organizes itself in response to an individual's experiences and acquired skills, which is a process that continues throughout the lifespan. For example, a neuroimaging study demonstrated that the rear hippocampus, a part of the brain that underlies spatial memory, increased in volume as London taxi-driver trainees learned the layout of the city streets.[47] While experience-expectant mechanisms refer to features of the environment that are (or should be) universal, experience-dependent mechanisms refer to aspects of the environment that are unique to the individual. These latter processes enable individuals to adapt to and thrive in their specific culture and environment.

Adequate nutrition can be considered an aspect of the environment that is expected by the brain for normal development.[48] An environment with poor quality and variety of sensory and social input impairs some of the same neurodevelopmental processes as nutrient deprivation during early development, including the complexity of dendritic branching and synaptic density (Table 1). The parallel influences of nutrient deficiency and stimulation from the environment on brain development may operate in several ways: additive effects, interacting effects, and mediating effects, all of which have been demonstrated in empirical studies. These are depicted in Figure 1 and discussed in greater detail below.

4.3.1.1 ADDITIVE EFFECTS

Nutrient deficiency and experiential input from the environment may have independent additive effects on brain development. In this case, in an at-risk population, one would expect children with both risk factors (nutrient deficiency and low stimulation) to perform at low levels, children with one risk factor (nutrient deficiency or low stimulation) to perform at average levels, and children with neither risk factor (sufficient nutrition and high stimulation) to perform at high levels in cognitive, motor, and socioemotional development. This pattern is shown in Figure 1a. In support of this hypothesis, several studies have shown that nutritional supplementation and psychosocial stimulation together result in greater improvements in child development than either intervention alone.[49, 50] In these studies, psychosocial stimulation consisted of periodic home visits during which community workers facilitated play sessions with mothers and children. The community workers conducted activities such as demonstrating play with homemade toys, emphasizing the quality of the verbal interactions between mothers and children, and teaching concepts such as color, shape, size, and number. Children in Costa Rica showed similar additive effects of iron-deficiency anemia in infancy and low socioeconomic status on cognitive scores at school age.[51]

4.3.1.2 INTERACTING EFFECTS

Alternatively, nutrient deficiency or intervention may affect some children but not others, depending on the amount and quality of stimulation they receive. For example, in Chile, low-birth-weight infants born into families with high socioeconomic status were at lower risk for poor developmental outcomes than those born into disadvantaged environments. [52] Similarly, in 6−8-year-old children in Vietnam, nutritional status was related to cognitive scores among children who did not participate in a preschool program at age 3−4 years, but not among those who did.[53] Thus, in some cases, stimulation from the environment can protect children from negative effects of undernutrition on development. This possibility is shown in Figure 1b. Conversely, undernourished children from disadvantaged homes where protective factors are lacking may show more of a developmental response to nutrition and other forms of interventions. For example, in Guatemala, the effect of a supplementary protein/energy drink on infant and preschool development was greatest among families of low socioeconomic status.[54] In Chile, 1 year of weekly home visits providing psychosocial stimulation increased cognitive and socioemotional scores in infants with iron-deficiency anemia (IDA), but not in infants without IDA.[55]

Another way that nutrition and stimulation may interact is that nutritional supplementation may only positively affect development among children who receive a certain amount of stimulation from the environment. If children do not receive any stimulation, improving nutrition alone may be insufficient to improve brain development. For example, in Jamaica, infants between the ages of 9 and 30 months who participated in a psychosocial stimulation intervention benefited from zinc supplementation, while those who did not receive psychosocial stimulation did not show any developmental benefit from supplementary zinc.[56] It is also possible that an intervention providing psychosocial stimulation may only benefit children who are adequately nourished. In an animal model of maternal choline deficiency, 7-month-old rodents were exposed to an environmental enrichment experience by being allowed to explore a maze once daily for 12 days. Rodents whose mothers had been given choline during gestation showed increased neurogenesis in the hippocampus through the enriching experience, while rodents whose mothers had been deprived of choline during gestation did not show altered neurogenesis.[57] This type of pattern is illustrated in Figure 1c.

4.3.1.3 MEDIATING EFFECTS

Finally, improving nutritional status may actually improve children's experiences and the stimulation they receive from the environment. Undernutrition affects physical growth, physical activity, and motor development, which may, in turn, influence brain development through two pathways. The first pathway is through caregiver behavior and the second is through child exploration of the environment[54, 58] (see Figure 2). First, caregivers may treat children who are small for their age as younger than they actually are, and thus not provide age-appropriate stimulation, which could result in altered brain development. Also, undernourished children may be frequently ill and therefore fussy, irritable, and withdrawn, leading caregivers to treat them more negatively than they would treat a happy, healthy child. Reduced activity due to undernutrition may limit the child's exploration of the environment and initiation of caregiver interactions, which could also lead to poor brain development.[59] Some evidence suggests that these mechanisms contribute to delayed motor and cognitive development in infants and children with IDA.[60, 61] However, in stunted Jamaican infants, nutritional supplementation affected cognitive development but not activity levels, and activity and development were not related to each other, suggesting that this mechanism did not mediate the effect of nutrition on cognitive development in this cohort.[62]

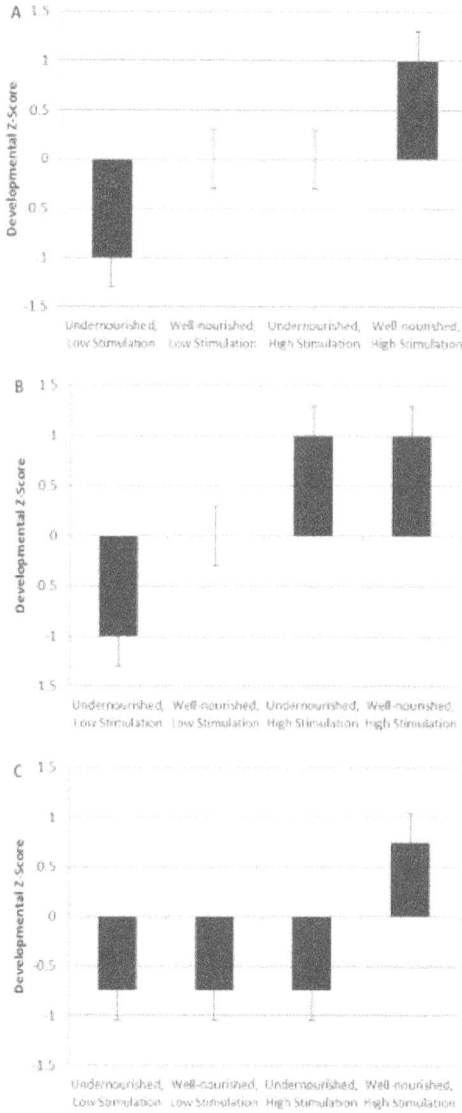

FIGURE 1: Three hypothetical scenarios in which the effects of undernutrition and a poor-quality environment may show additive or interacting effects on children's motor, cognitive, and socioemotional development. A Additive effects of undernutrition and poor-quality environment. B An enriched environment protects children from negative effects of undernutrition. C Nutrition intervention only affects children who have adequate stimulation, or stimulation intervention only affects children who have adequate nutrition.

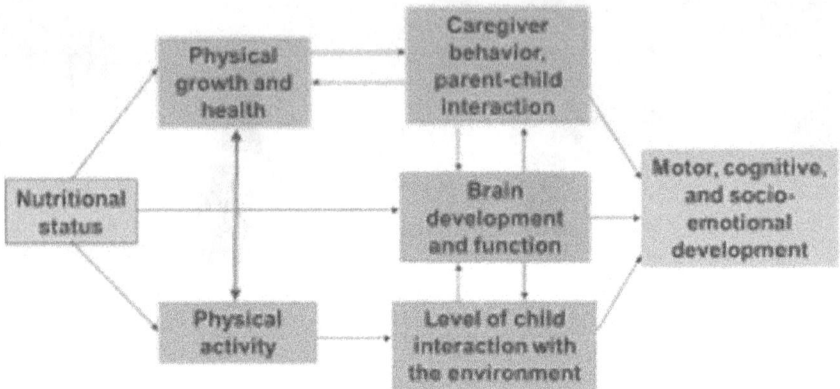

FIGURE 2: Hypothetical scenario in which the child's experience acts as a mediator between nutritional status and motor, cognitive, and socioemotional development. Adapted from Levitsky and Barnes[58] and Pollitt.[54]

Few studies have examined the potential additive, interacting, and mediating effects of nutrition and experiential input from the environment on child motor, cognitive, and socioemotional development. Studies that have tested all of these in a systematic way could not be located in the existing literature. In future research, datasets that allow the testing of each of these hypotheses are needed.

4.3.2 TIMING OF NUTRIENT DEPRIVATION OR SUPPLEMENTATION

Nutrient deficiency is more likely to impair brain development if the deficiency occurs during a time period when the need for that nutrient for neurodevelopment is high. Various nutrients are necessary for specific neurodevelopmental processes. Each process occurs in different, overlapping time periods in different brain areas. The timing of five key neurodevelopmental processes is presented in the first row of Table 1. Drawing links between specific nutrients, specific neurodevelopmental processes, and the time period of deprivation or supplementation allows specific hypotheses to be made concerning the effect of nutrient deprivation or supplementation on brain development.

For example, myelination of the brainstem auditory pathway occurs from week 26 of gestation until at least 1 year after birth.[63] Fatty acids such as docosahexaeonic acid (DHA) are necessary for myelination. This leads to the hypothesis that supplementation with DHA in the third trimester and the first year after birth may improve myelination of this auditory pathway. The latency of auditory-evoked potentials, which measure electrical activity in response to an auditory stimulus through electrodes placed on the scalp, is thought to reflect myelination, among other physiological aspects of brain function.[64] In support of the effect of DHA on myelination of the brainstem auditory pathway during the first few months after birth, a study in Turkey demonstrated that infants fed a formula containing DHA showed more rapid brainstem auditory-evoked potentials at age 16 weeks than infants fed a formula without DHA.[65] Future studies that examine precise hypotheses related to specific nutrients, neurodevelopmental processes, timing, and brain areas are needed to clarify the relationship between nutrition and brain development and its mechanisms. For a more complete discussion of the timing of neurodevelopmental processes and implications for measurement see Georgieff[66] and Wachs et al.[67]

4.3.3 DEGREE OF NUTRIENT DEFICIENCY

Much evidence shows that brain development may be compromised when nutrient deficiency is severe to moderate but spared when deficiency is mild to moderate. A number of homeostatic mechanisms protect the developing fetus and the developing brain from nutrient deficiency to a certain degree. For example, in the case of placental insufficiency, when insufficient nutrients and oxygen are available, fetal cardiac output is redistributed such that blood flow to the peripheral tissues decreases and blood flow to the brain, adrenal glands, and heart increases. This leads to brain sparing, or the sparing of brain growth even when overall fetal growth is reduced.[68] Another mechanism that protects the fetus from iron deficiency to a certain degree is the increased transfer of iron across the placenta as maternal levels decrease.[69] For each nutrient, there is likely to be a threshold at which deficiency results in impairment for the child. Exactly where this line is drawn is an important question which must be answered for each nutrient individually.

Several studies have shown that the effect of nutritional supplementation on brain development depends on initial nutritional status. For example, in Bangladesh and Indonesia, a positive effect of maternal multiple micronutrient supplementation during pregnancy and postpartum on child motor and cognitive development was found only in children of undernourished mothers.[70, 71] Similarly, in Chile, infants with low hemoglobin concentration at age 6 months showed improved cognition at age 10 years if they had been fed iron-fortified formula (compared to low-iron formula) during infancy, whereas children with high hemoglobin concentration at age 6 months performed better in cognitive tasks at age 10 years if they had received low-iron formula.[72] In summary, greater severity of nutritional deficiency increases both the likelihood of negative effects on brain development and the likelihood of positively responding to nutritional supplementation.

4.3.4 POSSIBILITY OF RECOVERY

Even if the timing and the degree of nutrient deficiency are sufficient to alter brain development, one important question is whether these changes can be subsequently corrected. If not, children undernourished in early life would show permanent developmental deficits. On the other hand, if some or all of these structural alterations can be corrected, children could partly or fully recover cognitive ability.

The brain's potential for recovery from early damage has been widely studied in the context of neurological injury during development. When a certain part of the brain is damaged during early life, recovery happens in three ways, depending on the timing of the injury and subsequent experience. First, there are changes in the organization of the remaining intact circuits in the brain that were left uninjured, involving the generation of new synapses in existing pathways. Second, new circuitry that did not exist before the injury develops. Third, neurons and glia are generated to replace the injured neurons and glia.[73] In the case of brain alterations caused by nutrient deficiency, recovery is plausible if nutrients become available during the time that the affected growth process is still occurring. In addition to nutrient repletion, enhanced sensory, linguistic, and social interactions may also facilitate recovery.

Data from a group of Korean orphans adopted by middle-class American families provided an opportunity to investigate the possibility of recovery. Children who were undernourished at the time of adoption (before age 2 years) did not score below the normal range on IQ tests at school age, but their scores were lower than those of Korean adoptees who had not been undernourished in infancy.[74] In addition, children adopted after age 2 years had lower IQ scores than those adopted before age 2 years, suggesting that improved conditions earlier rather than later in childhood provide a greater benefit.[75]

Other investigators have studied adults who were born during a period of famine in Holland during World War II when strict food rations were imposed on the entire Dutch population, including pregnant women. Children born during this period experienced nutrient deprivation in utero but adequate nutrition and health care thereafter. At age 19 years, their average IQ did not differ from that of a group whose mothers did not experience famine during pregnancy.[76] However, adults exposed to this famine in utero had increased risk of diagnosis of schizophrenia[77] and antisocial personality disorder,[78] as well as admittance to an addiction treatment program.[79] Together, this evidence suggests that some, but not all, of the negative effects of early undernutrition on brain development can be reversed through subsequent improvement in nutrition, health care, and enriched environments.

In these studies, the role of improved nutrition and the role of stimulation from the environment in recovery cannot be distinguished. Other evidence suggests that both of these can contribute to cognitive recovery after early undernutrition. In a large cohort of Peruvian children (n = 1,674), children who had been stunted before age 18 months but who were not stunted at age 4–6 years performed as well as children who had never been stunted in vocabulary and quantitative tests, while children who did not experience catch-up growth scored significantly lower.[80] In other studies, providing cognitive stimulation to children who suffered from an episode of severe acute malnutrition or IDA in early life improved mental and motor development.[55, 81] This type of evidence has led the World Health Organization to recommend structured activities to promote cognitive development as a component of the treatment of early childhood malnutrition, in addition to nutrition and healthcare.[82]

4.3.5 METHODOLOGICAL FACTORS

The selection of assessment tools and the age of assessment can also influence whether effects are found in nutrition studies. Global measures, such as the Bayley Scales of Infant Development (BSID) or IQ tests, are widely used but may be less sensitive to nutritional deficiency than tests of specific cognitive abilities.[83-85] In addition, using a test created in a high-income country in a low-income country without adaptation can lead to systematic bias.[86, 87] For a more complete discussion of assessing cognitive abilities in nutrition studies, see Isaacs and Oates.[84]

Detecting the effects of early nutrient deficiency can also depend on the age of cognitive assessment. For example, a group of children who experienced thiamine deficiency in infancy did not show neurological symptoms at the time of deficiency, but showed language impairment at age 5–7 years.[88] Similarly, in a randomized controlled trial, infants who received formula containing certain fatty acids (docosahexaenoic acid and arachidonic acid) showed higher vocabulary and IQ scores at age 5–6 years compared to infants who received formula without these fatty acids, even though they did not differ in vocabulary or BSID scores at age 18 months.[85] These examples show that long-term effects may be found even when immediate effects of early nutritional deficiency are not apparent.

In summary, the long-term effect of nutritional deficiency on brain development depends on the timing and degree of deficiency, as well as the quality of the child's environment. Recovery is possible with nutrient repletion during a time period when the affected neurodevelopmental process is ongoing and with enhanced interaction with caregivers and other aspects of the environment.

4.4 BRIEF REVIEW OF HUMAN STUDIES

As shown in Table 1, research in animals has demonstrated the effects of many specific nutrient deficiencies on the development of brain structure and function. However, studies examining the effect of mild to moderate undernutrition on brain development in free-living mothers and children have largely shown mixed or inconclusive results. The factors discussed such as the timing and degree of deficiency and interactions with the amount of stimulation children receive may account for some of these mixed results. In addition, in many studies, undernutrition is confounded by other factors such as poverty, unstimulating environments, little maternal education, poor healthcare, and preterm birth, which make it difficult to isolate the effects of nutrition. To do this, randomized controlled trials are needed, but few of these specifically examining neurobehavioral outcomes have been conducted. The following sections briefly review studies of the long-term consequences of undernutrition in early life, food and protein/energy supplementation, breastfeeding practices, essential fatty acids, and certain specific micronutrients, with a focus on studies from low- and middle-income countries.

4.4.1 LONG-TERM CONSEQUENCES OF UNDERNUTRITION IN EARLY LIFE

Many studies have compared school-age children who had suffered from an episode of severe acute malnutrition in the first few years of life to matched controls or siblings who had not. These studies generally showed that those who had suffered from early malnutrition had poorer IQ levels, cognitive function, and school achievement, as well as greater behavioral problems.[89] A recent study in Barbados showed that adults who had suffered from an episode of moderate to severe malnutrition in the first year of life showed more attention problems[90] and lower social status and standard of living[91] than matched controls, even after 37–43 years.

Chronic malnutrition, as measured by physical growth that is far below average for a child's age, is also associated with reduced cognitive and motor development. From the first year of life through school age, children who are short for their age (stunted) or underweight for their age score lower than their normal-sized peers (on average) in cognitive and motor tasks and in school achievement. Longitudinal studies that have followed children from infancy throughout childhood have also consistently shown that children who became stunted (height for age < -2 SD below norm values) before 2 years of age continued to show deficits in cognition and school achievement from the age of 5 years to adolescence.[92]

Growth faltering can begin before birth, and the evidence indicates that being born small for gestational age is associated with mild to moderately low performance in school during childhood and adolescence, and with lower psychological and intellectual performance in young adulthood. [93] However, recent studies in low- and middle-income countries that have examined the relationship between low birth weight ($<2,500$ g/5.5 lb) and IQ, behavior problems, and academic achievement in school-age children, with and without controlling for gestational age at birth, have shown mixed results.[94] In a large study in Taiwan, adolescents who were born at term with low birth weight scored slightly but significantly lower than those born at term with normal birth weight on language, math, and science tests.[95] However, no effects of full-term low birth weight on IQ or behavior problems were found between the ages of 6–12 years in recent studies in Jamaica, Brazil, and South Africa.[96-98]

As discussed earlier, certain protective factors after birth may reduce the risk of long-term effects of low birth weight, such as high socioeconomic status,[52] cognitive stimulation in early life,[81] catch-up growth in height, and increased duration of breastfeeding.[93] The mechanism of brain sparing, also discussed earlier, may also be a protective factor. One well-controlled study showed cognitive deficits at 7 years of age in children who had been low-birth-weight infants compared to their normal-birth-weight siblings only if head growth was also compromised.[99] Another study showed that the ratio of neonatal head circumference to birth weight (cephalization index) was a better predictor of IQ at 3 years of age (inverse association) than was birth weight (positive association).[100]

This evidence shows that severe acute malnutrition and chronic malnutrition are clearly associated with impaired cognitive development, while the effects of growth faltering before birth are less clear and may be amenable to cognitive recovery.

4.4.2 FOOD AND PROTEIN/ENERGY SUPPLEMENTATION

Children who experience severe acute malnutrition, chronic malnutrition, and low birth weight tend to face other disadvantages that also affect brain development, such as poverty, poor housing and sanitation, poor healthcare, and less stimulating home environments, making it difficult to draw a causal link from observational studies. The results of randomized trials of maternal and child food supplementation, which provide stronger evidence of causation, are mixed (Table 2). Such trials that provided supplements to both mothers during pregnancy and children throughout the first 2 years of life showed the strongest evidence for long-term positive effects regarding cognition. In a large trial in Guatemala, pregnant women and their children up to the age of 7 years were provided with a milk-based high protein and energy drink with micronutrients or a low protein and energy drink with micronutrients. Children who received the high protein and energy drink had higher cognitive scores at 4–5 years of age, higher scores on tests of numeracy (math), knowledge, vocabulary, and reading achievement at 11–18 years of age[54] and on reading and IQ scores (among women) at 22–29 years of age,[101] and a 46% increase in average wages (among men) at 26–42 years of age.[102] While some of the effects on school-age performance were found in the late exposure group (after the age of 2 years), most of these effects were only found among individuals who began supplementation before the age of 2 or 3 years, including the effect on average wages. In contrast, few long-term effects have been reported when supplementation was provided only to mothers or only to children, though some such trials have demonstrated short-term cognitive and motor effects (Table 2).

TABLE 2: Randomized trials of food supplementation with micronutrients and/or balanced protein and energy to mothers and/or children and their effect on brain development

Study location	Intervention	Age at intervention	Age at assessment	Results
New York City[103]	High protein and energy drink with increased amounts of micronutrients versus moderate protein and energy drink with standard amounts of micronutrients	Maternal supplementation throughout pregnancy until birth	12 months	No effect was found on the BSID mental or motor scores at age 12 months, but children whose mothers had received the high protein/energy drink scored higher on two information processing measures (visual habituation and dishabituation) and one of five measures of play (length of play episodes).
Taiwan[104, 105]	High protein and energy drink with micronutrients versus no protein, low energy drink with micronutrients	Maternal supplementation throughout pregnancy and lactation	8 months	A positive effect was found on BSID motor but not mental scores.
	No effect on IQ or mental age (mental ability expressed in years of age by comparison with a norm reference group).		5 years	
Guatemala[54, 101, 102]	High protein and energy drink with micronutrients versus no protein, low energy drink with micronutrients	Maternal and child supplementation throughout pregnancy and until age 7 years	11–18 years	Positive effects were found on tests of math and knowledge scores. Positive effects on vocabulary and reading achievement were found only in children who received supplementation before 2 years of age.
22–29 years (women)	A positive effect was found on reading and IQ scores.			
26–42 years (men)	The high protein and energy drink resulted in a 46% increase in average wages.			

TABLE 2: *Cont.*

Study location	Intervention	Age at intervention	Age at assessment	Results
Colombia[50, 106]	Families who were provided with food (e.g., oil, dried milk, and bread) versus families who did not receive food	Throughout pregnancy and until age 3 years	3 years	A positive effect was found on Griffith's Developmental Quotient.
5–8 years	A positive effect was found on reading readiness but not arithmetic or knowledge.			
Indonesia[107, 108]	Children in daycare centers who were provided with snacks containing protein and energy versus children in daycare centers not provided with snacks	Children between ages 6 and 20 months at enrollment for 3 months of intervention	9–23 months	A positive effect was found on BSID motor but not mental scores.
8–9 years	A positive effect was found on a test of working memory but not on reaction time, recall, emotionality, vocabulary, or arithmetic			
Indonesia[109, 110]	High protein and energy milk plus micronutrient tablet (treatment 1) versus low protein and energy milk plus micronutrient tablet (treatment 2) versus low protein and energy milk plus placebo (control)	Children age 12 or 18 months at enrollment for 12 months of intervention	24 or 30 months	Positive effects of the two treatments versus the control were found on several measures of motor development and activity levels. An effect of the high protein and energy milk was found on one of several measures of cognitive development.

TABLE 2: *Cont.*

Study location	Intervention	Age at intervention	Age at assessment	Results
Jamaica[49, 111-114]	Stunted children assigned to supplementation with high protein and energy milk or psychosocial stimulation or both supplementation and stimulation versus non-stunted controls	Children age 9–24 months at enrollment for 2 years of intervention	33–48 months	A positive effect of supplementation was found on Griffith's Developmental Quotient as well as the locomotor and performance subscales
7–8 years	No effect of supplementation on a battery of cognitive tests			
11–12 years	No effect of supplementation on a battery of cognitive tests			
17–18 years	No effect of supplementation on cognition or mental health			

Abbreviations: BSID, Bayley Scales of Infant Development.

Apart from the trial in Guatemala, only a trial in Jamaica[113] conducted longitudinal assessment at multiple time points throughout childhood and adolescence (Table 2). Although this trial did not show long-term effects of the nutrition component of the intervention, the psychosocial stimulation component resulted in sustained effects on IQ, language, and reading ability up to 18 years of age.[113] The authors suggested that the lack of sustained effects of the nutrition component may have been because beginning supplementation sometime between 9 and 24 months was too late or because the supplements may not have been consumed exclusively by the children. They indicated that beginning supplementation at an earlier age or achieving higher compliance with supplement consumption may have resulted in more lasting effects.[113]

Together, this evidence suggests that adequate nutrition during pregnancy and throughout infancy is necessary for optimal cognitive development. However, the most effective timing for nutritional supplementation is not yet clear, since few randomized trials have been conducted and even fewer have evaluated cognition and other outcomes in adolescence and adulthood.

4.4.3 BREASTFEEDING PRACTICES

Breastfeeding may improve cognitive development through several potential mechanisms, related both to the composition of breast milk and to the experience of breastfeeding. A suite of nutrients, growth factors, and hormones that are important for brain development are abundant in breastmilk, including critical building blocks such as DHA and choline. [115-117] Also, the physical act of breastfeeding may foster a positive mother-infant relationship and enhance mother-infant interaction, which are important for cognitive and socioemotional development. Breastfeeding also elicits a hormonal response in mothers during each feeding session, which may reduce stress and depression and thus improve infant caregiving and mother-infant interaction.[118]

In high-income countries, children who are breastfed as infants tend to have higher IQs at school-age than children fed with formula. Meta-analyses have yielded pooled estimates of 3–5 IQ points favoring children who had been breastfed,[119-121] with higher estimates among those born with low birth weight (5–8 IQ points).[120, 121] However, not all studies have found this positive relationship[122] and this relationship may be confounded by other factors, since mothers from higher socioeconomic backgrounds and with higher IQs are generally more likely to breastfeed in high-income countries.[123, 124]

This problem of confounding is less likely in low- and middle-income countries. For example, among a group of mothers in the Philippines, those from the poorest environments breastfed the longest[125] and in two separate cohorts in Brazil, socioeconomic status was unrelated to breastfeeding practices.[126, 127] The study in the Philippines showed that increased duration of breastfeeding was associated with better cognitive performance at age 8–11 years.[125] The first study in Brazil demonstrated that children who were breastfed for 9 months or more were ahead by 0.5 to 0.8 school grades at age 18 years relative to those breastfed for less than 1 month.[126] The second study in Brazil showed that higher IQ scores at age 4 years were associated with increased duration of breastfeeding, with children who were breastfed for 6 months or more scoring 6 IQ points higher than those breastfed for less than 1 month. Together, these positive associations between longer duration of breastfeeding and higher IQ and school achievement, after controlling for potential confounders, support the idea that a causal relationship exists.

The strongest evidence supporting the conclusion that breastfeeding is beneficial for brain development is from a large cluster-randomized trial in Belarus.[128] Clinics were randomly assigned to a breastfeeding promotion intervention or standard healthcare. Mothers in the breastfeeding promotion group had higher rates of any breastfeeding from birth to 12 months of age and higher rates of exclusive breastfeeding when the infants were 3 months of age. At a subsequent follow-up (mean age, 6.5 years), children in the breastfeeding promotion group had higher IQ scores and higher teacher ratings of reading and writing ability. This evidence indicates that promotion of breastfeeding can be an effective strategy to improve children's cognitive development.[59]

4.4.4 ESSENTIAL FATTY ACIDS

As shown in Table 1, essential fatty acids (EFA) and their derivatives are important for membrane function, synapse function, and myelination. Researchers have examined whether feeding infants formula containing these fatty acids positively affects cognitive development compared to standard formula that does not contain them. The authors of two recent papers, the first reporting a review[129] and the second a meta-analysis[130] of randomized controlled trials, concluded that EFA-containing formula does not affect general neurobehavioral development in full-term infants.[130] A positive effect among preterm infants, who are at risk for deficiency in certain fatty acids, including DHA, has been more frequently found.[129] Preterm infants are at risk because fatty acids accumulate rapidly in the brain during the third trimester of pregnancy.[131] Preterm birth interrupts this accumulation and puts the infant at risk for deficiency. However, in the report of Qawasmi et al.,[130] the pooled effect of EFA-containing formula on development among preterm infants was not significant. Note that most of the studies included in these two papers examined the effects on BSID scores. As discussed above, a recently published study showed a positive effect of EFA-containing formula on vocabulary and IQ at the age of 5–6 years even when no effect on 18-month BSID scores was found: this suggests the latter measure may not be sensitive enough to detect effects.

Supplementary EFA may benefit children in low- and middle-income countries whose diets may be lacking in EFA. However, very little research has been conducted in these countries. Studies in Turkey, Ghana, and China suggest that supplementation with EFA may affect infant neurodevelopment[65] and motor development.[132, 133] However, other trials in Africa did not find any difference in mental or motor development, e.g., in the Gambia, when fish oil was provided from 3 to 9 months,[134] and in Malawi, when complementary foods that differed in fatty acid content were provided from 6 to 18 months.[135] In the trial in the Gambia, the lack of effect is understandable, given that the infants were not deficient in fatty acids at baseline. Similarly, the latter trial was conducted in an area near Lake Malawi, where maternal fish consumption may result in relatively high levels of key fatty acids in breast milk, possibly masking any effects of supplementary EFA.

The effect of EFA on brain development during pregnancy is also not yet clear. While fatty acids are important for fetal neurodevelopment, randomized trials of maternal EFA supplementation have yielded mixed results. Gould et al.[136] recently conducted a systematic review and meta-analysis of randomized trials of maternal DHA supplementation. The meta-analysis on cognitive, language, and motor scores revealed no differences between supplemented and control children from birth to age 12 years, except for cognitive scores in children between the ages of 2 and 5 years. The authors concluded that methodological limitations in the 11 trials reviewed precluded confidence in the results; therefore, additional methodologically sound studies are needed, especially in children from disadvantaged or low-income backgrounds.[136]

4.4.5 MICRONUTRIENTS

Micronutrient deficiency is a critical concern for mothers and children throughout the world. It is estimated that 25% of the world's population suffers from IDA,[137] 33% have insufficient zinc intake,[138] and 30% have inadequate iodine intake.[139] Each of these micronutrients is involved in brain development (Table 1) and deficiencies are likely to impair cognitive, motor, and socioemotional abilities.

4.4.5.1 IRON

Iron is an essential structural component of the hemoglobin molecule, which transports oxygen to all the organs of the body, including the brain. IDA, that is, underproduction of hemoglobin due to iron deficiency, is a risk factor for both short-term and long-term cognitive impairment. IDA during infancy is associated with poor mental and motor development and during later childhood, with poor cognition and school achievement. Longitudinal studies have also consistently demonstrated that children who had been anemic before 2 years of age continued to show deficits in cognition and school achievement from 4 to 19 years of age.[140]

These long-term effects of infant IDA may persist even if iron treatment is provided during infancy. In longitudinal studies, adolescents who had been iron-deficient anemic in infancy continued to score lower than their non-anemic peers in IQ, social problems, and inattention, even though they were given iron treatment as infants.[141]

Prenatal iron supplementation may prevent some of these deficits. However, among three randomized trials of maternal iron supplementation during pregnancy that measured subsequent cognitive development of the children, only one showed positive results. In that trial, which was conducted in an area of Nepal with a high prevalence of IDA, children whose mothers had received iron, folic acid, and vitamin A performed better than those whose mothers had received vitamin A alone on tests of non-verbal intelligence, executive function, and motor ability at 7–9 years of age.[142] Two trials in China and Australia did not demonstrate effects of maternal iron supplementation on BSID scores at 3, 6, or 12 months of age[143] or on IQ at 4 years of age.[144]

Provision of iron to infants in low- and middle-income countries, where rates of iron deficiency are usually high, has consistently led to improved outcomes at the end of the intervention period. These trials are different from treatment trials in that all children are included, even if they have not been diagnosed with IDA, and the dose of iron is lower. Of five such trials, all showed positive effects on motor development, two on cognitive/language development, and three on socioemotional development.[141] These short-term results suggest that provision of iron to populations at risk for iron deficiency could have long-lasting positive effects. However, two recent follow-up studies reported no effect of iron supplementation in infancy on motor and cognitive ability at age 3.5 years in Sweden[145] and 7–9 years in Nepal.[146, 147] However, the study in Sweden found a significant impact on socioemotional development. Further long-term follow-up studies that examine cognitive, motor, and socioemotional skills are needed. Importantly, the provision of iron in malaria-endemic regions should be accompanied by adequate malaria surveillance and treatment.[148]

Taken as a whole, the evidence indicates that IDA during infancy is a strong risk factor for cognitive, motor, and socioemotional impairment in both the short and long term. Avoiding such consequences may require control of iron deficiency before it becomes severe or chronic, starting with adequate maternal iron intake before and during pregnancy and delayed cord clamping at birth.[149] Other elements of an appropriate strategy include preventing premature birth, feeding children iron-rich complementary foods, and providing postnatal services that promote responsive mother-infant interactions and early learning opportunities.[150]

4.4.5.2 IODINE

Iodine is necessary for the synthesis of thyroid hormones, which are essential for central nervous system development, including neurogenesis, neuronal migration, axon and dendrite growth, synaptogenesis, and myelination (Table 1). Pregnant women with severe iodine deficiency may underproduce thyroid hormones, leading to cretinism in the child. Cretinism is a disorder characterized by mental retardation, facial deformities, deaf-mutism, and severely stunted growth. Cretinism cannot be reversed after birth but can be prevented by the correction of iodine deficiency before conception.[151]

Even in the absence of overt cretinism, the evidence suggests that chronic iodine deficiency negatively affects intelligence. A meta-analysis showed a 13.5 IQ point difference between individuals living in iodine-sufficient and iodine-deficient areas.[152] Another more recent meta-analysis of studies in China indicated a similar estimated difference of 12.5 IQ points.[153] These results are equivalent to an effect size of 0.8–0.9 standard deviations. Although striking, these correlational studies may be confounded by uncontrolled factors, and randomized controlled trials of iodine supplementation in school-age children have yielded inconsistent results.[154]

Pregnancy seems to be a sensitive period with regard to the effects of iodine deficiency on neurodevelopment, since cretinism develops during this period. In an iodine-deficient region in China, 4–7-year-old children whose mothers were given iodine during pregnancy performed better on a psychomotor test than those who were supplemented beginning at 2 years of age.[155] A recent study in the United Kingdom suggests that even mild iodine deficiency in the first trimester of pregnancy can negatively affect children's cognition 8 years later. Among over 1,000 8-year-old children in the UK, those whose mothers had been iodine deficient in the first trimester of pregnancy were more likely to have scores in the lowest quartile for verbal IQ and reading comprehension.[156] Only two small randomized controlled trials of iodine supplementation during pregnancy have examined neurobehavioral outcomes, one among 72 mothers in Peru and another among 75 mothers in the Democratic Republic of Congo.[157] The average effect on the IQ scores of the children in these two trials at age 0–5 years was 10.2 IQ points.[157] Bougma et al.[157] also reviewed non-randomized iodine intervention studies and cohort studies in children age 5 years and under and found average effect sizes of 6.9–8.1 IQ points. The authors concluded that additional well-designed randomized controlled trials are needed to quantify more precisely the contribution of iodine deficiency to brain development in young children, including trials examining iodized salt.[157]

Though few well-designed controlled studies have been reported, adequate iodine intake is clearly necessary for normal brain development. Prevention of iodine deficiency, especially for pregnant mothers, is an important way to promote healthy brain development in children worldwide.

4.4.5.3 ZINC

Zinc is the fourth most abundant ion in the brain, where it contributes to brain structure and function through its role in DNA and RNA synthesis and the metabolism of protein, carbohydrates, and fat.[158] Although maternal and infant zinc deficiency in animals causes deficits in activity, attention, learning, and memory,[159] the evidence to date from human studies has not shown positive effects of zinc supplementation during pregnancy or infancy on child cognitive development.

Randomized trials of zinc supplementation during pregnancy in the United States, Peru, Nepal, and Bangladesh have shown no effects[142, 160, 161] or negative effects[162] of zinc compared to placebo or other micronutrients on the motor and cognitive abilities of children between the ages of 13 months and 9 years.

Similarly, infant zinc supplementation has not been demonstrated to improve cognitive development. Nine randomized controlled trials have provided zinc to infants beginning before the age of 2 years for at least 6 months and evaluated cognitive and/or motor development. Four of these provided zinc with or without iron or other micronutrients[147, 163-165] and one provided zinc with or without psychosocial stimulation.[56] Only one trial showed a positive effect of zinc on mental development and this benefit was found only in children who also received psychosocial stimulation; in the group who did not receive stimulation, there was no difference between the zinc and placebo groups.[56] One trial resulted in a negative effect of zinc supplementation on mental development compared to placebo.[166]

In these nine trials, positive effects on motor development were more commonly found. Four of the trials showed that zinc supplementation improved motor development,[56, 164, 167, 168] though one of these found an effect on the motor quality rating of the Bayley Behavior Rating Scale rather than on the Bayley Motor score,[168] and another showed an impact of zinc only when given in combination with iron.[164] In this latter study, iron and zinc together and iron and zinc in combination with other micronutrients, but not iron or zinc alone, affected motor development compared to placebo (riboflavin alone). Two other trials in India and Guatemala indicated that zinc supplementation in children under 2 years of age increased activity levels.[169, 170]

The available evidence suggests that zinc supplementation during pregnancy does not seem to improve childhood cognitive or motor development. Zinc supplementation during infancy may positively affect motor development and activity levels, but it does not seem to affect early cognitive ability. A 2009 meta-analysis of randomized controlled trials of zinc supplementation in infants did not find any evidence of impact on BSID mental or motor scores; however, the authors concluded that the number of available studies is still relatively small, and the duration of supplementation in these studies may be too short to permit detection of such effects.[171]

4.4.5.4 B-VITAMINS

Like zinc, B-vitamins, including thiamine, are important for brain development and function through many mechanisms. They play a role in carbohydrate metabolism (which helps to provide the brain's energy supply), membrane structure and function, and synapse formation and function.[172] Neurological symptoms typically characterize thiamine-deficiency disorders. In high-income countries, thiamine deficiency in infants has become a rare condition since food has been enriched with thiamine. However, recent evidence suggests that the prevalence of thiamine deficiency may be relatively high in some low-income countries. Of 778 infants who were admitted to a hospital in Laos without clinical signs of thiamine deficiency, 13.4% showed biochemical signs of thiamine deficiency based on analysis of their blood.[173] Moreover, a recent study in Israel demonstrated language deficits in 5–7-year-olds who had been fed a thiamine-deficient formula during infancy.[88] When doctors discovered that a certain manufacturer had mistakenly stopped adding thiamine to its infant formula in early 2003, they monitored the development of infants who had been fed that formula as high-risk patients. These children showed impaired language ability compared to control children at 5 years of age, even though they had not displayed any neurological symptoms during infancy.[88] The prevalence of thiamine deficiency and its effects on brain development require further research.[59]

Other observational studies have demonstrated associations between infant development and maternal niacin and vitamin B6 intake during pregnancy,[174] maternal riboflavin, niacin, and vitamin B6 intake during lactation,[175] and infant cobalamin and folate status.[176] Although randomized trials of supplementation with B-vitamins alone have not been conducted, many studies of multiple micronutrient supplementation included B-vitamins, as discussed below.

4.4.5.5 MULTIPLE MICRONUTRIENTS

Individuals who are deficient in one micronutrient are commonly at risk for deficiencies in others as well. Supplementation with any single micronutrient may not affect cognitive and motor development in individuals who are also deficient in other micronutrients. In these groups, supplementation with multiple micronutrients may be more beneficial than supplementation with a single micronutrient. The conversion of EFAs to DHA also depends on certain micronutrients and, thus, micronutrient deficiency may influence development through fatty acid status.[177]

Three randomized trials have reported positive effects of multiple micronutrient supplementation during pregnancy on child development between the ages of 6 and 18 months, including motor development in Bangladesh and Tanzania[70, 178] and cognitive development in China. [143] A trial in Indonesia showed positive effects of maternal multiple micronutrient supplementation on motor and cognitive development at age 3.5 years in the children of undernourished and anemic mothers.[71] In a fifth trial, 7–9-year-old children in Nepal whose mothers had received 15 micronutrients during pregnancy scored higher on a test of executive function than those whose mothers had received vitamin A alone.[142] However, this benefit was found for only one of six tests of motor and cognitive function. As described above, children of mothers in this same study in Nepal who received iron, folic acid, and vitamin A scored higher than those whose mothers received vitamin A alone on five of six cognitive and motor tests.

Studies of multiple micronutrient supplementation during infancy have shown some benefits immediately after the supplementation period. Three randomized trials in Ghana, China, and South Africa demonstrated positive effects on motor development in children between the ages of 12 and 18 months[132, 133, 179] and one trial also showed an effect on the overall developmental quotient.[133] In Mexico, infants between the ages of 8 and 12 months who had received multiple micronutrient supplementation for 4 months were more active than those who had not received supplementation.[180] However, a randomized trial in Bangladesh did not show an effect on mental or motor development in infants who received 16 micronutrients compared to infants who received one or two micronutrients. [164] Longer-term outcomes of these trials have not yet been reported.

4.5 CONCLUSION

When a child is adequately nourished from conception through infancy, the essential energy, protein, fatty acids, and micronutrients necessary for brain development are available during this foundational period, establishing the basis for lifetime brain function. The well-nourished child is also better able to interact with his or her caregivers and environment in a way that provides the experiences necessary for optimal brain development. Children who are not adequately nourished are at risk for failing to reach their developmental potential in cognitive, motor, and socioemotional abilities. These abilities are strongly linked to academic achievement and economic productivity. Therefore, preventing or reversing developmental losses in early childhood is crucial for fostering economic development in low- and middle-income countries as well as reducing economic disparities in high-income countries.

The evidence is clear that the following conditions are key risk factors for poor motor, cognitive, and socioemotional development: severe acute malnutrition (very low weight for height), chronic undernutrition (as evidenced by intrauterine growth retardation and linear growth retardation or stunting), IDA, and iodine deficiency. Preventing these conditions should be a global health priority.

The following interventions are examples of strategies that have been found to be effective in preventing or improving these conditions: salt iodization to prevent iodine deficiency,[181] provision of iron via home fortification (e.g., with micronutrient powders) to prevent IDA,[148] and educational interventions that include a strong emphasis on feeding nutrient-rich animal source foods, in conjunction with food supplementation in food-insecure populations.[182] With the exception of a few studies on food supplementation (Table 2), direct evidence of the impact of these strategies on brain development is scarce.

Strategies to promote exclusive breastfeeding during the first 6 months of life and continued breastfeeding thereafter, along with adequate complementary feeding, are also likely to improve cognitive development, though additional evidence for the effectiveness of these strategies is also needed.[94]

The following interventions are promising for preventing developmental loss: supplementation with iron and folic acid and/or multiple micronutrients during pregnancy, provision of multiple micronutrients (in addition to iron) during infancy, supplementation with essential fatty acids during pregnancy and infancy, fortified food supplements provided during pregnancy and infancy. However, additional robust research in low- and middle-income countries that evaluates the long-term effects of these interventions is needed.

The design and interpretation of further research should take into account the factors discussed above: the timing of nutrient deficiency or supplementation, the degree of deficiency, the possibility of recovery, and the potential for additive, interacting, or mediating effects with regard to the children's experiential input from the environment.

Interventions to improve the home environment and the quality of caregiver-infant interaction are also recommended to complement and enhance the effect of improved nutrition. These types of interventions are crucial to offset the negative effects of adverse environmental conditions (for example, poverty and low maternal education) that often coexist in populations in which undernutrition is common.

Integrated strategies targeting multiple risk factors, including nutrition, are necessary to reduce inequality and promote cognitive, motor, and socio-emotional development in disadvantaged children worldwide, ensuring that all children have the opportunity to fulfill their developmental potential.

REFERENCES

1. Black RE, Victora CG, Walker SP, et al. Maternal and child undernutrition and overweight in low-income and middle-income countries. Lancet. 2013;382:427–451.
2. Couperus JW, Nelson CA. Early brain development and plasticity. In: McCartney K , Phillips D , eds. The Blackwell Handbook of Early Childhood Development. Malden, MA: Blackwell Publsihing; 2006:85–105.
3. Johnson MH. Functional brain development in humans. Nat Rev Neurosci. 2001;2:475–483.
4. Sampaio RC, Truwit CL. Myelination in the developing human brain. In: Nelson CA , Luciana M , eds. Handbook of Developmental Cognitive Neuroscience. Cambridge, MA: MIT Press; 2001:35–44.
5. Oppenheim RW. Cell death during development of the nervous system. Annu Rev Neurosci. 1991;14:453–501.
6. Fugelstad A, Rao R, Georgieff MK. The role of nutrition in cognitive development. In: Nelson CA and Luciana M , ed. Handbook of Developmental Cognitive Neuroscience, 2nd ed. Cambridge, MA: MIT Press; 2008:623–641.
7. Tolsa CB, Zimine S, Warfield SK, et al. Early alteration of structural and functional brain development in premature infants born with intrauterine growth restriction. Pediatr Res. 2004;56:132–138.

8.   Winick M, Rosso P. The effect of severe early malnutrition on cellular growth of human brain. Pediatr Res. 1969;3:181–184.
9.   Cordero ME, D'Acuna E, Benveniste S, et al. Dendritic development in neocortex of infants with early postnatal life undernutrition. Pediatr Neurol. 1993;9:457–464.
10. Cordero ME, Valenzuela CY, Rodriguez A, et al. Dendritic morphology and orientation of pyramidal cells of the neocortex in two groups of early postnatal undernourished-rehabilitated rats. Brain Res Dev Brain Res. 2003;142:37–45.
11. Jones DG, Dyson SE. The influence of protein restriction, rehabilitation and changing nutritional status on synaptic development: a quantitative study in rat brain. Brain Res 1981;208:97–111.
12. Wiggins RC, Fuller G, Enna SJ. Undernutrition and the development of brain neurotransmitter systems. Life Sciences. 1984;35:2085–2094.
13. Hulshoff HE, Hoek HW, Susser E, et al. Prenatal exposure to famine and brain morphology in schizophrenia. Am J Psychiatry. 2000;157:1170–1172.
14. Antonow-Schlorke I, Schwab M, Cox LA, et al. Vulnerability of the fetal primate brain to moderate reduction in maternal global nutrient availability. Proc Natl Acad Sci U S A. 2011;108:3011–3016.
15. Coti Bertrand P, O'Kusky JR, Innis SM. Maternal dietary (n-3) fatty acid deficiency alters neurogenesis in the embryonic rat brain. J Nutr. 2006;136:1570–1575.
16. Uauy R, Dangour AD. Nutrition in brain development and aging: role of essential fatty acids. Nutr Rev. 2006;64(Suppl):S24–S33. discussion S72–91.
17. Miller SL, Klurfeld DM, Loftus B, et al. Effect of essential fatty acid deficiency on myelin proteins. Lipids. 1984;19:478–480.
18. McKenna MC, Campagnoni AT. Effect of pre- and postnatal essential fatty acid deficiency on brain development and myelination. J Nutr. 1979;109:1195–1204.
19. Rao R, Tkac I, Schmidt AT, et al. Fetal and neonatal iron deficiency causes volume loss and alters the neurochemical profile of the adult rat hippocampus. Nutr Neurosci. 2011;14:59–65.
20. Jorgenson LA, Wobken JD, Georgieff MK. Perinatal iron deficiency alters apical dendritic growth in hippocampal CA1 pyramidal neurons. Dev Neurosci. 2003;25:412–420.
21. Jorgenson LA, Sun M, O'Connor M, et al. Fetal iron deficiency disrupts the maturation of synaptic function and efficacy in area CA1 of the developing rat hippocampus. Hippocampus. 2005;15:1094–1102.
22. Beard JL, Connor JR. Iron status and neural functioning. Annu Rev Nutr. 2003;23:41–58.
23. Beard J. Recent evidence from human and animal studies regarding iron status and infant development. J Nutr. 2007;137(Suppl):524S–530S.
24. Kwik-Uribe CL, Gietzen D, German JB, et al. Chronic marginal iron intakes during early development in mice result in persistent changes in dopamine metabolism and myelin composition. J Nutr. 2000;130:2821–2830.
25. de Escobar GM, Obregon MJ, del Rey FE. Iodine deficiency and brain development in the first half of pregnancy. Public Health Nutr. 2007;10:1554–1570.
26. Chen ZP, Chen XX, Dong L, et al. The iodine deficient rat. In: Medeiros-Neto G, Maciel RMB, Halpern A, eds. Iodine Deficiency Diseases and Congenital Hypothyroidism. Sao Paolo: Ache Press; 1986:46–51.

27. Dussault JH, Ruel J. Thyroid hormones and brain development. Annu Rev Physiol. 1987;49:321–334.

28. Jia-Liu L, Zhong-Jie S, Yu-Bin T, et al. Morphologic study on cerebral cortex development in therapeutically aborted fetuses in an endemic goiter region in Guizhou. Chin Med J (Engl). 1984;97:67–72.

29. Sandstead HH. W.O. Atwater memorial lecture. Zinc: essentiality for brain development and function. Nutr Rev. 1985;43:129–137.

30. Walsh CT, Sandstead HH, Prasad AS, et al. Zinc: health effects and research priorities for the 1990s. Environ Health Perspect. 1994;2:5–46.

31. McNall AD, Etherton TD, Fosmire GJ. The impaired growth induced by zinc deficiency in rats is associated with decreased expression of the hepatic insulin-like growth factor I and growth hormone receptor genes. J Nutr. 1995;125:874–879.

32. Blusztajn JK, Cermak JM, Holler T, et al. Imprinting of hippocampal metabolism of choline by its availability during gestation: implications for cholinergic neurotransmission. J Physiol Paris. 1998;92:199–203.

33. Molloy AM, Kirke PN, Troendle JF, et al. Maternal vitamin B12 status and risk of neural tube defects in a population with high neural tube defect prevalence and no folic acid fortification. Pediatrics. 2009;123:917–923.

34. Chang SJ, Kirksey A, Moore DM. Effects of vitamin B6 deficiency on morphological changes in dendritic trees in Purkinje cells in developing cerebellum in rats. J Nutr. 1981;111:848–857.

35. Groziak SM, Kirksey A. Effects of maternal restriction of vitamin B6 on neocortex development in rats: neuron differentiation and synaptogenesis. J Nutr. 1990;120:485–492.

36. Guilarte T. Vitamin B6 and cognitive development: recent research findings from human and animal studies. Nutr Rev. 1993;51:193–198.

37. Guilarte TR, Wagner HN, Frost JJ. Effects of perinatal vitamin B6 deficiency on dopaminergic neurochemistry. J Neurochem. 1987;48:432–439.

38. Moore DM, Kirksey A, Das GD. Effects of vitamin B6 deficiency on the developing central nervous system of the rat. Myelination. J Nutr. 1978;108:1260–1265.

39. Kolb B, Whishaw IQ. Brain plasticity and behavior. Annu Rev Psychol. 1998;49:43–64.

40. Jacobs B, Schall M, Scheibel AB. A quantitative dendritic analysis of Wernicke's area in humans. II. Gender, hemispheric, and environmental factors. J Comp Neurol. 1993;327:97–111.

41. Greenough WT, Black JE. Induction of brain structure by experience: substrates for cognitive development. In: Gunnar MR , Nelson CA , eds. Developmental Behavioral Neuroscience. Hillsdale, NJ: Erlbaum; 1992:155–200.

42. Eluvathingal TJ, Chugani HT, Behen ME, et al. Abnormal brain connectivity in children after early severe socioemotional deprivation: a diffusion tensor imaging study. Pediatrics. 2006;117:2093–2100.

43. Bengtsson SL, Nagy Z, Skare S, et al. Extensive piano practicing has regionally specific effects on white matter development. Nat Neurosci. 2005;8:1148–1150.

44. Juraska JM, Kopcik JR. Sex and environmental influences on the size and ultrastructure of the rat corpus callosum. Brain Res. 1988;450:1–8.

45. Sanchez MM, Hearn EF, Do D, et al. Differential rearing affects corpus callosum size and cognitive function of rhesus monkeys. Brain Res. 1998;812:38–49.

46. Workman AD, Charvet CJ, Clancy B, et al. Modeling transformations of neurodevelopmental sequences across mammalian species. J Neurosci. 2013;33:7368–7383.

47. Woollett K, Maguire EA. Acquiring "the Knowledge" of London's layout drives structural brain changes. Curr Biol. 2011;21:2109–2114.

48. Nelson CA. A neurobiological perspective on early human deprivation. Child Dev Perspect. 2007;1:13–18.

49. Grantham-McGregor SM, Powell CA, Walker SP, et al. Nutritional supplementation, psychosocial stimulation, and mental development of stunted children: the Jamaican Study. Lancet. 1991;338:1–5.

50. Waber DP, Vuori-Christiansen L, Ortiz N, et al. Nutritional supplementation, maternal education, and cognitive development of infants at risk of malnutrition. Am J Clin Nutr. 1981;34(Suppl 4):807–813.

51. Lozoff B, Jimenez E, Smith JB. Double burden of iron deficiency in infancy and low socioeconomic status: a longitudinal analysis of cognitive test scores to age 19 years. Arch Pediatr Adolesc Med. 2006;160:1108–1113.

52. Torche F, Echevarria G. The effect of birthweight on childhood cognitive development in a middle-income country. Int J Epidemiol. 2011; 40:1008–1018.

53. Watanabe K, Flores R, Fujiwara J, et al. Early childhood development interventions and cognitive development of young children in rural Vietnam. J Nutr. 2005;135:1918–1925.

54. Pollitt E. Early supplementary feeding and cognition: effects over two decades. Monogr Soc Res Child Dev. 1993;58:1–99.

55. Lozoff B, Smith JB, Clark KM, et al. Home intervention improves cognitive and social-emotional scores in iron-deficient anemic infants. Pediatrics. 2010;126:e884–e894.

56. Gardner JM, Powell CA, Baker-Henningham H, et al. Zinc supplementation and psychosocial stimulation: effects on the development of undernourished Jamaican children. Am J Clin Nutr. 2005;82:399–405.

57. Glenn MJ, Gibson EM, Kirby ED, et al. Prenatal choline availability modulates hippocampal neurogenesis and neurogenic responses to enriching experiences in adult female rats. Eur J Neurosci. 2007;25:2473–2482.

58. Levitsky DA, Barnes RH. Nutrition and environmental interactions in the behavioural development of the rat: long-term effects. Science. 1972;176:68–71.

59. Prado EL, Dewey KG. Nutrition and brain development in early life. Alive & Thrive Technical Brief January 2012; (Issue 4).

60. Lozoff B, Klein NK, Nelson EC, et al. Behavior of infants with iron-deficiency anemia. Child Dev. 1998;69:25–36.

61. Corapci F, Radan AA, Lozoff B. Iron deficiency in infancy and mother-child interaction at 5 years. J Dev Behav Pediatr. 2006;27:371–378.

62. Meeks-Gardner J, Grantham-McGregor S, Chang S, et al. Activity and behavioral development in stunted and nonstunted children and response to nutritional supplementation. Child Dev. 1995;66:1785–1797.

63. Moore JK, Perazzo LM, Braun A. Time course of axonal myelination in the human brainstem auditory pathway. Hear Res. 1995;87:21–31.

64. Kerr CC, Rennie CJ, Robinson PA. Model-based analysis and quantification of age trends in auditory evoked potentials. Clin Neurophysiol. 2011;122:134–147.

65. Unay B, Sarici SU, Ulas UH, et al. Nutritional effects on auditory brainstem maturation in healthy term infants. Arch Dis Child Fetal Neonatal Ed. 2004;89:F177–F179.

66. Georgieff MK. Nutrition and the developing brain: nutrient priorities and measurement. Am J Clin Nutr. 2007;85(Suppl):614S–620S.

67. Wachs TD, Georgieff M, Cusick S, et al. Issues in the timing of integrated early interventions: contributions from nutrition, neuroscience and psychological research. Ann N Y Acad Sci. 2013;doi: 10.1111/nyas.12314.

68. Morrison JL. Sheep models of intrauterine growth restriction: fetal adaptations and consequences. Clin Exp Pharmacol Physiol. 2008;35:730–743.

69. O'Brien KO, Zavaleta N, Abrams SA, et al. Maternal iron status influences iron transfer to the fetus during the third trimester of pregnancy. Am J Clin Nutr. 2003;77:924–930.

70. Tofail F, Persson LA, Arifeen SE, et al. Effects of prenatal food and micronutrient supplementation on infant development: a randomized trial from the Maternal and Infant Nutrition Interventions, Matlab (MINIMat) study. Am J Clin Nutr 2008;87:704–711.

71. Prado EL, Alcock KJ, Muadz H, et al. Maternal multiple micronutrient supplements and child cognition: a randomized trial in Indonesia. Pediatrics. 2012;130:e536–e546.

72. Lozoff B, Castillo M, Clark KM, et al. Iron-fortified vs low-iron infant formula: developmental outcome at 10 years. Arch Pediatr Adolesc Med. 2012;166:208–215.

73. Kolb B, Gibb R. Early brain injury, plasticity, and behavior. In: Nelson CA, Luciana M, eds. Handbook of Developmental Neuroscience. Cambridge, MA: MIT Press; 2001:175–190.

74. Winick M, Meyer KK, Harris RC. Malnutrition and environmental enrichment by early adoption. Science. 1975;190:1173–1175.

75. Lien NM, Meyer KK, Winick M. Early malnutrition and "late" adoption: a study of their effects on the development of Korean orphans adopted into American families. Am J Clin Nutr. 1977;30:1734–1739.

76. Stein Z, Susser M, Saenger G, et al. Famine and Human Development: The Dutch Hunger Winter of 1944/45. New York: Oxford University Press; 1975.

77. Susser E, Hoek HW, Brown AS. Neurodevelopmental disorders after prenatal famine: the story of the Dutch famine study. Am J Epidemiol. 1998;147:213–216.

78. Neugebauer R, Hoek HW, Susser E. Prenatal exposure to wartime famine and development of antisocial personality disorder in early adulthood. JAMA. 1999;282:455–462.

79. Franzek EJ, Sprangers N, Janssens AC, et al. Prenatal exposure to the 1944–45 Dutch "hunger winter" and addiction later in life. Addiction. 2008;103:433–438.

80. Crookston BT, Penny ME, Alder SC, et al. Children who recover from early stunting and children who are not stunted demonstrate similar levels of cognition. J Nutr. 2010;140:1996–2001.

81. Engle PL, Fernald LC, Alderman H, et al. Strategies for reducing inequalities and improving developmental outcomes for young children in low-income and middle-income countries. Lancet. 2011; 378:1339–1353.

82. Ashworth A, Khanum S, Jackson A, et al. Guidelines for the Inpatient Treatment of Severely Malnourished Children. Geneva: World Health Organization; 2003.

83. Hughes D, Bryan J. The assessment of cognitive performance in children: considerations for detecting nutritional influences. Nutr Rev. 2003;61:413–422.

84. Isaacs E, Oates J. Nutrition and cognition: assessing cognitive abilities in children and young people. Eur J Nutr. 2008;47(Suppl 3):4–24.

85. Colombo J, Carlson SE, Cheatham CL, et al. Long-term effects of LCPUFA supplementation on childhood cognitive outcomes. Am J Clin Nutr. 2013;98:403–412.

86. Greenfield PM. You can't take it with you: why ability assessments don't cross cultures. Am Psychol. 1997;52:1115–1124.

87. Vierhaus M, Lohaus A, Kolling T, et al. The development of 3- to 9-month-old infants in two cultural contexts: Bayley longitudinal results for Cameroonian and German infants. Eur J Dev Psychol. 2011;8:349–366.

88. Fattal I, Friedmann N, Fattal-Valevski A. The crucial role of thiamine in the development of syntax and lexical retrieval: a study of infantile thiamine deficiency. Brain. 2011;134(Pt 6):1720–1739.

89. Grantham-McGregor S. A review of studies of the effect of severe malnutrition on mental development. J Nutr. 1995;125(Suppl 8):2233S–2238S.

90. Galler JR, Bryce CP, Zichlin ML, et al. Infant malnutrition is associated with persisting attention deficits in middle adulthood. J Nutr. 2012;142:788–794.

91. Galler JR, Bryce C, Waber DP, et al. Socioeconomic outcomes in adults malnourished in the first year of life: a 40-year study. Pediatrics. 2012;130:e1–e7.

92. Grantham-McGregor S, Baker-Henningham H. Review of evidence linking protein and energy to mental development. Public Health Nutr. 2005;8(7A):1191–1201.

93. Lundgren EM, Tuvemo T. Effects of being born small for gestational age on long-term intellectual performance. Best Pract Res Clin Endocrinol Metab. 2008;22:477–488.

94. Walker SP, Wachs TD, Grantham-McGregor S, et al. Inequality in early childhood: risk and protective factors for early child development. Lancet. 2011; 378:1325–1338.

95. Wang WL, Sung YT, Sung FC, et al. Low birth weight, prematurity, and paternal social status: impact on the basic competence test in Taiwanese adolescents. J Pediatr. 2008;153:333–338.

96. Walker SP, Chang SM, Younger N, et al. The effect of psychosocial stimulation on cognition and behaviour at 6 years in a cohort of term, low-birthweight Jamaican children. Dev Med Child Neurol. 2010;52:e148–e154.

97. Emond AM, Lira PI, Lima MC, et al. Development and behaviour of low-birthweight term infants at 8 years in northeast Brazil: a longitudinal study. Acta Paediatr. 2006;95:1249–1257.

98. Sabet F, Richter LM, Ramchandani PG, et al. Low birthweight and subsequent emotional and behavioural outcomes in 12-year-old children in Soweto, South Africa: findings from Birth to Twenty. Int J Epidemiol. 2009;38:944–954.

99. Strauss RS, Dietz WH. Growth and development of term children born with low birth weight: effects of genetic and environmental factors. J Pediatr. 1998;133:67–72.

100. Fattal-Valevski A, Leitner Y, Kutai M, et al. Neurodevelopmental outcome in children with intrauterine growth retardation: a 3-year follow-up. J Child Neurol. 1999;14:724–727.

101. Li H, Barnhart HX, Stein AD, et al. Effects of early childhood supplementation on the educational achievement of women. Pediatrics. 2003;112:1156–1162.
102. Hoddinott J, Malussio JA, Behrman JR, et al. Effect of a nutrition intervention during early childhood on economic productivity in Guatemalan adults. Lancet. 2008;371:411–416.
103. Rush D. The behavioral consequences of protein-energy deprivation and supplementation in early life: an epidemiological perspective. In: Galler J , ed. Human Nutrition: A Comprehensive Treatise. New York/London: Plenum Press; 1984:119–154.
104. Joos SK, Pollitt E, Mueller WH, et al. The Bacon Chow study: maternal nutritional supplementation and infant behavioral development. Child Dev. 1983;54:669–676.
105. Hsueh AM, Meyer B. Maternal dietary supplementation and 5 year old Stanford Binet IQ test on the offspring in Taiwan. Fed Proc. 1981;40:897.
106. Super CM, Herrera MG. Cognitive outcomes of early nutritional intervention in the Bogota study. Paper presented at the meeting of the Society for Research in Child Development, Seattle, WA. 1991.
107. Husaini MA, Karyadi L, Husaini YK, et al. Developmental effects of short-term supplementary feeding in nutritionally at-risk Indonesian infants. Am J Clin Nutr. 1991;54:799–804.
108. Pollitt E, Watkins WE, Husaini MA. Three-month nutritional supplementation in Indonesian infants and toddlers benefits memory function 8 y later. Am J Clin Nutr 1997;66:1357–1363.
109. Pollitt E, Saco-Pollitt C, Jahari A, et al. Effects of an energy and micronutrient supplement on mental development and behavior under natural conditions in undernourished children in Indonesia. Eur J Clin Nutr. 2000;54(Suppl):S80–S90.
110. Aitchison TC, Durnin JV, Beckett C, et al. Effects of an energy and micronutrient supplement on growth and activity, correcting for non-supplemental sources of energy input in undernourished children in Indonesia. Eur J Clin Nutr. 2000;54(Suppl):S69–S73.
111. Grantham-McGregor S, Walker S, Chang S, et al. Effects of early childhood supplementation with and without stimulation on later development in stunted Jamaican children. Am J Clin Nutr. 1997;66:247–253.
112. Walker S, Grantham-McGregor S, Powell C, et al. Effects of stunting in early childhood on growth, IQ and cognition at age 11–12 years and the benefits of nutritional supplementation and psychological stimulation. J Pediatr. 2000;137:36–41.
113. Walker SP, Chang SM, Powell CA, et al. Effects of early childhood psychosocial stimulation and nutritional supplementation on cognition and education in growth-stunted Jamaican children: prospective cohort study. Lancet. 2005;366:1804–1807.
114. Walker SP, Chang SM, Powell CA, et al. Early childhood stunting is associated with poor psychological functioning in late adolescence and effects are reduced by psychosocial stimulation. J Nutr. 2007;137:2464–2469.
115. Innis SM. Human milk and formula fatty acids. J Pediatr. 1992;120(4 Pt 2):S56–S61.
116. Kunz C, Rudloff S, Baier W, et al. Oligosaccharides in human milk: structural, functional, and metabolic aspects. Annu Rev Nutr. 2000;20:699–722.
117. Zeisel SH. Choline: needed for normal development of memory. J Am Coll Nutr. 2000;19(Suppl 5):528S–531S.

118. Reynolds A. Breastfeeding and brain development. Pediatr Clin North Am. 2001;48:159–171.
119. Jain A, Concato J, Leventhal JM. How good is the evidence linking breastfeeding and intelligence? Pediatrics. 2002;109:1044–1053.
120. Anderson JW, Johnstone BM, Remley DT. Breast-feeding and cognitive development: a meta-analysis. Am J Clin Nutr. 1999;70:525–535.
121. Drane DL, Logemann JA. A critical evaluation of the evidence on the association between type of infant feeding and cognitive development. Paediatr Perinat Epidemiol. 2000;14:349–356.
122. Walfisch A, Sermer C, Cressman A, et al. Breast milk and cognitive development – the role of confounders: a systematic review. BMJ Open. 2013;3:e003259.
123. Der G, Batty GD, Deary IJ. Effect of breast feeding on intelligence in children: prospective study, sibling pairs analysis, and meta-analysis. BMJ. 2006;333:945–949.
124. Ip S, Chung M, Raman G, et al. Breastfeeding and maternal and infant health outcomes in developed countries. Evid Rep Technol Assess (Summ) 2007;153:1–186.
125. Daniels MC, Adair LS. Breast-feeding influences cognitive development in Filipino children. J Nutr. 2005;135:2589–2595.
126. Victora CG, Barros FC, Horta BL, et al. Breastfeeding and school achievement in Brazilian adolescents. Acta Paediatr. 2005;94:1656–1660.
127. Brion MJ, Lawlor DA, Matijasevich A, et al. What are the causal effects of breast-feeding on IQ, obesity and blood pressure? Evidence from comparing high-income with middle-income cohorts. Int J Epidemiol. 2011; 40:670–680.
128. Kramer MS, Aboud F, Mironova E, et al. Breastfeeding and child cognitive development: new evidence from a large randomized trial. Arch Gen Psychiatry. 2008;65:578–584.
129. Makrides M, Collins CT, Gibson RA. Impact of fatty acid status on growth and neurobehavioural development in humans. Matern Child Nutr. 2011;7(Suppl 2):80–88.
130. Qawasmi A, Landeros-Weisenberger A, Leckman JF, et al. Meta-analysis of long-chain polyunsaturated fatty acid supplementation of formula and infant cognition. Pediatrics. 2012;129:1141–1149.
131. Martinez M. Developmental profiles of polyunsaturated fatty acids in the brain of normal infants and patients with peroxisomal diseases: severe deficiency of docosahexaenoic acid in Zellweger's and pseudo-Zellweger's syndromes. World Rev Nutr Diet. 1991;66:87–102.
132. Adu-Afarwuah S, Lartey A, Brown KH, et al. Randomized comparison of 3 types of micronutrient supplements for home fortification of complementary foods in Ghana: effects on growth and motor development. Am J Clin Nutr. 2007;86:412–420.
133. Wang YY, Wang FZ, Wang K, et al. Effects of nutrient fortified complementary food supplements on development of infants and young children in poor rural area of Gansu Province. Wei Sheng Yan Jiu. 2006;35:772–774.
134. van der Merwe LF, Moore SE, Fulford AJ, et al. Long-chain PUFA supplementation in rural African infants: a randomized controlled trial of effects on gut integrity, growth, and cognitive development. Am J Clin Nutr. 2013;97:45–57.
135. Phuka JC, Gladstone M, Maleta K, et al. Developmental outcomes among 18-month-old Malawians after a year of complementary feeding with lipid-based nutrient supplements or corn-soy flour. Matern Child Nutr. 2012;8:239–248.

136. Gould JF, Smithers LG, Makrides M. The effect of maternal omega-3 (n-3) LCPUFA supplementation during pregnancy on early childhood cognitive and visual development: a systematic review and meta-analysis of randomized controlled trials. Am J Clin Nutr. 2013;97:531–544.

137. World Health Organization, Centers for Disease Control and Prevention. Worldwide Prevalence of Anaemia 1993–2005. WHO Global Database on Anaemia. Geneva: World Health Organization; 2008.

138. Brown KH, Rivera JA, Bhutta Z, et al. International Zinc Nutrition Consultative Group (IZiNCG) technical document #1. Assessment of the risk of zinc deficiency in populations and options for its control. Food Nutr Bull. 2004;25(Suppl 2):S99–203.

139. de Benoist B, McLean E, Andersson M, et al. Iodine deficiency in 2007: global progress since 2003. Food Nutr Bull. 2008;29:195–202.

140. Lozoff B, Beard J, Connor J, et al. Long-lasting neural and behavioral effects of iron deficiency in infancy. Nutr Rev. 2006;64(Suppl):S34–S43.

141. Walker SP, Wachs TD, Meeks-Gardner JM, et al. Child development: risk factors for adverse outcomes in developing countries. Lancet. 2007;369:145–157.

142. Christian P, Murray-Kolb LE, Khatry SK, et al. Prenatal micronutrient supplementation and intellectual and motor function in early school-aged children in Nepal. JAMA. 2010;304:2716–2723.

143. Li Q, Yan H, Zeng L, et al. Effects of maternal micronutrient supplementation on the mental development of infants in rural western China: follow-up evaluation of a double-blind, randomized, controlled trial. Pediatrics. 2009;123:e685–e692.

144. Zhou SJ, Gibson RA, Crowther CA, et al. Effect of iron supplementation during pregnancy on the intelligence quotient and behavior of children at 4 y of age: long-term follow-up of a randomized controlled trial. Am J Clin Nutr. 2006;83:1112–1117.

145. Berglund SK, Westrup B, Hagglof B, et al. Effects of iron supplementation of LBW infants on cognition and behavior at 3 years. Pediatrics. 2013;131:47–55.

146. Christian P, Morgan ME, Murray-Kolb L, et al. Preschool iron-folic acid and zinc supplementation in children exposed to iron-folic acid in utero confers no added cognitive benefit in early school-age. J Nutr. 2011;141:2042–2048.

147. Murray-Kolb LE, Khatry SK, Katz J, et al. Preschool micronutrient supplementation effects on intellectual and motor function in school-aged Nepalese children. Arch Pediatr Adolesc Med. 2012;166:404–410.

148. World Health Organization. Guideline: Use of Multiple Micronutrient Powders for Home Fortification of Foods Consumed by Infants and Children 6–23 Months of Age. Geneva: World Health Organization; 2011.

149. Dewey KG, Chaparro CM. Session 4: mineral metabolism and body composition iron status of breast-fed infants. Proc Nutr Soc. 2007;66:412–422.

150. Black MM, Quigg AM, Hurley KM, et al. Iron deficiency and iron-deficiency anemia in the first two years of life: strategies to prevent loss of developmental potential. Nutr Rev. 2011;69(Suppl 1):S64–S70.

151. Pharoah POD, Buttfield IH, Hetzel BS. Neurological damage to the fetus resulting from severe iodine deficiency during pregnancy. Lancet. 1971;1:308–310.

152. Bleichrodt N, Born MP. A metaanalysis of research on iodine and its relationship to cognitive development. In: Stanbury JB, ed. The Damaged Brain of Iodine Deficiency. New York: Cognizant Communication Corporation; 1994:195–200.

153. Qian M, Wang D, Watkins WE, et al. The effects of iodine on intelligence in children: a meta-analysis of studies conducted in China. Asia Pac J Clin Nutr. 2005;14:32–42.

154. Melse-Boonstra A, Jaiswal N. Iodine deficiency in pregnancy, infancy and childhood and its consequences for brain development. Best Pract Res Clin Endocrinol Metab. 2010;24:29–38.

155. O'Donnell KJ, Rakeman MA, Zhi-Hong D, et al. Effects of iodine supplementation during pregnancy on child growth and development at school age. Dev Med Child Neurol. 2002;44:76–81.

156. Bath SC, Steer CD, Golding J, et al. Effect of inadequate iodine status in UK pregnant women on cognitive outcomes in their children: results from the Avon Longitudinal Study of Parents and Children (ALSPAC). Lancet. 2013; 382:331–337.

157. Bougma K, Aboud FE, Harding KB, et al. Iodine and mental development of children 5 years old and under: a systematic review and meta-analysis. Nutrients. 2013;5:1384–1416.

158. Sandstead HH, Frederickson CJ, Penland JG. History of zinc as related to brain function. J Nutr. 2000;130(Suppl 2):496S–502S.

159. Golub MS, Keen CL, Gershwin ME, et al. Developmental zinc deficiency and behavior. J Nutr. 1995;125(Suppl 8):2263S–2271S.

160. Caulfield LE, Putnick DL, Zavaleta N, et al. Maternal gestational zinc supplementation does not influence multiple aspects of child development at 54 mo of age in Peru. Am J Clin Nutr. 2010;92:130–136.

161. Tamura T, Goldenberg RL, Chapman VR, et al. Folate status of mothers during pregnancy and mental and psychomotor development of their children at five years of age. Pediatrics. 2005;116:703–708.

162. Hamadani JD, Fuchs GJ, Osendarp SJ, et al. Zinc supplementation during pregnancy and effects on mental development and behavior of infants: a follow up study. Lancet. 2002;360:290–294.

163. Lind T, Lonnerdal B, Stenlund H, et al. A community-based randomized controlled trial of iron and zinc supplementation in Indonesian infants: effects on growth and development. Am J Clin Nutr. 2004;80:729–736.

164. Black MM, Baqui AH, Zaman K, et al. Iron and zinc supplementation promote motor development and exploratory behavior among Bangladesh infants. Am J Clin Nutr. 2004;80:903–910.

165. Katz J, Khatry SK, Leclerq SC, et al. Daily supplementation with iron plus folic acid, zinc, and their combination is not associated with younger age at first walking unassisted in malnourished preschool children from a deficient population in rural Nepal. J Nutr. 2010;140:1317–1321.

166. Hamadani JD, Fuchs GJ, Osendarp SJ, et al. Randomized controlled trial of the effect of zinc supplementation on the mental development of Bangladeshi infants. Am J Clin Nutr. 2001;74:381–386.

167. Friel JK, Andrews WL, Matthew JD, et al. Zinc supplementation in very-low-birthweight infants. J Pediatr Gastroenterol Nutr. 1993;17:97–104.

168. Castillo-Duran C, Perales CG, Hertampf ED, et al. Effect of zinc supplementation on development and growth of Chilean infants. J Pediatr. 2001;138:229–235.

169. Sazawal S, Bentley M, Black RE, et al. Effect of zinc supplementation on observed activity in low socioeconomic Indian preschool children. Pediatrics. 1996;98:1132–1137.

170. Bentley ME, Caulfield LE, Ram M, et al. Zinc supplementation affects the activity patterns of rural Guatemalan infants. J Nutr. 1997;127:1333–1338.

171. Brown KH, Peerson JM, Baker SK, et al. Preventive zinc supplementation among infants, preschoolers, and older prepubertal children. Food Nutr Bull. 2009;30(Suppl 1):S12–S40.

172. Butterworth RF. Thiamin deficiency and brain disorders. Nutr Res Rev. 2003;16:277–283.

173. Khounnorath S, Chamberlain K, Taylor AM, et al. Clinically unapparent infantile thiamin deficiency in Vientiane, Laos. PLoS Negl Trop Dis. 2011;5:e969.

174. Kirksey A, Wachs TD, Yunis F, et al. Relation of maternal zinc nutriture to pregnancy outcome and infant development in an Egyptian village. Am J Clin Nutr. 1994;60:782–792.

175. Rahmanifar A, Kirksey A, Wachs TD, et al. Diet during lactation associated with infant behavior and caregiver-infant interaction in a semirural Egyptian village. J Nutr. 1993;123:164–175.

176. Strand TA, Taneja S, Ueland PM, et al. Cobalamin and folate status predicts mental development scores in North Indian children 12–18 mo of age. Am J Clin Nutr. 2013;97:310–317.

177. Huffman SL, Harika RK, Eilander A, et al. Essential fats: how do they affect growth and development of infants and young children in developing countries? A literature review. Matern Child Nutr. 2011;7(Suppl 3):44–65.

178. McGrath N, Bellinger D, Robins J, et al. Effect of maternal multivitamin supplementation on the mental and psychomotor development of children who are born to HIV-1-infected mothers in Tanzania. Pediatrics. 2006;117:e216–e225.

179. Faber M, Kvalsvig JD, Lombard CJ, et al. Effect of a fortified maize-meal porridge on anemia, micronutrient status, and motor development of infants. Am J Clin Nutr. 2005;82:1032–1039.

180. Aburto NJ, Ramirez-Zea M, Neufeld LM, et al. The effect of nutritional supplementation on physical activity and exploratory behavior of Mexican infants aged 8–12 months. Eur J Clin Nutr. 2010;64:644–651.

181. Delange F, de Benoist B, Alnwick D. Risks of iodine-induced hyperthyroidism after correction of iodine deficiency by iodized salt. Thyroid. 1999;9:545–556.

182. Dewey KG, Adu-Afarwuah S. Systematic review of the efficacy and effectiveness of complementary feeding interventions in developing countries. Matern Child Nutr. 2008;4(Suppl 1):24–85.

CHAPTER 5

GENOMIC AND EPIGENOMIC INSIGHTS INTO NUTRITION AND BRAIN DISORDERS

MARGARET JOY DAUNCEY

5.1 INTRODUCTION

Advances in genomics and epigenomics are revolutionizing understanding of mechanisms underlying brain disorders [1,2,3,4]. Considerable evidence suggests that many neuropsychiatric, neurodevelopmental and neurodegenerative disorders are linked with multiple complex interactions between genetic factors and environmental variables, such as nutrition [5,6,7]. Indeed, numerous diets, foods and nutrients are implicated in optimal and sub-optimal brain health throughout the life-cycle [8,9,10,11,12,13,14,15,16].

Nutrition affects multiple aspects of neuroscience including neurodevelopment, neurogenesis and functions of neurons, synapses and neural networks in specific brain regions [17]. Nutrition-gene interactions play a critical role in these responses, leading in turn to major effects on brain health, dysfunction and disease [5,6,7,18]. Individual differences in multiple gene variants, including mutations, single nucleotide polymorphisms (SNPs) and copy number variants (CNVs), significantly modify

Genomic and Epigenomic Insights into Nutrition and Brain Disorders. © *Dauncey MJ, licensee MDPI, Basel, Switzerland,* Nutrients, *5,3 (2013). doi:10.3390/nu5030887. Licensed under Creative Commons Attribution 3.0 Unported License, http://creativecommons.org/licenses/by/3.0/.*

the effects of nutrition on gene expression. A further layer of regulation is added by differences in the epigenome, and nutrition is one of many epigenetic regulators that can modify gene expression without changes in DNA sequence.

Epigenetic mechanisms play a major role in developmental, physiological and pathological processes [19,20]. They include DNA methylation and hydroxymethylation, histone modifications and higher order chromatin remodelling, and non-coding RNA (ncRNA) regulation. Activation of these mechanisms affects the expression of multiple genes involved in cell development, signalling and function [4,5,6,7,21,22,23]. Numerous epigenetic regulators, including environmental factors, interact with multiple gene variants to produce striking individual differences in responses to nutrition. Critical interactions also exist between specific dietary components, and between nutrition and other environmental variables such as stress, infections, social interactions, season of birth and stage of development [5,6,7,24,25,26,27]. These epigenetic regulators, together with multiple genetic factors, comprise a sophisticated control network that plays a central role in brain function.

The current review highlights the significance of advances in genomics and epigenomics to an understanding of the role of nutrition in brain disorders. Studies using genome-wide analysis of multiple genes and comprehensive analysis of specific genes are together elucidating mechanisms underlying responses of the brain to nutrition. This is a vast field of research, involving many hundreds of publications every month. The present review therefore focuses on recent progress in four key areas (Figure 1): First, a short overview is given of significant advances in genomic and epigenomic technologies over the last few years. These are revolutionizing our ability to evaluate mechanisms underlying neurological responses to nutrition, and hence to determine outcomes in relation to health or disease. Second, to illustrate the potential of these technological advances, the role of ncRNAs, and especially microRNAs (miRNAs) and long non-coding RNAs (lncRNAs), is addressed because of their emergence as critical regulators of transcription, epigenetic processes and gene silencing. Third, novel approaches to nutrition, epigenetics and neuroscience are discussed, especially in relation to the role of exogenous factors in determining neurological phenotype and disorders.

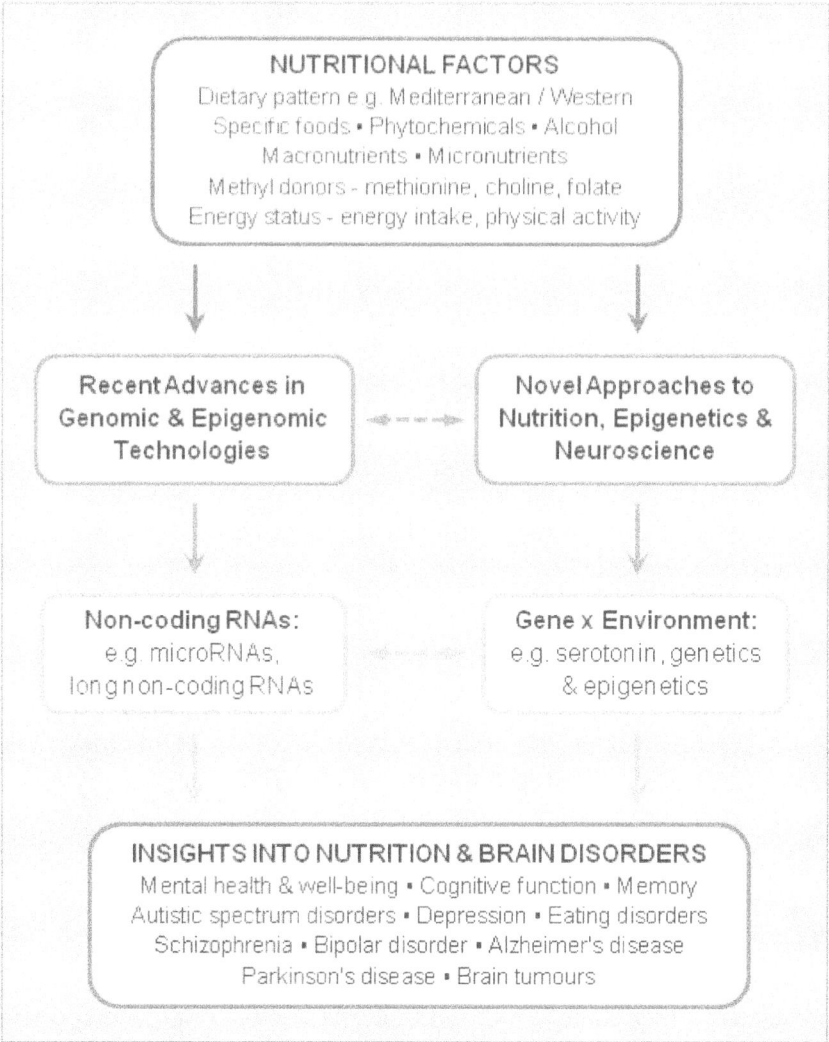

NUTRITIONAL FACTORS
Dietary pattern e.g. Mediterranean / Western
Specific foods • Phytochemicals • Alcohol
Macronutrients • Micronutrients
Methyl donors - methionine, choline, folate
Energy status - energy intake, physical activity

Recent Advances in Genomic & Epigenomic Technologies

Novel Approaches to Nutrition, Epigenetics & Neuroscience

Non-coding RNAs: e.g. microRNAs, long non-coding RNAs

Gene x Environment: e.g. serotonin, genetics & epigenetics

INSIGHTS INTO NUTRITION & BRAIN DISORDERS
Mental health & well-being • Cognitive function • Memory
Autistic spectrum disorders • Depression • Eating disorders
Schizophrenia • Bipolar disorder • Alzheimer's disease
Parkinson's disease • Brain tumours

FIGURE 1: Nutrition-gene interactions and brain disorders: Outline of current review.

Finally, the relevance of these novel approaches is addressed in relation to gene-environment interactions in the serotonergic system, as an example of just one of the multiple neural signalling pathways that are affected in neuropsychiatric and neurological disorders. Current and future advances in these four areas should contribute significantly to the prevention and treatment of multiple devastating brain disorders.

5.2 RECENT ADVANCES IN GENOMIC AND EPIGENOMIC TECHNOLOGIES

During the last few years, major advances in DNA sequencing technology have revolutionized understanding of the mechanisms underlying complex biological problems and multifactorial diseases [28,29]. Compared with methods used by the Human Genome Project [30], modern sequencers are 50,000-fold faster and have dramatically reduced the cost of DNA sequencing by a factor of more than 50,000. These new technologies have thus enabled major advances in understanding of human genomics and epigenomics. Especially significant are new insights into individual genetic variability, and the critical role of non-coding RNAs (ncRNAs) in epigenetics and gene regulation.

5.2.1 WHOLE GENOME STRATEGIES, NEXT-GENERATION DNA SEQUENCING AND BRAIN DISORDERS

Successful and early completion of the human genome sequence in 2001 was based on the classic electrophoretic Sanger sequencing method [30]. However, this method was unsuitable for studying genetic variability. Instead, individual genotypes were assessed using specific DNA sequence probes targeted at known SNP positions. At this time, it could not have been predicted that next-generation sequencing technology would enable the complete analysis of all the functional elements and variations in the human genome. By contrast with the limited scalability of the Sanger method, this new approach uses image-based massively parallel sequencing-by-synthesis platforms. Together with a marked increase in analytical throughput, this has catapulted genome-sequencing into a multi-purpose tool for mapping epigenetic modifications of the genome, and the complete assessment of protein-coding and non-coding RNA transcripts. In the longer term, further advances in data assessment may enable complete analysis of the relation between genomic variation and phenotype.

Over the past five years, new technologies have provided an overview of both common and rare genetic variability across the whole genome that has significantly improved understanding of many brain disorders [1,2]. These include Alzheimer's disease, schizophrenia, bipolar disorder, major depressive disorder, autistic spectrum disorders, attention-deficit hyperactivity disorder, anorexia nervosa, alcohol dependence and nicotine dependence. Data on structural variants, rare exonic variants, and an increasing number of common variants have helped to identify risk factors for the development of several complex disorders. Moreover, they support novel hypotheses related, for example, to (a) cholesterol metabolism and the innate immune response in Alzheimer's disease, (b) a network involving the microRNA miR-137 in schizophrenia, (c) calcium signalling in bipolar disorder and schizophrenia, and (d) chromatin remodelling in autism.

Genome-wide association studies (GWAS) involve many thousands of patients and control subjects, to overcome problems associated with the huge number of interrogated genetic variants. This approach has been used with considerable success to identify many disease-predisposing variants. For example, recent studies have identified: a low-frequency variant in the amyloid-β precursor protein (APP) that protects against Alzheimer's disease and age-related cognitive decline [31], a common variant conferring risk of psychosis [32], common SNPs and rare copy number variants (CNVs) that may confer risk to anorexia nervosa [33], and susceptibility loci for the most common form of migraine, a disabling episodic neurovascular brain disorder affecting 12% of the general population [34]. Despite these significant advances, it is now appreciated that future studies aimed at identifying disease-associated low-frequency and rare variants may need to involve even larger sample sizes than those currently used in GWAS, in order to achieve the necessary statistical power [35,36]. This approach should prove especially rewarding in the study of many complex brain disorders that result from both genetic and environmental factors, including Alzheimer's disease, autism, schizophrenia and eating disorders. Moreover, when complemented by a systems genetics approach the outcome will be particularly informative. Systems genetics is a specialized version of systems biology that seeks to reveal multiple complex connections from genetic variation, through intermediate phenotypes such as gene coexpression networks, to overlying systems level phenotypes [37,38,39,40]. The importance of an integrative approach to understanding the mechanisms linking genetic variability, nutrition-gene interactions and phenotypic diversity is illustrated in Section 5 of this review.

Current knowledge suggests that assessing multiple forms of genetic variation is likely to yield many new findings in neuroscience. The challenge for nutritionists is to coordinate these findings with novel approaches to assessing the role of interactions between environmental factors and genotype. Recent findings from two key projects that are currently providing new understanding of genetic variability and epigenetic mechanisms, The 1000 Genomes Project and ENCODE, are therefore discussed in the following paragraphs.

5.2.2 GENETIC VARIATION AND THE 1000 GENOMES PROJECT

Genetic variability underlies not only individual differences in responses to nutrition but also the propensity of individuals for specific brain disorders. Major advances in gene sequencing technology have enabled characterization of the vast majority of human SNPs and many structural variants, including CNVs, across the human genome. The 1000 Genomes Project is an international sequencing collaboration launched in 2008 to produce an extensive catalogue of all types of human genetic variation. The project published pilot data in 2010 [41], and will have sequenced the genomes of approximately 2500 people from 25 global populations when complete.

The three studies in the pilot phase involved low-coverage whole-genome sequencing of 179 people from four populations, high-coverage sequencing of two mother-father-child trios, and exon-targeted sequencing of 697 people from seven populations [41]. The results described the location, allele frequency and local haplotype structure of approximately 15 million SNPs, 1 million short insertions and deletions, and 20,000 structural variants, most of which had not been described previously. Each person was found to carry approximately 250–300 loss-of-function variants in annotated genes, and 50–100 variants previously implicated in inherited disorders.

More than 95% of common (>5% frequency) variants were discovered in the pilot phase of the 1000 Genomes Project, thus paving the way for investigation of the links between genotype and phenotype. However, lower-frequency variants, especially those outside the exome, remained poorly characterized. Nevertheless, it was appreciated that low-frequency variants are enriched for potentially functional mutations, and that characterizing such variants, for both point mutations and structural changes, was likely to identify many functionally important variants and be crucial for interpreting individual genome sequences. Highly significant progress has recently been made in this area.

In November 2012, following extensive genomic assessment of 1092 people from 14 populations world-wide, an integrated map of human genetic variation was published [42]. This provides an exceptional resource describing human genomic variability. It encompasses a haplotype map of 38 million SNPs, 1.4 million short insertions and deletions, and more than 14,000 larger deletions. Profiles of rare and common variants differ between populations, and low-frequency variants show substantial geographic differentiation. Moreover, each person contains hundreds of rare non-coding variants at conserved sites, such as motif-disrupting changes in transcription factor binding site. The considerable significance of these non-coding variants to brain disorders is discussed in Section 3 of the current review.

5.2.3 ENCODE: AN ENCYCLOPEDIA OF DNA ELEMENTS IN THE HUMAN GENOME

A series of articles by ENCODE, the Encyclopedia of DNA Elements, in September 2012 has critical implications for providing insights into the organization and regulation of our genes and genome [3]. ENCODE is an international research consortium launched in 2003 and funded by the National Human Genome Research Institute to identify all functional elements in the human genome sequence, i.e., all regions of transcription,

transcription factor association, chromatin structure and histone modification. Their data now enable biochemical functions to be assigned to 80% of the genome, in particular outside the well-studied protein-coding regions.

ENCODE's massive enterprise has involved the production and initial analysis of 1640 data sets, and integration of results from studies involving 147 cell types and data from other resources including genome-wide association studies (GWAS). Key findings indicate that (a) most of the human genome takes part in at least one biochemical RNA- and/or chromatin-associated event in at least one cell type; (b) classifying the genome into seven chromatin states indicates an initial set of 399,124 regions with enhancer-like features and 70,292 regions with promoter-like features; (c) promoter functionality can explain most of the variation in RNA expression; (d) the number of non-coding variants in individual genome sequences is at least as large as those within protein-coding regions; (e) SNPs associated with disease are enriched with non-coding functional elements, and in many cases the disease phenotypes are associated with a specific cell type or transcription factor.

The significance of these findings is immense and of profound relevance to future investigations on the role of nutrition-gene interactions in health and disease. In the words of the head of the team working on the GENCODE sub-project [43,44]: "If the Human Genome Project was the baseline for genetics, ENCODE is the baseline for biology, and GENCODE are the parts that make the human biological machine work. Our list is essential to all those who would fix the human machine."

5.2.4 EPIGENOMICS AND NEW TECHNOLOGIES

Approximately 70% of all abstracts featuring "epigenome" have been published within the last three years [45]. This proliferation of investigations on epigenomics, i.e., the dynamic regulatory layers that modulate expression of the genome's static DNA sequence, has been possible because of major advances in high-throughput technologies. These enable the analysis and positioning of epigenetic markers such as DNA methylation, histone modifications and chromatin states within the biological context of the whole genome.

Epigenome core technologies are now largely standardized, although advances in sensitivity and resolution are still being made [46]. The standard assay for transcription factor binding, and mapping genome-wide distribution of histone modifications, is chromatin immunoprecipitation followed by sequencing (ChIP-seq). Similarly, techniques for DNA methylation use methylated DNA immunoprecipitation, to enrich the methylated DNA sequences, followed by high-throughput sequencing (MeDIP-seq). Methods are now tending to converge on whole genome bisulphite sequencing because of its high resolution combined with reduced costs. The desire to map the entire methylome is driving further developments in large-scale DNA methylation profiling methods. Comparison of MeDIP-seq with the targeted approach of the Infinium HumanMethylation450 BeadChip has revealed strengths and weaknesses in both methods [47]. In particular, the former technique allows the detection of almost twice as many differentially methylated regions as the latter, including thousands of non-RefSeq genes and repetitive elements that may be important in disease.

Data from epigenome studies are providing information of far greater significance than simply mapping specific epigenetic marks to a given cell type. Key applications are related to genome annotation, cell identity and disease [46]. As the ENCODE project has demonstrated [3], investigations based on the primary DNA sequence alone cannot provide a comprehensive understanding of the mammalian genome. Chromatin signatures, for example, enable efficient and precise genome annotation of regulatory elements and can locate functional or cell type-specific regions of interest. Epigenomic maps provide more information than is gained from gene expression data alone. Precise chromatin states can clarify a gene's activity status, which in turn has consequences for how specific gene loci behave in normal development and disease. Moreover, epigenomic maps are playing an important role in studies of brain disorders, and are clarifying affected pathways and identifying novel prognostic methylation biomarkers, for example in neuroblastomas [48,49].

Especially powerful is the combination of epigenome-wide association studies with genome-wide association studies (GWAS) to locate disease-relevant regulatory elements [3,50]. This combined approach will prove especially valuable for providing further insights into the multiple roles of nutrition in brain development and function. The relevance of combining studies on genotype and epigenotype is highlighted in Figure 2 and is discussed further in the following sections.

5.3 NON-CODING RNAS (NCRNAS), GENE REGULATION AND NEUROSCIENCE

The Human Genome Project provided ground-breaking information on the human genome sequence [30], and this was followed by considerable advances in identifying protein-coding genes. However, understanding of the genome, especially with respect to ncRNAs, alternatively spliced transcripts and regulatory sequences remained far from complete. Indeed, since only 2.2% of human genomic DNA is protein-coding, the rest was sometimes termed "junk DNA" [51]. The possibility existed, however, that these non-coding regions may have a functional role in complex regulatory processes, thus explaining the relatively low number of protein-coding genes in humans, an evolutionarily advanced species. Significant advances in the last few years have shown that this is indeed the case.

5.3.1 GENOMIC AND EPIGENOMIC REGULATION BY NCRNAS

During the decade following publication of the human genome sequence, the centrally held paradigm of gene expression, that DNA is transcribed into messenger RNA (mRNA) which is then translated into protein, has been gradually undermined. Advances in new technologies have enabled the unexpected discovery of multiple classes of RNAs that are not translated into protein, i.e., non-coding RNAs (ncRNAs), and yet play key roles in transcription, epigenetics and gene function [3,52,53]. The complexity of gene regulation is further revealed by the discovery that most of the genome is transcribed in both the sense and antisense directions. Natural antisense transcripts (NATs) are transcribed from the opposite strand of protein-coding and non-protein-coding genes and act as epigenetic regulators of chromatin remodelling and gene expression [54].

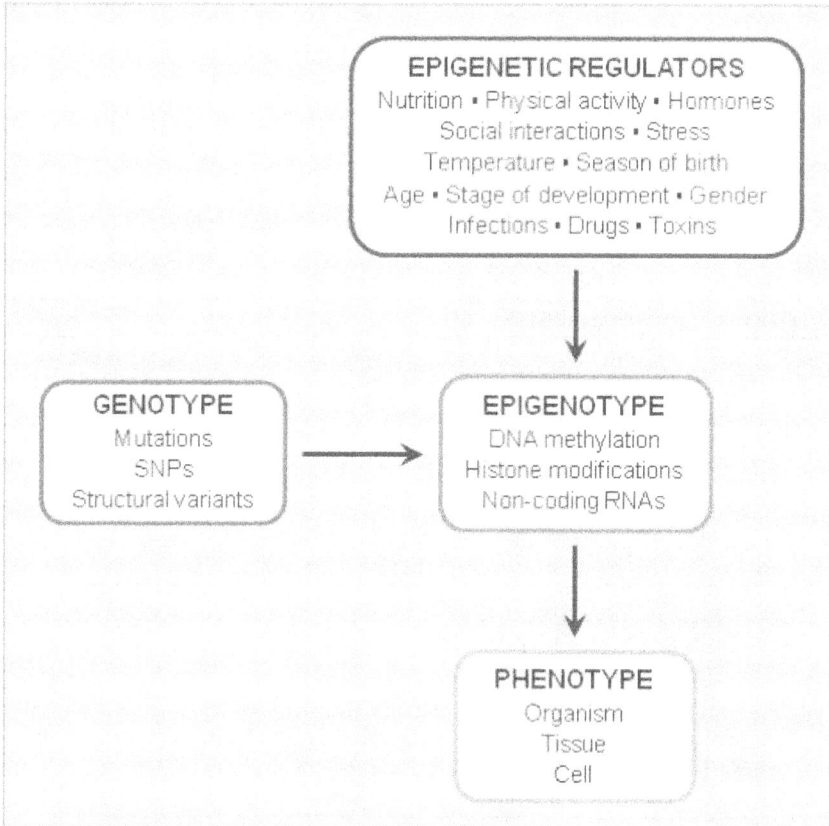

FIGURE 2: Interactions between genotype, epigenotype and phenotype.

The multiple types of ncRNA are often classified according to size as small or long (Table 1). Several years ago, the role of small ncRNAs in developmental gene regulation was discovered but only recently has the significance of the abundant and versatile long ncRNAs (lncRNAs) been appreciated. They have a broad range of functions, including roles in transcriptional and epigenetic mechanisms v,ia recruitment of transcription factors and chromatin-modifying complexes to specific nuclear and genomics sites, post-translational RNA modifications, nuclear-cytoplasmic shuttling, and translational control.

TABLE 1: Examples of non-coding RNAs (ncRNAs) and their molecular functions (for further details, see [55,56]).

Small ncRNAs (<200/400 nucleotides)
• MicroRNAs (miRNAs): Mainly induce translational repression; involved in post-transcriptional gene silencing, or deadenylation and degradation
• Endogenous small interfering RNAs (endo-siRNAs): Induce degradation or heterochromatin formation
• PIWI-interacting RNAs (piRNA): Epigenetic and possibly translational control via complementarity with DNA or RNA sequences
• Transcription initiation RNAs (tiRNAs): Possibly promote transcription via epigenetic regulation

Long ncRNAs (>200/400 nucleotides, sometimes >100,000 nucleotides)
• Long intergenic ncRNAs (lincRNAs): Epigenetic regulation
• Natural antisense transcripts (NATs): mRNA transcription, splicing, stability and translation; epigenetic modifications; precursors of endo-siRNAs
• Expressed non-coding regions (ENORs): Transcriptional regulation, genomic imprinting, precursors of other short and long ncRNAs
• Enhancer RNAs (eRNAs): Transcriptional regulation

5.3.2 NCRNAS AND BRAIN DISORDERS

Dramatic progress in RNA biology over recent years is of particular significance to brain disorders because neurons are highly transcriptionally active and demonstrate strong expression of ncRNAs. Indeed, many ncRNAs play a vital role in normal brain function, and are involved in neural development, plasticity, memory and cognition [55,56,57]. Epigenetic processes are often involved, suggesting key interactions between ncRNAs and environmental factors such as nutrition.

Initial studies on the relevance of ncRNAs to disease tended to focus on the disruption of miRNA expression in cancer. These have provided new insights into the molecular basis of disease and suggested novel approaches to investigation of brain disorders, including brain tumours. In the central nervous system, balanced expression of miRNAs plays an important role in preventing neurodegeneration, and misregulation of miRNA pathways appears to be essential in the pathogenesis of several age-dependent neurodegenerative disorders [58]. Indeed, dysregulation of numerous types of ncRNA is linked with many diseases [59,60], and especially significant is evidence that ncRNAs are involved in the pathophysiology of every major class of neurological and neuropsychiatric disorder [55,56,61].

Considerable evidence suggests central roles for ncRNAs in Alzheimer's disease. Two of the most important proteins linked with Alzheimer's, amyloid precursor protein and BACE-1, are extensively controlled by multiple miRNAs, NATs and other ncRNAs [56,62]. Alzheimer's disease brains are deficient in brain-derived neurotrophic factor (BDNF), a key regulator of synaptic plasticity and memory, and of major significance is the recent finding that miRNA-dependent dysregulation of BDNF participates in the pathogenesis of Alzheimer's [63]. In postmortem brain samples from a mouse model and humans with Alzheimer's, miR-206 is upregulated. The concomitant decrease in BDNF expression is restored by the antagomir AM206, a neutralizing inhibitor of miR-206. Moreover, the increase in brain BDNF levels with AM206 enhances hippocampal synatophysin expression and neurogenesis in the mouse model, suggesting that it can improve cognitive function. The effects of food intake and physical activity on brain health are mediated in part via BDNF [5,6,7,8,64]. This suggests the possibility that miR-206 plays a role not only in Alzheimer's but also in mediating energy status-BDNF interactions in healthy individuals. The relevance of these findings is discussed further in Section 5 of this review.

Evidence also links miRNAs with the second most prevalent neurodegenerative disorder, Parkinson's disease [56,65]. For example, a miRNA pathway regulates dopaminergic neuron development and function, and expression of α-synuclein, a protein linked with Parkinson's pathology, is affected by several miRNAs. Especially important is the finding that genetic polymorphisms of miRNA related sequences confers risk for Parkinson's disease.

The risk of brain disorders is influenced by genetic variation not only in protein-coding genes but also in ncRNAs and their targets. In Parkinson's disease, a SNP in the 3' untranslated region of the fibroblast growth factor 20 gene (FGF20) disrupts a binding site for miR-433, increasing translation of FGF20 [66]. This increase is correlated with increased α-synuclein, which can lead to Parkinson's disease. Moreover, miRNAs contribute to retinoic acid induced differentiation in neuroblastoma [67]: miR-10a and miR-10b play a key role in neural cell differentiation through direct targeting of nuclear receptor corepressor 2 and concomitant downregulation of MYCN, a potent oncoprotein in neuroblastoma. Epigenetic deregulation of many ncRNA genes is also associated with brain disorders. Large-scale cancer genomics projects are profiling hundreds of tumours at multiple molecular layers including miRNA expression, with the long-term possibility of developing small RNA therapeutics specific for subtype or individual [68]. For example, overexpression in neurospheres of two predicted proneural drivers, miR-124 and miR-132, leads to partial reversal of tumour expression changes.

5.3.3 NCRNAS, NUTRITION AND THE BRAIN

The non-coding transcriptome has extraordinary functional diversity and environmental responsiveness, and the expression of ncRNAs is controlled by numerous transcriptional and epigenetic factors, including nutrition. NcRNAs, together with their associated regulatory networks, in turn have critical influences on the brain via their multiple neurobiological functions (Figure 3).

In recent years there has been increasing interest in nutritional modulation of miRNAs, throughout the life cycle. Significant advances have been made in relation to nutritional regulation of miRNAs in cancer [69]. Dietary factors including folate, choline, retinoic acid, vitamin D, vitamin E, selenium, omega-3 fatty acids, butyrate, phytochemicals and resveratrol modify miRNA expression and their mRNA targets in several cancer processes. These include apoptosis, cell cycle regulation, differentiation, inflammation, angiogenesis, metastasis and stress response pathways. The extent to which nutrition-gene interactions may modulate miRNAs associated with risk of brain tumours remains to be established.

Polyphenols are the most abundant antioxidants in the human diet and occur widely in fruits, tea, coffee, cocoa and red wine [9]. Epidemiological, clinical and animal studies suggest a role for polyphenols in cognitive function and neurodegenerative disorders [12,70]. Gene variants of the apolipoprotein apoE are linked with risk of Alzheimer's: apoE4 increases risk whereas apoE2 may protect against Alzheimer's [5,6,7]. Of particular interest, therefore, is the recent finding that dietary polyphenols modulate hepatic miRNA expression in apoE deficient mice [71]. Polyphenols appear to counteract the modulation of miRNAs induced by knock-out of the apoE gene. Five of the differentially expressed miRNAs were regulated in common by all nine of the different polyphenols investigated, suggesting a common mode of action for polyphenols. Precise functions and roles of these miRNAs, and the extent to which the apoE genotype may modulate the action of polyphenols on miRNA expression remain to be investigated. However, taken together, these studies suggest that dietary polyphenols exert beneficial effects on brain function by influencing cellular energy metabolism, miRNAs and signalling pathways of key molecules in neural plasticity such as BDNF.

Much remains to be discovered about the nutritional modulation of ncRNAs, especially in relation to cell-specific responses and interactions with other epigenetic regulators. Physical activity, for example, plays a key role in regulating miRNAs and DNA methylation [72,73,74]: following acute exhaustive exercise, there are unique and dynamic alterations in circulating-miRNAs, suggesting that they may serve important endocrine functions. Moreover, future studies on the role of nutrition in regulating long non-coding RNAs (lncRNAs) may be especially beneficial to understanding of mechanisms underlying brain disorders.

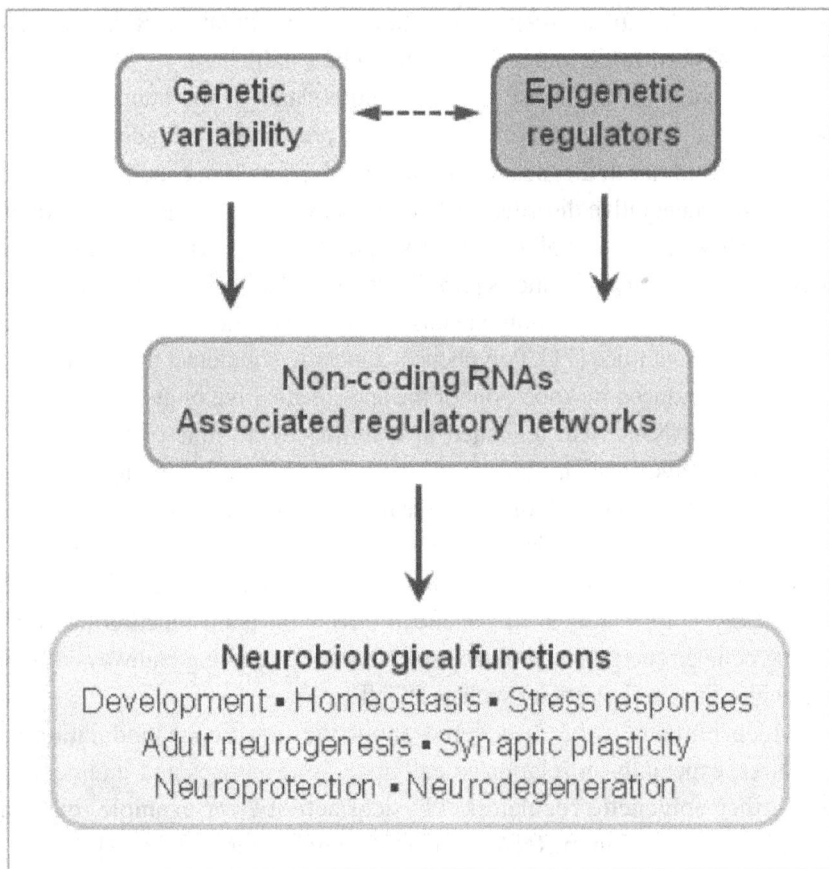

FIGURE 3: Regulation and neurobiological functions of non-coding RNAs.

5.4 NOVEL APPROACHES TO NUTRITION, EPIGENETICS AND NEUROSCIENCE

Serendipity plays a significant role in advancing scientific knowledge and an open, informed mind is essential for optimal progress in the biomedical sciences. Concomitant with progress in genomic and epigenomic technologies, significant advances are being made using novel approaches to the study of nutrition-gene interactions and neuroscience.

The development, homeostasis and plasticity of the central nervous system are mediated by epigenetic mechanisms that regulate gene expression, without changes in DNA sequence, in response to endogenous and exogenous environmental variables. Substantial evidence also implicates epigenetic mechanisms in numerous neuropsychiatric and neurological disorders including schizophrenia, bipolar disorders, Alzheimer's disease, Parkinson's disease and primary brain tumours [4,5,6,7,20,75,76].

Nutrition has a major influence on the epigenome although its precise role is difficult to establish because of multiple interactions between dietary components, and with other epigenetic regulators and specific genotypes [5,6,7,77,78]. Recent advances in two novel species, honey bees and locusts, are discussed in this section of the review because of their unique ability to provide insights into mechanisms underlying epigenetic regulation of phenotype and hence the propensity for disease.

5.4.1 GENOTYPE, EPIGENOTYPE AND PHENOTYPE

It has long been recognized that genotype does not necessarily determine phenotype, i.e., observable traits or characteristics. In 1911, Johannsen suggested "Supposing that some organisms of identical genotypical constitution are developing under different external conditions, then these differences will produce more or less differences as to the personal qualities of the individual organisms" [79]. Environmental temperature, nutrition and interactions between these variables profoundly affect multiple aspects of mammalian development, morphology, physiology, behaviour, endocrinology, cell biology and molecular biology [80,81]. Indeed, the changes induced postnatally are so great that they could be mistakenly perceived as being due to genetic differences. Ultimately, these effects are mediated by epigenetic mechanisms, with numerous endogenous and exogenous regulators modifying gene expression via changes in epigenotype.

Phenotypic plasticity is common across species, and is the differential expression of alternative phenotypes from a single genotype depending on environmental conditions [82]. Changes occur at the level of organism, tissue or cell and this epigenetic remodelling allows individuals to respond and adapt to specific factors in the environment such as nutrition, temperature and social interactions (see Figure 2). In the nervous system, for example, epigenetic remodelling can significantly affect learning and memory. Marked structural and functional plasticity occurs in the brain during development and in adults. Whether epigenetic regulators are beneficial or harmful holds profound implications for phenotypic outcome in terms of brain function. Precise mechanisms underlying brain and neuronal plasticity are thus of considerable relevance and are providing new insights into mechanisms underlying neurological function.

5.4.2 NUTRITION, HONEYBEES AND EPIGENETICS

Recent research suggests that the honeybee *Apis mellifera* may be an especially useful model for understanding the basis of learning, memory and cognition [83]. This species exhibits complex social, navigational and communication behaviours, and an impressive cognitive repertoire. These functions are undertaken by a brain containing only 1 million neurons compared with 100 billion in the human brain. Moreover, neural networks in the honeybee are limited in size and complexity, enabling the tracing of neural plasticity to specific neural circuits and single neurons.

A major focus of studies on nutritional regulation of epigenetic markers is DNA methylation. Level of food intake and multiple specific nutrients affect DNA methylation patterns in a diverse range of species [84,85,86,87,88]. In honeybee colonies, whether an individual becomes a queen or a worker depends not on genotype but on its diet during development. Female honeybee larvae develop into either a queen or worker phenotype, and determination of phenotype is due entirely to dietary-induced

DNA methylation by royal jelly. This mixture of proteins, sugars and fatty acids, including 10-hydroxydecanoic acid and phenyl butyrate, reduces DNA methyltransferase 3 expression, leading to altered DNA methylation patterns that induce the queen bee phenotype [89].

Recent studies have shown that epigenetic mechanisms are important not only in development but also in behavioural changes during adult life [90]. Worker bees can be either nurses or foragers, depending on the needs of the hive for care of larvae versus collection of food and water. By contrast with the queen and worker castes, the phenotype of these subcastes is reversible. Whole genome bisulphite sequencing and comprehensive high-throughput array-based methylation analysis was used to compare methylomes in the distinct honeybee phenotypes. Especially important was the finding of reversible switching between epigenetic states in the two types of worker bee. Over 100 differentially methylated regions were found in nurse compared with forager bees, whereas there were no such differences in DNA methylation between the irreversible queen and worker castes. Similarly, there were marked differences in methylated regions when foragers were induced to revert to nursing. Regions of the genome involved in this response contained genes linked with development, ATP-binding, learning and axon migration, via transcriptional control and chromatin remodelling.

Current studies comparing long-lived queen and short-lived worker phenotype are proving useful for the study of diet-induced epigenetic effects on lifespan [91]. Further advances would undoubtedly result from investigation of the nutritional regulation of epigenotype in specific neurons and regions of the brain. These should provide novel insights into the role of nutrition in neurological development and function.

5.4.3 PHENOTYPIC PLASTICITY, LOCUSTS AND NEUROLOGICAL FUNCTION

One of the most dramatic forms of phenotypic plasticity occurs in locusts [82,92]. They can change reversibly between two extreme forms, and transformation between the solitarious form and the swarming gregarious form is driven by changes in population density and concomitant social interactions. These two forms of locust differ so extensively in appearance, morphology, physiology, neurochemistry and behaviour, that they were once thought to be two distinct species. For example, solitary locusts walk with a slow, creeping gait, fly mainly at night, have a restricted diet and avoid other locusts. By contrast, gregarious locusts have a rapid, upright gait, fly during the day, have a broad diet and are attracted to other locusts.

The locust thus makes an outstanding model system in which to study epigenetic regulation of neurological phenotype. Brain size, structure and function are quite different in the two phenotypic forms of locust. The gregarious locust is smaller than the solitary form but its brain is some 30% larger. Moreover, marked differences in size of specific brain regions are related to function. Numerous differences also occur in individual neurons, neuronal connections and neurochemistry. Of considerable significance is the finding that serotonin (5 hydroxytryptamine, 5-HT), an evolutionarily conserved mediator of neuronal plasticity, is responsible for the extreme phenotypic transformation in the desert locust *Schistocerca gregaria* [82,92]. In the two phenotypic forms, marked differences occur in many neurotransmitters and neuromodulators, including dopamine, taurine, arginine, glycine and glutamate. However, it is serotonin alone that is both necessary and sufficient to induce the initial gregarious behaviour in locusts.

Genomic approaches have advanced understanding of many mechanistic aspects of phenotypic plasticity in locusts. Genome-wide gene expression profiling during switching between solitary and gregarious forms of the migratory locust *Locusta migratoria* has revealed changes in genes related to chemosensory proteins, the catecholamine pathway, and dopamine synthesis and synaptic release [93,94]. Very little is known about the specific epigenetic mechanisms involved in the phenotypic change of locusts. Studies in the migratory locust have, however, shown that it possesses genes that putatively encode methylation machinery, i.e., DNA methyl transferases and a methyl-binding domain protein, and it exhibits genomic methylation, some of which appears to be localized to repetitive regions of the genome [95].

Taken together, these findings in locusts suggest that it could make an excellent model for investigating interactions between social and nutritional factors in regulating the epigenome and neurological phenotype.

5.5 GENE-ENVIRONMENT INTERACTIONS: THE SEROTONERGIC SYSTEM AND BRAIN DISORDERS

Elucidation of mechanisms underlying gene-environment interactions is central to an understanding of brain function and dysfunction. Many neurotransmitters and their associated pathways are implicated in brain disorders and their precise roles continue to be the subject of considerable discussion and controversy. To illustrate advances made in this field and the complexity of the multiple interacting processes involved, this section discusses gene-environment interactions in the serotonergic system, as a paradigm of the multiple key molecules and signalling pathways that are affected in brain disorders.

Serotonin is implicated in many forms of behavioural plasticity associated with social interactions. These range from marked behavioural differences in locusts to emotional well-being, depression and anxiety in humans [92]. Serotonin plays a key role in cognition and memory, and a dysfunctional serotonergic system is implicated in the pathophysiology of many neuropsychiatric and neurological disorders, including schizophrenia, Alzheimer's disease and vascular dementia [96,97]. Recent progress in identifying mechanisms involved in these disorders suggests important roles for gene variants and epigenetic factors in modifying the serotonergic system. In addition, they suggest important interactions between the serotonergic system, other neurotransmitters including GABA and glutamine, and neuromodulators such as BDNF and glucocorticoids. An indication of the many critical interactions between genes, nutrition and stress in relation to neurological function and brain disorders is discussed in this section of the review and illustrated in Figure 4.

5.5.1 DIETARY TRYPTOPHAN AND BRAIN SEROTONIN

In mammals, the essential amino acid tryptophan is the precursor for serotonin and the extent to which nutrition interacts with the serotonergic system is therefore of considerable interest. Changes in brain tryptophan concentration rapidly influence the rate of neuronal serotonin synthesis.

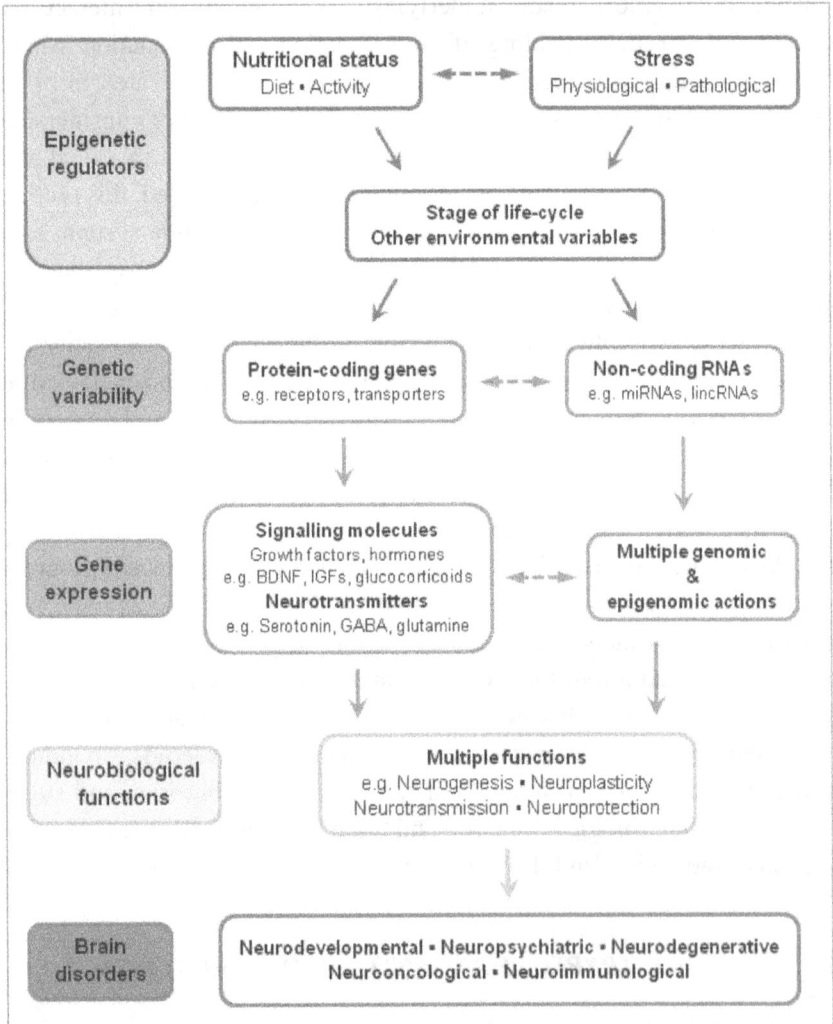

FIGURE 4: Nutrition-stress-gene interactions and brain disorders.

However, tryptophan is transported across the blood-brain barrier in competition with other large neutral amino acids (LNAA). Therefore serotonin levels do not necessarily reflect dietary tryptophan intake; instead there are complex interactions with the protein and amino acid content of the diet. This explains the impact of meals containing little or no protein on serotonin production. High-carbohydrate meals induce a striking difference in plasma tryptophan-LNAA acid ratios compared with high-protein meals, and may therefore affect brain tryptophan concentrations and serotonin synthesis [98]. Such meals also have distinct effects on the plasma tyrosine-LNAA ratio and hence have the potential to modify brain catecholamine synthesis.

Serotonin synthesis from tryptophan occurs in presynaptic neurons and is vitamin B6 dependent [99]. After its release from synaptic vesicles, it acts via seven types of postsynaptic cell-membrane bound receptors (5-HTR) to modulate neurological function in multiple processes including cognition, learning, memory, mood and appetite. Actions of serotonin are terminated by its reuptake from the synaptic cleft into the presynaptic neurons. This occurs via a specific transmembrane transporter (SERT, 5-HTT). Key drugs for treatment of several neuropsychiatric disorders therefore target the serotonergic system, e.g., monoamine oxidase inhibitors prevent serotonin breakdown, and selective serotonin reuptake inhibitors (SSRIs) ensure that serotonin stays longer in the synaptic cleft.

Of particular interest in the present context is the finding that both SSRIs and herbal treatments increase BDNF in the hippocampus, a brain region critical for memory and cognition, while also reducing circulating glucocorticoids [100]. The aim was to compare a novel herbal treatment for anxiety disorder with conventional treatment using SSRIs. In a mouse model, the herbal treatment reduced anxiety-like behaviours, possibly via a reduction in circulating corticosterone and increase in BDNF levels in the hippocampus.

5.5.2 BRAIN PLASTICITY: BDNF, GLUCOCORTICOIDS AND SEROTONIN

Numerous growth factors, hormones and their specific receptors play a central role in mediating the effects of energy status on brain plasticity and function [5,6,7,8,64]. Especially relevant, therefore, are recent findings on the intimate cross-talk between glucocorticoids, BDNF and other trophic factors, especially in relation to dynamic brain plasticity [101,102,103].

Glucocorticoids and BDNF do not function alone as modulators of plasticity. Their effects are dependent on signals from many other neurotransmitters and intracellular molecules [101] Multiple lines of evidence suggest that BDNF plays a pivotal role in the pathophysiology of major depressive disorder, a common, chronic, recurrent mental illness that affects 10%–20% of the population [104]. Serum levels of mature BDNF, but not its precursor proBDNF, are decreased in patients with major depressive disorder [105]. Both BDNF and agonists of its receptor, TrkB, have antidepressant effects in animal models. This suggests a crucial role of the BDNF-TrkB signalling pathway in the therapeutic action of antidepressants such as SSRIs [104].

Neural plasticity in response to stress involves not only an increase in glucocorticoids but also requires numerous molecules including BDNF [101]. BDNF levels are highly dynamic in response to stress and vary across brain regions and over time. The transglutaminase 2 (TG2) inhibitor cysteamine is neuroprotective and increases TrkB signalling in the brain. Chronic administration of cysteamine ameliorates the decreases in TrkB in the frontal cortex and hippocampus and the anxiety/depression-like behaviours induced in mice by glucocorticoid treatment [106]. This indicates that BDNF-TrkB signalling plays an important role in the beneficial effects of cysteamine, suggesting that it would be a novel therapeutic drug for glucocorticoid-related symptoms of neuropsychiatric disorders. Moreover, TG2 may be a factor in the serotonin deficiency associated with major depressive disorder: increased levels of TG2 probably convert serotonin to Rac1, resulting in decreased levels of serotonin and BDNF that are associated with major depressive disorder [104].

5.5.3 SEROTONERGIC SYSTEM: GENE VARIABILITY, EPIGENETICS AND BRAIN DISORDERS

Studies on the role of gene-environment interactions in neuropsychiatric disorders suggest that genetic and epigenetic changes in serotonin receptors (*5-HTR*) and transporter (*5-HTT, SERT*) are involved [107]. In peripheral blood leukocytes from patients with schizophrenia and bipolar disorder, DNA methylation in the promoter region of the serotonin type 1A gene (*5HTR1A*) is increased [108]. This would reduce gene expression and, if similar changes occur in the brain, would explain the decrease in receptor mRNA in these disorders. Support for this conclusion comes from the study of another serotonin receptor gene (*5HTR2A*): in post-mortem frontal brain samples from patients with schizophrenia and bipolar disorder compared with matched controls, genotype and DNA methylation interacted to fine-tune *5HTR2A* expression, and epigenetic down-regulation of *5HTR2A* was associated with early onset of disease [109].

Another focus of considerable interest and controversy in the field of gene-environment actions is the link between the serotonin transporter gene (*5HTT, SLC6A4*), stress and the *BDNF* gene in the risk of depression [110,111,112,113]. Recent evidence suggests a link between a functional deletion/insertion polymorphism, *5-HTTLPR,* in the serotonin transporter gene and environmental stresses over time, and especially during childhood and adolescence [114]. Adolescents homozygous for the short allele (SS) and exposed to early childhood adversities have a marked inability to process emotional information; a response linked with increased risk of depression and anxiety. Controversy exists in part because a description of the functional mechanisms involved has been lacking. However, findings on the functional anatomy of the serotonergic dorsal raphe nucleus suggest that genetic variation in serotonin uptake may affect the stress response and risk of depression through critical brain circuitry underlying stressor reactivity and regulation of emotion [115].

The precise role of the serotonergic system in brain disorders remains highly controversial. Nevertheless, these findings on genotype-epigenotype modifications of serotonin receptors and transporter suggest possibilities for novel therapeutic approaches based on the downstream effects of serotonin.

5.5.4 NUTRITION-STRESS-GENE INTERACTIONS AND BRAIN DISORDERS

The present discussion of the serotonergic system's role in brain disorders provides insight into the complexities, difficulties and potential benefits of elucidating the many signalling pathways and neural networks involved in gene-environment regulation of brain function. Multiple interactions occur between the serotonergic system and other neurotransmitter, neuromodulator and neurotrophic systems. Moreover, nutrition interacts with numerous environmental factors to determine overall impact on the epigenome of specific brain regions and cell types throughout the life-cycle. Stress is one such factor. Indeed, it is probable that individual differences in stress responses are modified by nutrition, and this in turn determines outcome in relation to the adverse effects of stress on multiple brain disorders [20,116].

Physiological stress can be defined as any external or internal condition that challenges the homeostasis of the cell or organism, and includes environmental stress, intrinsic development and aging [117]. The effects of the stress response can be beneficial or harmful, depending on the type and intensity of stress, its timing and duration, and individual differences in coping with stress [20,118]. Exposure to physiological and psychological stressors activates the hypothalamic-pituitary-adrenal axis (HPA), resulting in increased secretion of glucocorticoids. Moreover, variants of the glucocorticoid receptor gene (NR3C1) are linked with schizophrenia and bipolar disorder [119]. By contrast with its actions on glucocorticoids, stress down-regulates neurotrophins such as BDNF, thus contributing to the pathophysiology of brain disorders including depression, Alzheimer's and Parkinson's disease. Moreover, variants of the BDNF gene are linked with risk of neuropsychiatric disorders, including depression, eating disorders and schizophrenia [5,6,7,110,120].

Epigenetic mechanisms affect both short-term and long-term responses to stress and may even be inter-generational [121]. Compared with healthy controls, adult patients with psychosis have higher rates of childhood trauma, impairments in cognitive performance and smaller amygdala volume, a brain region important in emotional processing and higher functions such as working memory [122]. Considerable evidence suggests a key role for early-life nutrition, and especially prenatal maternal undernutrition, in risk of neurodevelopmental and neuropsychiatric disorders such as schizophrenia [5,6,7,123,124,125].

The central nervous system has a major role in metabolic control, and this is especially apparent in stressful events such as catabolic states and hormone deficiencies that mimic starvation [126]. Various nutrient, energetic and hormonal cues function in the hypothalamus to control glucose and lipid metabolism and overall energy balance. Hormones with nuclear receptors that act as transcription factors are especially potent mediators of nutrition-gene interactions [21,22]. Glucocorticoids, for example, mediate many of the effects of stress via epigenetic events involving DNA methylation, histone modifications and ncRNAs [127]. The growth arrest-specific 5 (Gas5) ncRNA is a riborepressor of the glucocorticoid receptor, and influences cell survival and metabolic activity during starvation by modulating the transcriptional activity of the receptor [128]. Moreover, the methylation states of many hormones and their receptors are modified by nutrition throughout the life-cycle. In humans, maternal intake of the methyl donor choline alters placental epigenomic marks and the epigenetic state of key modulators of placental and fetal HPA axis reactivity [129]. The possibility, therefore, is that maternal choline intake could be used to prevent the adverse effects of prenatal stress on subsequent neurological and neuropsychiatric disorders.

Deeper understanding of the genomic and epigenomic mechanisms underlying nutrition-stress interactions in the central nervous system should help to suggest novel approaches for prevention, treatment and alleviation of the multiple disorders associated with stress and sub-optimal nutrition, including cognitive impairment, dementia, depression, anxiety, schizophrenia, Alzheimer's disease and Parkinson's disease.

5.6 CONCLUSIONS

The current review has shown that knowledge of individual genetic variability and epigenetic regulation of gene expression underpins the understanding of nutritional regulation of optimal and sub-optimal brain health. Recent advances are providing insights into disorders ranging from cognitive impairment, depression and eating disorders to Alzheimer's disease, schizophrenia and brain tumours. Future advances will involve very large-scale investigations of the whole genome and epigenomes of specific cell types, together with focused assessment of specific regulatory factors including protein-coding genes and non-coding RNAs (ncRNAs).

Considerable effort is now being made by large scale consortia to cope with the enormous sample sizes and vast amounts of data being generated by advances in genomics and epigenomics. The development of genome-wide association studies (GWAS) is enabling significant advances in identifying common disease-predisposing gene variants. However, the robust detection of disease-associated low-frequency alleles in complex diseases will require even larger study samples than those used in GWAS [36]. Moreover, studies combining GWAS with a systems genetics approach will undoubtedly advance understanding of the complex pathways linking genetics, environment and disease [37,38,130].

The International Human Epigenome Consortium (IHEC) incorporates inputs from scientists in North America, Europe, Australia, Japan and South Korea. Its primary goal is to provide free access to high-resolution reference human epigenome maps to the research community. A range of 21 normal and disease cell types are being investigated, including those from the fetal and adult nervous system. Epigenomic maps can be used to trace the origin of cells, dissect affected pathways and identify predictive biomarkers [46]. The hope is that these maps will have an impact on the understanding, treatment and management of many diseases. Underpinning these advances is the need for a global biobanking strategy to harmonize the multiple interests of organizations, initiatives, resources and stakeholders, including patients [131].

Technological advances cannot in themselves provide solutions to all problems associated with the aetiology and treatment of brain disorders. Future studies using innovative approaches and novel systems will also help to advance understanding of the links between nutrition and neuroscience. Some of these are highlighted in the present review. Evolutionary complexity is linked with increasingly large proportions of non-protein-coding sequences in the genome. Indeed, recent studies implicate ncRNAs in mediating changes in neural gene expression during evolution. They also suggest that the expansion of ncRNAs was in part responsible for the emergence of vertebrate complexity, especially in the brain, together with the increased cognitive and behavioural repertories of higher organisms [55]. Comparative genomic and epigenomic studies in a wide range of species will therefore be of particular benefit in elucidating mechanisms underlying brain disorders [86,132,133,134]. Key studies in development and neuroscience have been undertaken in many species including the fruit fly *Drosophila melanogaster*, zebra fish, frog and mouse. *Drosophila* has long been used as a model organism for studying diseases ranging from cancer to neurodegenerative disorders. Its versatile genetics and the ability to quickly generate multiple genetic variants could be of particular value in studying complex neuropsychiatric disorders such as autism and schizophrenia [134]. Moreover, studies in a range of species is currently enabling significant progress in understanding the role of the Wnt/β-catenin cell signalling pathway in many neurological and neuropsychiatric disorders, including Alzheimer's, schizophrenia and the devastating brain cancer glioma [133].

In addition to the epigenetic studies in honeybees and locusts discussed in the current review, further novel approaches could, for example, involve molecular evolutionary studies of dietary selection. These should provide new insights into eating behaviours and disorders in humans. The giant panda *Ailuropoda melanoleuca* has a highly specialized bamboo diet that is quite different from the carnivorous or omnivorous diets of other bears. Comprehensive sequence analysis of the genes involved in the appetite-reward system suggests a complex genetic background, possibly involving miRNAs and deficiencies in dopamine metabolism, behind the panda's dietary switch [135]. Progress in elucidating the complex role of nutrition in brain disorders will benefit considerably from future studies on ncRNAs. The predicted exponential rise in understanding of the role of ncRNAs in the central nervous system, combined with the versatility and relative simplicity of RNA chemistry, should make translation into diagnostic and therapeutic applications a reasonable possibility [56].

It is probable that genomic and epigenomic technologies will continue to advance significantly, resulting in reduced costs and increased opportunities. This should enable large numbers of individual genomes and epigenomes to be analysed throughout the life-cycle in relation to multiple environmental variables including specific diets, nutrients, energy intake and physical activity. In the long-term, outcomes should include major benefits in relation to optimization of life-style and ameliorating any underlying genetic propensity for disease. However, major cautions and caveats must also be mentioned. Current concern with respect to the ethical use of personal data will only increase as the functions of millions of newly identified gene variants are elucidated. Moreover, it is essential that nutritionists and dietitians are involved at all stages of such investigations. Significant advances are now being made in relation to two highly relevant areas: the accurate assessment of dietary intake and life-style, and the education of professional nutritionists in the molecular and cellular basis of health and disease.

In summary, future advances in genomics and epigenomics will continue to provide new insights into the mechanisms that underpin the nutritional regulation of gene expression in the brain. Technological progress cannot in itself provide solutions to all biomedical problems. Innovative approaches combined with state-of-the-art techniques should suggest possibilities for preventing, ameliorating and treating the multiple complex brain disorders associated with adverse genetic and environmental factors.

REFERENCES

1. Bras, J.; Guerreiro, R.; Hardy, J. Use of next-generation sequencing and other whole-genome strategies to dissect neurological disease. Nat. Rev. Neurosci. 2012, 13, 453–464, doi:10.1038/nrn3271.

2. Sullivan, P.F.; Daly, M.J.; O'Donovan, M. Genetic architectures of psychiatric disorders: The emerging picture and its implications. Nat. Rev. Genet. 2012, 13, 537–551, doi:10.1038/nrg3240.

3. Dunham, I.; Kundaje, A.; Aldred, S.F.; Collins, P.J.; Davis, C.A.; Doyle, F.; Epstein, C.B.; Frietze, S.; Harrow, J.; Kaul, R.; et al. An integrated encyclopedia of DNA elements in the human genome. Nature 2012, 489, 57–74.

4. Qureshi, I.A.; Mehler, M.F. Epigenetic mechanisms governing the process of neurodegeneration. Mol. Aspects Med. 2012. in press.

5. Dauncey, M.J. Recent advances in nutrition, genes and brain health. Proc. Nutr. Soc. 2012, 71, 581–591, doi:10.1017/S0029665112000237.

6. Dauncey, M.J. Novos conhecimentos sobre nutrição, genes e saúde do cérebro. Nutr. Pauta 2012, 115, 3–10.

7. Dauncey, M.J. Novos conhecimentos sobre nutrição, genes e doenças do cérebro. Nutr. Pauta 2012, 116, 3–12.

8. Gomez-Pinilla, F. Brain foods: The effects of nutrients on brain function. Nat. Rev. Neurosci. 2008, 9, 568–578, doi:10.1038/nrn2421.

9. Nurk, E.; Refsum, H.; Drevon, C.A.; Tell, G.S.; Nygaard, H.A.; Engedal, K.; Smith, A.D. Intake of flavonoid-rich wine, tea, and chocolate by elderly men and women is associated with better cognitive test performance. J. Nutr. 2009, 139, 120–127.

10. Dauncey, M.J. New insights into nutrition and cognitive neuroscience. Proc. Nutr. Soc. 2009, 68, 408–415, doi:10.1017/S0029665109990188.

11. Dauncey, M.J. Recentes avanços em nutrição e neurociência cognitiva. Nutr. Pauta 2009, 97, 4–13.
12. Gomez-Pinilla, F.; Nguyen, T.T. Natural mood foods: The actions of polyphenols against psychiatric and cognitive disorders. Nutr. Neurosci. 2012, 15, 127–133.
13. Milte, C.M.; Parletta, N.; Buckley, J.D.; Coates, A.M.; Young, R.M.; Howe, P.R. Eicosapentaenoic and docosahexaenoic acids, cognition, and behavior in children with attention-deficit/hyperactivity disorder: A randomized controlled trial. Nutrition 2012, 28, 670–677, doi:10.1016/j.nut.2011.12.009.
14. Morris, M.S. The role of B vitamins in preventing and treating cognitive impairment and decline. Adv. Nutr. 2012, 3, 801–812, doi:10.3945/an.112.002535.
15. Sinn, N.; Milte, C.M.; Street, S.J.; Buckley, J.D.; Coates, A.M.; Petkov, J.; Howe, P.R. Effects of n-3 fatty acids, EPA v. DHA, on depressive symptoms, quality of life, memory and executive function in older adults with mild cognitive impairment: A 6-month randomised controlled trial. Br. J. Nutr. 2012, 107, 1682–1693, doi:10.1017/S0007114511004788.
16. Susser, E.; Kirkbride, J.B.; Heijmans, B.T.; Kresovich, J.K.; Lumey, L.H.; Stein, A.D. Maternal prenatal nutrition and health in grandchildren and subsequent generations. Ann. Rev. Anthropol. 2012, 41, 577–610, doi:10.1146/annurev-anthro-081309-145645.
17. Dauncey, M.J.; Bicknell, R.J. Nutrition and neurodevelopment: Mechanisms of developmental dysfunction and disease in later life. Nutr. Res. Rev. 1999, 12, 231–253, doi:10.1079/095442299108728947.
18. Dauncey, M.J.; Astley, S. Genômica nutricional: Novos estudos sobre as interações entre nutrição e o genoma humano. Nutr. Pauta 2006, 77, 4–9.
19. Hackett, J.A.; Zylicz, J.J.; Surani, M.A. Parallel mechanisms of epigenetic reprogramming in the germline. Trends Genet. 2012, 28, 164–174, doi:10.1016/j.tig.2012.01.005.
20. Babenko, O.; Kovalchuk, I.; Metz, G.A. Epigenetic programming of neurodegenerative diseases by an adverse environment. Brain Res. 2012, 1444, 96–111, doi:10.1016/j.brainres.2012.01.038.
21. Dauncey, M.J.; White, P.; Burton, K.A.; Katsumata, M. Nutrition-hormone receptor-gene interactions: Implications for development and disease. Proc. Nutr. Soc. 2001, 60, 63–72, doi:10.1079/PNS200071.
22. Dauncey, M.J.; White, P. Nutrition and cell communication: Insulin signalling in development, health and disease. Rec. Res. Dev. Nutr. 2004, 6, 49–81.
23. Park, L.K.; Friso, S.; Choi, S.W. Nutritional influences on epigenetics and age-related disease. Proc. Nutr. Soc. 2012, 71, 75–83, doi:10.1017/S0029665111003302.
24. Dauncey, M.J. From early nutrition and later development to underlying mechanisms and optimal health. Br. J. Nutr. 1997, 78, S113–S123, doi:10.1079/BJN19970226.
25. Dauncey, M.J. Interações precoces nutrição-hormônios: Implicações nas doenças degenerativas de adultos. Nutr. Pauta 2004, 66, 30–35.
26. Langie, S.A.; Lara, J.; Mathers, J.C. Early determinants of the ageing trajectory. Best Pract. Res. Clin. Endocrinol. Metab. 2012, 26, 613–626, doi:10.1016/j.beem.2012.03.004.
27. Robinson, S.; Fall, C. Infant nutrition and later health: A review of current evidence. Nutrients 2012, 4, 859–874, doi:10.3390/nu4080859.

28. Liu, G.E. Recent applications of DNA sequencing technologies in food, nutrition and agriculture. Rec. Pat. Food Nutr. Agric. 2011, 3, 187–195, doi:10.2174/221279 8411103030187.

29. Kilpinen, H.; Barrett, J.C. How next-generation sequencing is transforming complex disease genetics. Trends Genet. 2013, 29, 23–30, doi:10.1016/j.tig.2012.10.001.

30. Lander, E.S.; Linton, L.M.; Birren, B.; Nusbaum, C.; Zody, M.C.; Baldwin, J.; Devon, K.; Dewar, K.; Doyle, M.; FitzHugh, W.; et al. Initial sequencing and analysis of the human genome. Nature 2001, 409, 860–921, doi:10.1038/35057062.

31. Jonsson, T.; Atwal, J.K.; Steinberg, S.; Snaedal, J.; Jonsson, P.V.; Bjornsson, S.; Stefansson, H.; Sulem, P.; Gudbjartsson, D.; Maloney, J.; et al. A mutation in APP protects against Alzheimer's disease and age-related cognitive decline. Nature 2012, 488, 96–99.

32. Steinberg, S.; de Jong, S.; Mattheisen, M.; Costas, J.; Demontis, D.; Jamain, S.; Pietilainen, O.P.; Lin, K.; Papiol, S.; Huttenlocher, J.; et al. Common variant at 16p11.2 conferring risk of psychosis. Mol. Psychiatry 2012, doi:10.1038/mp.2012.157.

33. Wang, K.; Zhang, H.; Bloss, C.S.; Duvvuri, V.; Kaye, W.; Schork, N.J.; Berrettini, W.; Hakonarson, H. A genome-wide association study on common SNPs and rare CNVs in anorexia nervosa. Mol. Psychiatry 2011, 16, 949–959, doi:10.1038/mp.2010.107.

34. Freilinger, T.; Anttila, V.; de Vries, B.; Malik, R.; Kallela, M.; Terwindt, G.M.; Pozo-Rosich, P.; Winsvold, B.; Nyholt, D.R.; van Oosterhout, W.P.; et al. Genome-wide association analysis identifies susceptibility loci for migraine without aura. Nat. Genet. 2012, 44, 777–782, doi:10.1038/ng.2307.

35. Boraska, V.; Davis, O.S.; Cherkas, L.F.; Helder, S.G.; Harris, J.; Krug, I.; Liao, T.P.; Treasure, J.; Ntalla, I.; Karhunen, L.; et al. Genome-wide association analysis of eating disorder-related symptoms, behaviors, and personality traits. Am. J. Med. Genet. B Neuropsychiatr. Genet. 2012, 159, 803–811.

36. Palotie, A.; Widen, E.; Ripatti, S. From genetic discovery to future personalized health research. N. Biotechnol. 2012. in press.

37. Nadeau, J.H.; Dudley, A.M. Genetics. Systems genetics. Science 2011, 331, 1015–1016, doi:10.1126/science.1203869.

38. Kalupahana, N.S.; Moustaid-Moussa, N. Overview of symposium "Systems genetics in nutrition and obesity research". J. Nutr. 2011, 141, 512–514, doi:10.3945/jn.110.130104.

39. Voy, B.H. Systems genetics: A powerful approach for gene-environment interactions. J. Nutr. 2011, 141, 515–519, doi:10.3945/jn.110.130401.

40. Vidal, M.; Cusick, M.E.; Barabasi, A.L. Interactome networks and human disease. Cell 2011, 144, 986–998, doi:10.1016/j.cell.2011.02.016.

41. Abecasis, G.R.; Altshuler, D.; Auton, A.; Brooks, L.D.; Durbin, R.M.; Gibbs, R.A.; Hurles, M.E.; McVean, G.A. A map of human genome variation from population-scale sequencing. Nature 2010, 467, 1061–1073, doi:10.1038/nature09534.

42. Abecasis, G.R.; Auton, A.; Brooks, L.D.; DePristo, M.A.; Durbin, R.M.; Handsaker, R.E.; Kang, H.M.; Marth, G.T.; McVean, G.A. An integrated map of genetic variation from 1092 human genomes. Nature 2012, 491, 56–65.

43. Harrow, J.; Frankish, A.; Gonzalez, J.M.; Tapanari, E.; Diekhans, M.; Kokocinski, F.; Aken, B.L.; Barrell, D.; Zadissa, A.; Searle, S.; et al. GENCODE: The refer-

ence human genome annotation for The ENCODE Project. Genome Res. 2012, 22, 1760–1774, doi:10.1101/gr.135350.111.

44. Human Genome Far More Active Than Thought. GENCODE Consortium Discovers Far More Genes Than Previously Thought. Available online: http://www.sanger. ac.uk/about/press/2012/120905.html (accessed on 10 December 2012).

45. Attar, N. The allure of the epigenome. Genome Biol. 2012, 13, 419, doi:10.1186/ gb-2012-13-10-419.

46. Meissner, A. What can epigenomics do for you? Genome Biol. 2012, 13, 420, doi:10.1186/gb-2012-13-10-420.

47. Clark, C.; Palta, P.; Joyce, C.J.; Scott, C.; Grundberg, E.; Deloukas, P.; Palotie, A.; Coffey, A.J. A comparison of the whole genome approach of MeDIP-Seq to the targeted approach of the Infinium HumanMethylation450 BeadChip® for methylome profiling. PLoS One 2012, 7, e50233.

48. Davies, M.N.; Volta, M.; Pidsley, R.; Lunnon, K.; Dixit, A.; Lovestone, S.; Coarfa, C.; Harris, R.A.; Milosavljevic, A.; Troakes, C.; et al. Functional annotation of the human brain methylome identifies tissue-specific epigenetic variation across brain and blood. Genome Biol. 2012, 13, R43, doi:10.1186/gb-2012-13-6-r43.

49. Decock, A.; Ongenaert, M.; Hoebeeck, J.; De Preter, K.; Van Peer, G.; Van Criekinge, W.; Ladenstein, R.; Schulte, J.H.; Noguera, R.; Stallings, R.L.; et al. Genome-wide promoter methylation analysis in neuroblastoma identifies prognostic methylation biomarkers. Genome Biol. 2012, 13, R95, doi:10.1186/gb-2012-13-10-r95.

50. Ernst, J.; Kheradpour, P.; Mikkelsen, T.S.; Shoresh, N.; Ward, L.D.; Epstein, C.B.; Zhang, X.; Wang, L.; Issner, R.; Coyne, M.; et al. Mapping and analysis of chromatin state dynamics in nine human cell types. Nature 2011, 473, 43–49.

51. Huttenhofer, A.; Schattner, P.; Polacek, N. Non-coding RNAs: Hope or hype? Trends Genet. 2005, 21, 289–297, doi:10.1016/j.tig.2005.03.007.

52. Derrien, T.; Johnson, R.; Bussotti, G.; Tanzer, A.; Djebali, S.; Tilgner, H.; Guernec, G.; Martin, D.; Merkel, A.; Knowles, D.G.; et al. The GENCODE v7 catalog of human long noncoding RNAs: Analysis of their gene structure, evolution, and expression. Genome Res. 2012, 22, 1775–1789, doi:10.1101/gr.132159.111.

53. Rinn, J.L.; Chang, H.Y. Genome regulation by long noncoding RNAs. Annu. Rev. Biochem. 2012, 81, 145–166, doi:10.1146/annurev-biochem-051410-092902.

54. Magistri, M.; Faghihi, M.A.; St Laurent, G., III; Wahlestedt, C. Regulation of chromatin structure by long noncoding RNAs: Focus on natural antisense transcripts. Trends Genet. 2012, 28, 389–396, doi:10.1016/j.tig.2012.03.013.

55. Qureshi, I.A.; Mehler, M.F. Emerging roles of non-coding RNAs in brain evolution, development, plasticity and disease. Nat. Rev. Neurosci. 2012, 13, 528–541, doi:10.1038/nrn3234.

56. Salta, E.; de Strooper, B. Non-coding RNAs with essential roles in neurodegenerative disorders. Lancet Neurol. 2012, 11, 189–200, doi:10.1016/S1474-4422(11)70286-1.

57. Qureshi, I.A.; Mattick, J.S.; Mehler, M.F. Long non-coding RNAs in nervous system function and disease. Brain Res. 2010, 1338, 20–35, doi:10.1016/j. brainres.2010.03.110.

58. Gascon, E.; Gao, F.B. Cause or effect: Misregulation of microRNA pathways in neurodegeneration. Front. Neurosci. 2012, 6, 48.

59. Esteller, M. Non-coding RNAs in human disease. Nat. Rev. Genet. 2011, 12, 861–874, doi:10.1038/nrg3074.

60. Gutschner, T.; Diederichs, S. The hallmarks of cancer: A long non-coding RNA point of view. RNA Biol. 2012, 9, 703–719, doi:10.4161/rna.20481.

61. Spadaro, P.A.; Bredy, T.W. Emerging role of non-coding RNA in neural plasticity, cognitive function, and neuropsychiatric disorders. Front. Genet. 2012, 3, 132.

62. Tan, L.; Yu, J.T.; Hu, N.; Tan, L. Non-coding RNAs in Alzheimer's Disease. Mol. Neurobiol. 2013, 47, 382–393, doi:10.1007/s12035-012-8359-5.

63. Lee, S.T.; Chu, K.; Jung, K.H.; Kim, J.H.; Huh, J.Y.; Yoon, H.; Park, D.K.; Lim, J.Y.; Kim, J.M.; Jeon, D.; et al. miR-206 regulates brain-derived neurotrophic factor in Alzheimer disease model. Ann. Neurol. 2012, 72, 269–277, doi:10.1002/ana.23588.

64. Gomez-Pinilla, F. The combined effects of exercise and foods in preventing neurological and cognitive disorders. Prev. Med. 2011, 52, S75–S80, doi:10.1016/j.ypmed.2011.01.023.

65. Harraz, M.M.; Dawson, T.M.; Dawson, V.L. MicroRNAs in Parkinson's disease. J. Chem. Neuroanat. 2011, 42, 127–130, doi:10.1016/j.jchemneu.2011.01.005.

66. Wang, G.; van der Walt, J.M.; Mayhew, G.; Li, Y.J.; Zuchner, S.; Scott, W.K.; Martin, E.R.; Vance, J.M. Variation in the miRNA-433 binding site of FGF20 confers risk for Parkinson disease by overexpression of alpha-synuclein. Am. J. Hum. Genet. 2008, 82, 283–289, doi:10.1016/j.ajhg.2007.09.021.

67. Foley, N.H.; Bray, I.; Watters, K.M.; Das, S.; Bryan, K.; Bernas, T.; Prehn, J.H.; Stallings, R.L. MicroRNAs 10a and 10b are potent inducers of neuroblastoma cell differentiation through targeting of nuclear receptor corepressor 2. Cell. Death Differ. 2011, 18, 1089–1098, doi:10.1038/cdd.2010.172.

68. Setty, M.; Helmy, K.; Khan, A.A.; Silber, J.; Arvey, A.; Neezen, F.; Agius, P.; Huse, J.T.; Holland, E.C.; Leslie, C.S. Inferring transcriptional and microRNA-mediated regulatory programs in glioblastoma. Mol. Syst. Biol. 2012, 8, 605.

69. Ross, S.A.; Davis, C.D. MicroRNA, nutrition, and cancer preventio. Adv. Nutr. 2011, 2, 472–485, doi:10.3945/an.111.001206.

70. Kesse-Guyot, E.; Fezeu, L.; Andreeva, V.A.; Touvier, M.; Scalbert, A.; Hercberg, S.; Galan, P. Total and specific polyphenol intakes in midlife are associated with cognitive function measured 13 years later. J. Nutr. 2012, 142, 76–83, doi:10.3945/jn.111.144428.

71. Milenkovic, D.; Deval, C.; Gouranton, E.; Landrier, J.F.; Scalbert, A.; Morand, C.; Mazur, A. Modulation of miRNA expression by dietary polyphenols in apoE deficient mice: A new mechanism of the action of polyphenols. PLoS One 2012, 7, e29837.

72. Baggish, A.L.; Hale, A.; Weiner, R.B.; Lewis, G.D.; Systrom, D.; Wang, F.; Wang, T.J.; Chan, S.Y. Dynamic regulation of circulating microRNA during acute exhaustive exercise and sustained aerobic exercise training. J. Physiol. 2011, 589, 3983–3994, doi:10.1113/jphysiol.2011.213363.

73. Fernandes-Silva, M.M.; Carvalho, V.O.; Guimarães, G.V.; Bacal, F. Physical exercise and microRNAs: New frontiers in heart failure. Arq. Bras. Cardiol. 2012, 98, 459–466, doi:10.1590/S0066-782X2012000500012.

74. Barrès, R.; Yan, J.; Egan, B.; Treebak, J.T.; Rasmussen, M.; Fritz, T.; Caidahl, K.; Krook, A.; O'Gorman, D.J.; Zierath, J.R. Acute exercise remodels promoter meth-

ylation in human skeletal muscle. Cell. Metab. 2012, 15, 405–411, doi:10.1016/j. cmet.2012.01.001.

75. Habibi, E.; Masoudi-Nejad, A.; Abdolmaleky, H.M.; Haggarty, S.J. Emerging roles of epigenetic mechanisms in Parkinson's disease. Funct. Integr. Genomics 2011, 11, 523–537, doi:10.1007/s10142-011-0246-z.

76. Labrie, V.; Pai, S.; Petronis, A. Epigenetics of major psychosis: Progress, problems and perspectives. Trends Genet. 2012, 28, 427–435, doi:10.1016/j.tig.2012.04.002.

77. Jimenez-Chillaron, J.C.; Diaz, R.; Martinez, D.; Pentinat, T.; Ramon-Krauel, M.; Ribo, S.; Plosch, T. The role of nutrition on epigenetic modifications and their implications on health. Biochimie 2012, 94, 2242–2263, doi:10.1016/j.biochi.2012.06.012.

78. Khandaker, G.M.; Zimbron, J.; Lewis, G.; Jones, P.B. Prenatal maternal infection, neurodevelopment and adult schizophrenia: A systematic review of population-based studies. Psychol. Med. 2013, 43, 239–257, doi:10.1017/S0033291712000736.

79. Johannsen, W. The genotype conception of heredity. Am. Nat. 1911, 45, 129–159.

80. Dauncey, M.J.; Ingram, D.L. Acclimatization to warm or cold temperatures and the role of food intake. J. Therm. Biol. 1986, 11, 89–93, doi:10.1016/0306-4565(86)90025-2.

81. Dauncey, M.J. From whole body to molecule: An integrated approach to the regulation of metabolism and growth. Thermochim. Acta 1995, 250, 305–318, doi:10.1016/0040-6031(94)01967-L.

82. Anstey, M.L.; Rogers, S.M.; Ott, S.R.; Burrows, M.; Simpson, S.J. Serotonin mediates behavioral gregarization underlying swarm formation in desert locusts. Science 2009, 323, 627–630, doi:10.1126/science.1165939.

83. Menzel, R. The honeybee as a model for understanding the basis of cognition. Nat. Rev. Neurosci. 2012, 13, 758–768, doi:10.1038/nrn3357.

84. Wakeling, L.A.; Ions, L.J.; Ford, D. Could Sirt1-mediated epigenetic effects contribute to the longevity response to dietary restriction and be mimicked by other dietary interventions? Age (Dordr.) 2009, 31, 327–341, doi:10.1007/s11357-009-9104-5.

85. McKay, J.A.; Mathers, J.C. Diet induced epigenetic changes and their implications for health. Acta Physiol. (Oxf.) 2011, 202, 103–118, doi:10.1111/j.1748-1716.2011.02278.x.

86. Singh, K.; Molenaar, A.J.; Swanson, K.M.; Gudex, B.; Arias, J.A.; Erdman, R.A.; Stelwagen, K. Epigenetics: A possible role in acute and transgenerational regulation of dairy cow milk production. Animal 2012, 6, 375–381.

87. Weiner, S.A.; Toth, A.L. Epigenetics in social insects: a new direction for understanding the evolution of castes. Genet. Res. Int. 2012, 2012, 609810.

88. Gerhauser, C. Cancer chemoprevention and nutri-epigenetics: State of the art and future challenges. Top. Curr. Chem. 2013, 329, 73–132, doi:10.1007/128_2012_360.

89. Kucharski, R.; Maleszka, J.; Foret, S.; Maleszka, R. Nutritional control of reproductive status in honeybees via DNA methylation. Science 2008, 319, 1827–1830, doi:10.1126/science.1153069.

90. Herb, B.R.; Wolschin, F.; Hansen, K.D.; Aryee, M.J.; Langmead, B.; Irizarry, R.; Amdam, G.V.; Feinberg, A.P. Reversible switching between epigenetic states in honeybee behavioral subcastes. Nat. Neurosci. 2012, 15, 1371–1373, doi:10.1038/nn.3218.

91. Ford, D. Honeybees and cell lines as models of DNA methylation and aging in response to diet. Exp. Gerontol. 2012, doi:10.1016/j.exger.2012.07.010.

92. Burrows, M.; Rogers, S.M.; Ott, S.R. Epigenetic remodelling of brain, body and behaviour during phase change in locusts. Neural. Syst. Circuits 2011, 1, 11, doi:10.1186/2042-1001-1-11.

93. Guo, W.; Wang, X.; Ma, Z.; Xue, L.; Han, J.; Yu, D.; Kang, L. CSP and takeout genes modulate the switch between attraction and repulsion during behavioral phase change in the migratory locust. PLoS Genet. 2011, 7, e1001291, doi:10.1371/journal.pgen.1001291.

94. Ma, Z.; Guo, W.; Guo, X.; Wang, X.; Kang, L. Modulation of behavioral phase changes of the migratory locust by the catecholamine metabolic pathway. Proc. Natl. Acad. Sci. USA 2011, 108, 3882–3887.

95. Robinson, K.L.; Tohidi-Esfahani, D.; Lo, N.; Simpson, S.J.; Sword, G.A. Evidence for widespread genomic methylation in the migratory locust, Locusta migrat oria (Orthoptera: Acrididae). PLoS One 2011, 6, e28167.

96. Geyer, M.A.; Vollenweider, F.X. Serotonin research: Contributions to understanding psychoses. Trends Pharmacol. Sci. 2008, 29, 445–453, doi:10.1016/j.tips.2008.06.006.

97. Rodriguez, J.J.; Noristani, H.N.; Verkhratsky, A. The serotonergic system in ageing and Alzheimer's disease. Prog. Neurobiol. 2012, 99, 15–41, doi:10.1016/j.pneurobio.2012.06.010.

98. Wurtman, R.J.; Wurtman, J.J.; Regan, M.M.; McDermott, J.M.; Tsay, R.H.; Breu, J.J. Effects of normal meals rich in carbohydrates or proteins on plasma tryptophan and tyrosine ratios. Am. J. Clin. Nutr. 2003, 77, 128–132.

99. Le Floc'h, N.; Otten, W.; Merlot, E. Tryptophan metabolism, from nutrition to potential therapeutic applications. Amino Acids 2011, 41, 1195–1205, doi:10.1007/s00726-010-0752-7.

100. Doron, R.; Lotan, D.; Rak-Rabl, A.; Raskin-Ramot, A.; Lavi, K.; Rehavi, M. Anxiolytic effects of a novel herbal treatment in mice models of anxiety. Life Sci. 2012, 90, 995–1000, doi:10.1016/j.lfs.2012.05.014.

101. Gray, J.D.; Milner, T.A.; McEwen, B.S. Dynamic plasticity: The role of glucocorticoids, brain-derived neurotrophic factor and other trophic factors. Neuroscience 2012. in press.

102. Numakawa, T.; Adachi, N.; Richards, M.; Chiba, S.; Kunugi, H. Brain-derived neurotrophic factor and glucocorticoids: Reciprocal influence on the central nervous system. Neuroscience 2012. in press.

103. Suri, D.; Vaidya, V.A. Glucocorticoid regulation of brain-derived neurotrophic factor: Relevance to hippocampal structural and functional plasticity. Neuroscience 2012. in press.

104. Hashimoto, K. Understanding depression: Linking brain-derived neurotrophic factor, transglutaminase 2 and serotonin. Expert Rev. Neurother. 2013, 13, 5–7, doi:10.1586/ern.12.140.

105. Yoshida, T.; Ishikawa, M.; Niitsu, T.; Nakazato, M.; Watanabe, H.; Shiraishi, T.; Shiina, A.; Hashimoto, T.; Kanahara, N.; Hasegawa, T.; et al. Decreased serum levels of mature brain-derived neurotrophic factor (BDNF), but not its precursor proBDNF, in patients with major depressive disorder. PLoS One 2012, 7, e42676.

106. Kutiyanawalla, A.; Terry, A.V., Jr.; Pillai, A. Cysteamine attenuates the decreases in TrkB protein levels and the anxiety/depression-like behaviors in mice induced by corticosterone treatment. PLoS One 2011, 6, e26153, doi:10.1371/journal.pone.0026153.

107. Pidsley, R.; Mill, J. Research highlights: Epigenetic changes to serotonin receptor gene expression in schizophrenia and bipolar disorder. Epigenomics 2011, 3, 537–538, doi:10.2217/epi.11.87.

108. Carrard, A.; Salzmann, A.; Malafosse, A.; Karege, F. Increased DNA methylation status of the serotonin receptor 5HTR1A gene promoter in schizophrenia and bipolar disorder. J. Affect. Disord. 2011, 132, 450–453, doi:10.1016/j.jad.2011.03.018.

109. Abdolmaleky, H.M.; Yaqubi, S.; Papageorgis, P.; Lambert, A.W.; Ozturk, S.; Sivaraman, V.; Thiagalingam, S. Epigenetic dysregulation of HTR2A in the brain of patients with schizophrenia and bipolar disorder. Schizophr. Res. 2011, 129, 183–190, doi:10.1016/j.schres.2011.04.007.

110. Kaufman, J.; Yang, B.Z.; Douglas-Palumberi, H.; Grasso, D.; Lipschitz, D.; Houshyar, S.; Krystal, J.H.; Gelernter, J. Brain-derived neurotrophic factor-5-HTTLPR gene interactions and environmental modifiers of depression in children. Biol. Psychiatry 2006, 59, 673–680, doi:10.1016/j.biopsych.2005.10.026.

111. Kalueff, A.V.; Wheaton, M.; Ren-Patterson, R.; Murphy, D.L. Brain-derived neurotrophic factor, serotonin transporter, and depression: Comment on Kaufman et al.. Biol. Psychiatry 2007, 61, 1112–1113; author reply 1113–1115.

112. Van Den Hove, D.L.; Jakob, S.B.; Schraut, K.G.; Kenis, G.; Schmitt, A.G.; Kneitz, S.; Scholz, C.J.; Wiescholleck, V.; Ortega, G.; Prickaerts, J.; et al. Differential effects of prenatal stress in 5-Htt deficient mice: Towards molecular mechanisms of gene × environment interactions. PLoS One 2011, 6, e22715.

113. Bellani, M.; Nobile, M.; Bianchi, V.; van Os, J.; Brambilla, P. G × E interaction and neurodevelopment II. Focus on adversities in paediatric depression: the moderating role of serotonin transporter. Epidemiol. Psychiatr. Sci. 2012, 22, 21–28.

114. Owens, M.; Goodyer, I.M.; Wilkinson, P.; Bhardwaj, A.; Abbott, R.; Croudace, T.; Dunn, V.; Jones, P.B.; Walsh, N.D.; Ban, M.; Sahakian, B.J. 5-HTTLPR and early childhood adversities moderate cognitive and emotional processing in adolescence. PLoS One 2012, 7, e48482, doi:10.1371/journal.pone.0048482.

115. Jasinska, A.J.; Lowry, C.A.; Burmeister, M. Serotonin transporter gene, stress and raphe-raphe interactions: A molecular mechanism of depression. Trends Neurosci. 2012, 35, 395–402, doi:10.1016/j.tins.2012.01.001.

116. Heim, C.; Binder, E.B. Current research trends in early life stress and depression: Review of human studies on sensitive periods, gene-environment interactions, and epigenetics. Exp. Neurol. 2012, 233, 102–111, doi:10.1016/j.expneurol.2011.10.032.

117. Kagias, K.; Nehammer, C.; Pocock, R. Neuronal responses to physiological stress. Front. Genet. 2012, 3, 222.

118. Vedhara, K.; Metcalfe, C.; Brant, H.; Crown, A.; Northstone, K.; Dawe, K.; Lightman, S.; Smith, G.D. Maternal mood and neuroendocrine programming: Effects of time of exposure and sex. J. Neuroendocrinol. 2012, 24, 999–1011, doi:10.1111/j.1365-2826.2012.02309.x.

119. Sinclair, D.; Fullerton, J.M.; Webster, M.J.; Shannon Weickert, C. Glucocorticoid receptor 1B and 1C mRNA transcript alterations in schizophrenia and bipolar disorder, and their possible regulation by GR gene variants. PLoS One 2012, 7, e31720.

120. Carrard, A.; Salzmann, A.; Perroud, N.; Gafner, J.; Malafosse, A.; Karege, F. Genetic association of the phosphoinositide-3 kinase in schizophrenia and bipolar disorder and interaction with a BDNF gene polymorphism. Brain Behav. 2011, 1, 119–124, doi:10.1002/brb3.23.

121. Nestler, E.J. Epigenetics: Stress makes its molecular mark. Nature 2012, 490, 171–172, doi:10.1038/490171a.

122. Aas, M.; Navari, S.; Gibbs, A.; Mondelli, V.; Fisher, H.L.; Morgan, C.; Morgan, K.; MacCabe, J.; Reichenberg, A.; Zanelli, J.; et al. Is there a link between childhood trauma, cognition, and amygdala and hippocampus volume in first-episode psychosis? Schizophr. Res. 2012, 137, 73–79, doi:10.1016/j.schres.2012.01.035.

123. Nosarti, C.; Reichenberg, A.; Murray, R.M.; Cnattingius, S.; Lambe, M.P.; Yin, L.; MacCabe, J.; Rifkin, L.; Hultman, C.M. Preterm birth and psychiatric disorders in young adult life. Arch. Gen. Psychiatry 2012, 69, E1–E8.

124. Meredith, R.M.; Dawitz, J.; Kramvis, I. Sensitive time-windows for susceptibility in neurodevelopmental disorders. Trends Neurosci. 2012, 35, 335–344, doi:10.1016/j.tins.2012.03.005.

125. Kirkbride, J.B.; Susser, E.; Kundakovic, M.; Kresovich, J.K.; Davey Smith, G.; Relton, C.L. Prenatal nutrition, epigenetics and schizophrenia risk: Can we test causal effects? Epigenomics 2012, 4, 303–315, doi:10.2217/epi.12.20.

126. Myers, M.G., Jr.; Olson, D.P. Central nervous system control of metabolism. Nature 2012, 491, 357–363, doi:10.1038/nature11705.

127. Hunter, R.G. Epigenetic effects of stress and corticosteroids in the brain. Front. Cell. Neurosci. 2012, 6, 18, doi:10.3389/fncel.2012.00018.

128. Kino, T.; Hurt, D.E.; Ichijo, T.; Nader, N.; Chrousos, G.P. Noncoding RNA Gas5 is a growth arrest and starvation-associated repressor of the glucocorticoid receptor. Sci. Signal. 2010, 3, ra8, doi:10.1126/scisignal.2000568.

129. Jiang, X.; Yan, J.; West, A.A.; Perry, C.A.; Malysheva, O.V.; Devapatla, S.; Pressman, E.; Vermeylen, F.; Caudill, M.A. Maternal choline intake alters the epigenetic state of fetal cortisol-regulating genes in humans. FASEB J. 2012, 26, 3563–3574, doi:10.1096/fj.12-207894.

130. Nakaoka, H.; Cui, T.; Tajima, A.; Oka, A.; Mitsunaga, S.; Kashiwase, K.; Homma, Y.; Sato, S.; Suzuki, Y.; Inoko, H.; Inoue, I. A systems genetics approach provides a bridge from discovered genetic variants to biological pathways in rheumatoid arthritis. PLoS One 2011, 6, e25389, doi:10.1371/journal.pone.0025389.

131. Harris, J.R.; Burton, P.; Knoppers, B.M.; Lindpaintner, K.; Bledsoe, M.; Brookes, A.J.; Budin-Ljosne, I.; Chisholm, R.; Cox, D.; Deschenes, M.; et al. Toward a roadmap in global biobanking for health. Eur. J. Hum. Genet. 2012, 20, 1105–1111, doi:10.1038/ejhg.2012.96.

132. Groenen, M.A.; Archibald, A.L.; Uenishi, H.; Tuggle, C.K.; Takeuchi, Y.; Rothschild, M.F.; Rogel-Gaillard, C.; Park, C.; Milan, D.; Megens, H.J.; et al. Analyses of pig genomes provide insight into porcine demography and evolution. Nature 2012, 491, 393–398.

133. Al-Harthi, L. Wnt/beta-catenin and its diverse physiological cell signaling pathways in neurodegenerative and neuropsychiatric disorders. J. Neuroimmune Pharmacol. 2012, 7, 725–730, doi:10.1007/s11481-012-9412-x.

134. Van Alphen, B.; van Swinderen, B. Drosophila strategies to study psychiatric disorders. Brain Res. Bull. 2013, 92, 1–11, doi:10.1016/j.brainresbull.2011.09.007.
135. Jin, K.; Xue, C.; Wu, X.; Qian, J.; Zhu, Y.; Yang, Z.; Yonezawa, T.; Crabbe, M.J.; Cao, Y.; Hasegawa, M.; et al. Why does the giant panda eat bamboo? A comparative analysis of appetite-reward-related genes among mammals. PLoS One 2011, 6, e22602, doi:10.1371/journal.pone.0022602.

174. Van Alfena, D; van Spijker, H. Dmoeginia should be a study by online effect S. evidence-based med. 2013, 98, 1–11 (vol. 10-101-24) ... hodgoi: 10.011/

175. ... ... T. ... Z. Olanzate flu. 983 ... ... May ...

176. ... ... signal-relevant ... ... Plos ... 14(2)
... ... Journal ... 00.2006/5.4

CHAPTER 6

NUTRITION AS AN IMPORTANT MEDIATOR OF THE IMPACT OF BACKGROUND VARIABLES ON OUTCOME IN MIDDLE CHILDHOOD

PATRICIA KITSAO-WEKULO, PENNY HOLDING,
H. GERRY TAYLOR, AMINA ABUBAKAR, JANE KVALSVIG,
AND KEVIN CONNOLLY

6.1 INTRODUCTION

While the literature provides evidence that the negative effects of early malnutrition persist to school-age (Pollitt et al., 1996), there are several significant knowledge gaps. First, despite evidence that the impact of nutrition varies across different neurocognitive domains, there have been few studies investigating this area, especially in middle childhood. And yet at school age, children are exposed to more differential experiences and acquire more sophisticated abilities across various cognitive domains (Fischer and Bullock, 1984). Second, there is a complex inter-related relationship between poverty, nutritional status and neurocognitive outcomes.

Nutrition as an Important Mediator of the Impact of Background Variables on Outcome in Middle Childhood. © Kitsao-Wekulo P, Holding P, Taylor HG, Abubakar A, Kvalsvig J, and Connolly K. Frontiers in Human Neuroscience, 7,713 (2013). doi:10.3389/fnhum.2013.00713. Licensed under Creative Commons Attribution 3.0 Unported License, http://creativecommons.org/licenses/by/3.0/.

Not only do the constraints of low income in deprived settings create practical barriers to good nutrition; additional socio-environmental factors reinforce the effects of this deprivation (Engle and Black, 2008). Poor nutritional status at this age may have long-term negative consequences and restrict development of a child's full potential. This is therefore a critical period for investigating the link between malnutrition and developmental outcomes, especially within a multiple risk context.

In many developing countries, particularly in sub-Saharan Africa, linear growth retardation, or stunting, a manifestation of chronic protein-energy malnutrition (PEM), is highly prevalent, with rates as high as 38% (de Onis et al., 2012). Various individual and environmental variables have been associated with an elevated risk of experiencing poor nutritional status. Important differences have been highlighted in the prevalence of stunting among boys and girls (Badenhorst et al., 1993; Lwambo et al., 2000; Semproli and Gualdi-Russo, 2007; Acham et al., 2008; Omigbodun et al., 2010; Goon et al., 2011; Senbanjo et al., 2011) although there are substantial variations in regional trends. Moreover, patterns observed among school-age populations are similar to those reported at younger ages (Wamani et al., 2007). With regard to age, several studies have reported a dramatic increase in stunting among older children (Stoltzfus et al., 1997; Lwambo et al., 2000; Goon et al., 2011; Senbanjo et al., 2011) demonstrating that linear growth continues to falter throughout the school-age years (The Partnership for Child Development, 1998). Mendez and Adair (1999) found that children who started school at earlier ages (5 or 6 years) were substantially taller than children who started school later (7 or 8 years) so it may be that better-off children enroll in school at earlier ages. And although children in low income settings may all suffer the effects of deprivation, those from the least wealthy households in low income settings are more likely to be malnourished (Sigman et al., 1989; Brooks-Gunn and Duncan, 1997; Bradley and Corwyn, 2002; Abubakar et al., 2008; Ndukwu et al., 2013). Rural residence (Hautvast et al., 2000; Nabag, 2011) and a reduced likelihood of attending school (Ivanovic et al., 2012) have also been related to poor nutritional status. Over childhood, these risk factors have been known to alter the profile of undernutrition (protecting against or accentuating the risk of undernutrition) in a population (Pollitt et al., 1996), as well as being recognized as adversely affecting cognitive functioning independently of nutritional status.

Undernutrition has been shown to negatively impact on various developmental and cognitive domains including motor development (Pollitt et al., 1994; Chang-Lopez, 2007; Olney et al., 2007), language functioning (Wachs, 1995; Duc, 2009), IQ (Mendez and Adair, 1999) as well as memory and executive functions (Kar et al., 2008). This latter study observed that malnourished children showed poor performance on tests of higher cognitive functions but not on motor performance. Moreover, the impact of malnutrition on specific skills seems to vary according to diverse child-related and environmental variables. For instance, among the various gender-patterned deficits documented through an Indian study (Bhandari and Ghosh, 1980), malnutrition affected a wider range of aspects of immediate memory of boys than that of girls.

The effects and outcomes of nutritional status are correlated with environmental factors, the most salient of which is socioeconomic status (Bradley and Corwyn, 2002). Low SES leads to poor dietary intake which in turn impacts on brain and mental development eventually causing developmental deficits. School attendance has also been associated with better cognitive scores among both stunted and non-stunted children (Mendez and Adair, 1999). And as we have reiterated earlier on, rural children have a substantially higher risk of poor nutrition (Fox and Heaton, 2012) as well as poor cognitive outcomes.

In recent times, there have been efforts to investigate the complex relationship between background variables, nutritional status and developmental outcomes (Wachs, 1995). And in Kenya, a recent study investigated the direct and indirect effects of economic poverty on child outcomes (Abubakar et al., 2008). The results suggested that in infancy, impaired psychomotor development is associated directly with undernutrition, while the effect of poverty is mediated entirely through nutritional status (Abubakar et al., 2008). These results are similar to what had been earlier reported from Indonesia where nutritional influences mediated the relationship between poverty-related variables (e.g., SES) and child outcomes (Pollitt et al., 1994). As far as our literature search has revealed, the majority of studies exploring the relationship between undernutrition, co-occurring risk factors and other aspects of impaired child outcome has largely concentrated on children under the age of 5 years (Kariger et al., 2005; Abubakar et al., 2008; Olney et al., 2009, 2007; McDonald et al., 2013). We would like to build up on earlier work and extend the lines of research by focussing on school-age children.

Given the co-occurrence of malnutrition and multiple risk factors within this setting, are the adverse effects of these variables on neurocognitive outcomes related to their impact on nutritional status? Based on a model modified from Wachs (1995), we hypothesized that, (a) sociodemographic and biological factors make a unique contribution to nutritional status, and, (b) nutritional status is a strong predictor of various outcomes in school-age children. Because cognitive skills are more differentiated at this stage, we were able to explore the relationship between chronic malnutrition and developmental outcome across several outcomes. To delineate these effects and to investigate these relationships simultaneously required advanced statistical modeling. The main aim of this study was therefore to establish if diverse background characteristics created variations in nutritional status. We also sought to compare the relative strength of the effects of poor nutritional status on language skills, motor abilities, and cognitive functioning at school age. This information will enable the identification of points of intervention for those most at risk.

6.2 MATERIALS AND METHODS

The study was cross-sectional in nature.

6.2.1 STUDY SETTING

The study was conducted in Kilifi District, Kenya, among a predominantly rural community. The majority (66.8%) of the population lives below the poverty line and is therefore unable to access basic needs due to geographical, economic, and sociocultural barriers (Kahuthu et al., 2005). The district is a food deficit region relying on trade with other districts to meet the food gap—however, income-generating opportunities are few and unsustainable (FAO Kenya, 2007). Malnutrition remains rampant due to variability in crop production; and high illiteracy levels increase the population's vulnerability to food insecurity [Kenya National Bureau of Statistics (KNBS) and ICF Macro, 2010].

6.2.2 STUDY SAMPLE

Children between the ages of 8 and 11 years were recruited from the catchment areas of five local primary schools distributed across neighborhoods ranging from sparsely populated rural areas to more densely populated semi-urban areas. The total sample of 308 children comprised both schooling and non-schooling children. Their first language was Mijikenda, the local vernacular or Kiswahili, the lingua franca and national language.

The Ten Questions Questionnaire (Mung'ala-Odera et al., 2004) was administered to parents to determine the presence of any impairments or serious health problems in children. When the parent was not able to determine if the child had any impairments (visual, auditory, or motor) or in cases where only milder concerns were reported, testing was attempted. Children who were physically unable to perform the tasks were excluded.

6.2.3 ETHICAL CONSIDERATIONS

The Kenya Medical Research Institute/National Ethics Review Committee (KEMRI/NERC) provided ethical clearance for the study. Permission to visit schools was obtained from the District Education Office. We explained the purpose of the study to the head teachers of selected schools and then sought their permission to recruit children. We also held meetings with community leaders, elders, and parents (and guardians) of selected pupils to explain the purpose of the study. After each meeting, a screening questionnaire was administered to establish if selected children met the study's eligibility criteria. We presented information on the study to parents in the language with which they were most familiar. We then obtained written informed consent for their children's participation. All the selected children assented to their participation in the study.

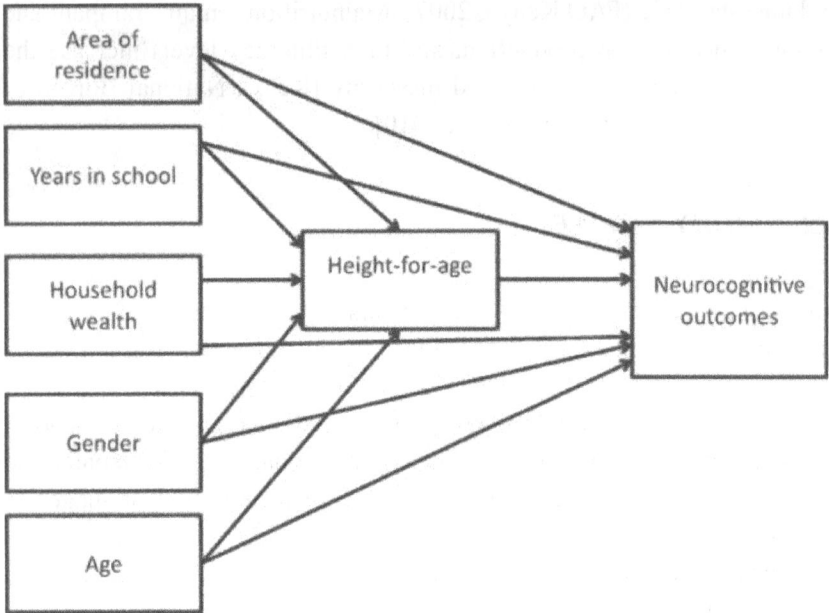

FIGURE 1: Hypothesized model for testing the mediating influence of nutritional status on child neurocognitive outcomes.

6.2.4 MEASUREMENT OF VARIABLES

Building on the extant research literature, our analysis included age, gender, area of residence, school attendance and household wealth as underlying biological and environmental influences, nutritional status as a mediating variable and language skills, motor abilities and two factor scores of cognitive function as child outcomes. In order to test the various hypothesized relationships, we developed the model presented in Figure Figure11.

In the full model which included all the explanatory variables, the use of structural equation modeling (SEM) allowed the disaggregation of the total effect of the explanatory variables into direct effects (effects that go directly from one variable to another) and indirect effects (effects between two variables that are mediated by at least one intervening variable) (Bollen, 1989). We hypothesized that the effects of area of residence, school attendance, household wealth, age, and gender on child outcomes are experienced directly. Additionally, we hypothesized that the influence of these variables has an indirect effect on child outcomes through their influence on nutritional status. The model also took into account possible correlations among the five background variables. We fitted separate models for language skills, motor abilities, verbal memory, and executive function to see if there were differences among the four child outcomes.

6.2.5 BACKGROUND CHARACTERISTICS

Information on child gender, age, school attendance (number of years that child has attended school), and household wealth was collected using a standard questionnaire. Birth records were used, where available, to confirm the child's date of birth. In the cases where records were not available, the procedure outlined by Kitsao-Wekulo et al. (2012) was followed. For the purpose of this study, an age variable in 6-month increments was created. An index of household wealth that divided the sample into three approximately equal groups—least wealthy (Level 1), moderately wealthy (Level 2), and the most wealthy (Level 3)—was derived from six socioeconomic indicators: maternal and paternal education, maternal, and paternal occupation, type of windows in the child's dwelling and ownership of small livestock. Area of residence was characterized as rural or peri-urban according to the most common settlement within the school catchment area.

6.2.6 MEDIATING FACTOR

Children's heights were measured to the nearest centimetre using a stadiometer and height-for-age indices were calculated using EpiInfo (Centers for Disease Control, Atlanta, GA). Growth retardation was defined as height that was more than 2 standard deviations below levels predicted for age according to the World Health Organization reference curves for school-aged children (World Health Organization, 2007).

TABLE 1: Description of sample characteristics, N = 308.

Variable	Stunted		Not stunted	
	N	%	N	%
GENDER				
Boys	31	20.9	117	79.1
Girls	43	26.9	117	73.1
AREA OF RESIDENCE				
Rural	65	26.5	180	73.5
Peri-urban	9	14.3	54	85.7
AGE (YEARS)				
≤8.0	11	15.3	61	84.7
8.5–9.0	19	17.6	89	82.4
≥9.5	44	34.4	84	65.6
SCHOOL EXPOSURE				
0 years	22	62.9	13	37.1
1–2 years	21	20.8	80	79.2
>2years	31	18	141	82
HOUSEHOLD WEALTH				
Level 1	39	31.7	84	68.3
Level 2	21	22.3	73	77.7
Level 3	14	15.4	77	84.6

6.2.7 CHILD OUTCOMES

A battery of neuropsychological tests was used to assess children's language skills, motor abilities, and cognitive functioning.

Language skills. The Kilifi Naming Test (KNT), a test of confrontation naming, was used to assess expressive vocabulary (Kitsao-Wekulo et al., in preparation). In the KNT, the child was asked to spontaneously give one-word responses when presented with a black and while line drawing of a familiar object. Correct responses were coded "1." A stimulus cue was provided when no response was given, the child stated that they did not know the name of the item or the item was perceived incorrectly. If the child did not provide a correct response after the stimulus cue, the word that was provided was recorded verbatim. The test was discontinued after six incorrectly named consecutive items. The final score was calculated by summing the number of spontaneously correct items and the number of correct items following a stimulus cue. These scores were standardized enabling the direct comparison of children's performance across tests.

Motor abilities. Children's motor abilities were assessed using five tests of gross motor abilities covering two areas of motor performance—static and dynamic balance—and three timed tests of fine motor coordination and manual dexterity (Kitsao-Wekulo et al., under review). Age-corrected scores were obtained by computing differences between observed and predicted scores in units of standard error of the estimate (i.e., in z-score units). Maximum likelihood factor analysis with oblique rotation was then applied to the z-scores to reduce the multiple motor scores to ability composites (Ackerman and Cianciolo, 2000). Factor analysis yielded support for a two-factor solution; four tests loaded on the Motor-Co-ordination factor while the remaining four tests loaded on the Static and Dynamic Balance factor. Factor scores were defined as the mean of the z-scores for the tests loading on each factor. An Overall Motor Index was defined as the mean of the two factor scores.

Cognitive functioning. We administered eight tests of cognitive functioning. These included:

1. a non-verbal Tower Test of executive function to measure problem-solving and planning ability;
2. the Self-Ordered Pointing Test (SOPT) to assess verbal/visual selective reminding in terms of the capacity to initiate a sequence of responses, retain the responses and monitor the consequences of behavior;
3. Verbal List Learning (VLL) in which five serial verbal presentations of a 15-item word list were used to test learning and working memory;

4. Dots, a non-verbal test of memory where the child was required to point at a special dot on a sheet;
5. a Contingency Naming Test of executive function designed to assess response inhibition, attentional shift and cognitive flexibility;
6. Score, a test of auditory sustained and selective attention in which the child was required to place beads on one of two plates only after a special sound was heard from a cassette tape;
7. the People Search, a test of visual sustained and selective attention in which the child was required to cross out compete figures as quickly as possible on a stimulus sheet comprising complete and incomplete stick figures;
8. the Coloured Progressive Matrices (CPM) in which matrices of abstract patterns with a missing piece were presented and the child was required to complete the pattern with one from a choice of four pieces. This test assessed non-verbal reasoning and was administered to rule out impairment in global mental functioning.

A detailed description of the tests is presented elsewhere (Kitsao-Wekulo et al., 2012).

To reduce the test battery to a smaller set of ability composites, z-scores for each measure were subjected to principal component factor analysis with Varimax rotation. Based on factor content, skill composites were labeled Executive Function and Verbal Memory. Skill composites of the z-scores comprising each factor were computed based on factor weightings.

6.2.8 DATA COLLECTION PROCEDURES

All the tests were administered at a school near the child's home. Each child was tested individually in a quiet area within sight of other children, and in familiar surroundings to minimize test anxiety. Observations by the assessors suggested that none of the children was unduly anxious during the test sessions.

6.2.9 DATA ANALYSIS

Independent samples t-tests, Chi-square tests and univariate analysis were undertaken to determine group differences in nutritional status and outcomes. Pearson product-moment correlation coefficients were used to examine the relationship between the background variables and cognitive outcomes, language skills, motor abilities, and nutritional status. AMOS version 20 (SPSS) was used to test the fit of the overall model and to examine the relationships among the variables. SEM was used to examine the relationships between background characteristics, child nutritional status and child outcomes. We developed and tested a path analysis model (Figure (Figure1)1) based on logic and theory about how background variables co-vary with nutritional status, and how they influence child outcomes directly and indirectly. In the full model which included all the explanatory variables, this format allowed us to test the mechanisms through which each of the background variables influenced various child outcomes directly and indirectly though a mediated path. An independent disturbance term that represented unexplained variance was estimated for each endogenous variable.

In fitting the Structural Equation Models, missing information was taken into account using the Maximum Likelihood (ML) Estimates. The ML technique assumes data are missing at random for continuous, binary, and categorical variables. All direct and indirect paths were tested and each of the four child outcomes was analyzed in isolation. Specific procedures for model development were to remove non-significant paths ($p = 0.05$) and use modification indices as suggested by the AMOS SEM program (Arbuckle, 1988) to add paths or correlations that would improve model fit. Chi-square analysis was conducted in initial examination of the goodness of fit to insure non-significance. However, because this method is sensitive to sample size, other indices of goodness of fit included the Tucker Lewis Index (TLI), Comparative Fit Index (CFI), and Root Mean Square Error of Approximation (RMSEA) (Bentler and Chou, 1987; Browne and Cudeck, 1993). Acceptable fit was defined as TLI and CFI >0.90 and RMSEA <0.08 and an excellent fit as TLI and CFI >0.95 and RMSEA <0.05.

6.3 RESULTS

6.3.1 DESCRIPTIVE STATISTICS

The study involved 308 boys and girls. The prevalence of linear growth retardation in this study population was high. Approximately 24% (N = 74) of all the children were stunted. Table Table11 portrays a summary of the sample characteristics. The proportion of stunted children residing in rural areas was significantly higher than that of their counterparts in peri-urban areas, χ^2 (1, N = 308) = 4.12, p = 0.04. A higher proportion of girls than boys was stunted but these differences were not significant, χ^2 (1, N = 308) = 1.48, p = 0.22.

More than one-third of the oldest children (aged 9.5 years or more) compared to 15.3% in the youngest group (aged 8 years or less) and 17.6% among those aged between 8.5 and 9 years were stunted. These differences were significant, χ^2 (2, N = 308) = 12.98, p = 0.002. Among children who did not attend school, a very high proportion was stunted compared to their counterparts who had attended school for at least 1 year and those with more than 2 years of school exposure. These differences were highly significant, χ^2 (2, N = 308) = 32.89, p < 0.001. In terms of household wealth, the highest proportion of stunted children was found among those in the sample who were least wealthy (Level 1). The differences in prevalence of stunting among the three groups were significant, χ^2 (2, N = 308) = 7.85, p = 0.02.

6.3.2 CORRELATIONS

Variable intercorrelations are presented in Table Table2.2. As can be seen from the table, more schooling and higher age were the most frequently correlated with household wealth, stunting, and child outcomes. These correlations provide some initial evidence that school attendance and age have moderate to strong associations with nutritional status, which in turn is associated with children's language functioning and motor skills.

TABLE 2: Correlations among variables in the models.

	1	2	3	4	5	6	7	8	9
Area of residence	1								
Gender	−0.012	1							
Age	−0.025	0.019	1						
Years in school	0.313**	−0.084	0.041	1					
HAZ	0.130*	−0.006	−0.300**	0.272**	1				
Household wealth	0.135*	−0.067	−0.240**	0.391**	0.146*	1			
Language scores	0.045	−0.166**	0.318**	0.427**	0.127*	0.048	1		
Motor scores	0.060	0.074	0.402**	0.318**	0.106	0.017	0.499**	1	
Verbal memory	−0.010	0.134*	0.182**	0.125*	0.043	−0.009	0.259**	0.311**	1
Executive function	0.213**	−0.082	0.28**	0.519**	0.240**	0.107	0.554**	0.614**	0.397**

*$p < 0.05$; **$p < 0.01$.*

TABLE 3: Differences in outcomes.

	Stunted (N = 74)		Not stunted (N = 234)		Cohen's d
	Mean	SD	Mean	SD	
Language skills	−0.26	1.09	0.08	0.95	0.333
Motor abilities	−0.06	0.72	0.03	0.57	0.140
Verbal memory	−0.03	0.89	0.01	1.03	0.042
Executive function	−0.26	1.04	0.08	0.83	0.364

6.3.3 DIFFERENCES IN OUTCOMES

Children who were stunted performed more poorly than their counter-parts who were not stunted on all the outcomes tested (Table (Table3).3). These differences were significant for the tests of language, $t_{(306 equal\ variances)}$ = −2.627, p = 0.009, and executive function, $t_{(100 unequal\ variances)}$ = −2.490, p =

0.014. (Levene's test indicated unequal variances (F = 5.572, p = 0.019), so degrees of freedom were adjusted from 306 to 100 for executive function). Medium effect sizes were seen for language and executive function tests.

6.3.4 MODEL MODIFICATION

For each outcome, the initial model did not have a good fit. The steps in developing the individual path models involved making several revisions by deleting non-significant paths and covariances (Table (Table4).4). (Non-significant paths in initial models are' indicated with dashed lines). Modification indices did not suggest the need for additional paths or correlations. The final models for the four child outcomes provided a good fit to the data. In order to simplify the output, only significant standardized path coefficients are shown in the final models (Figures 2A–D).

TABLE 4: Maximum likelihood estimates of covariances for initial model.

Covariance	Covariance estimate	Standard error	Correlation estimate	p-value
Years in school ↔ Area of residence	0.212	0.041	0.313	<0.001
Age ↔ Household wealth	−1.049	0.257	−0.240	<0.001
Area of residence ↔ Household wealth	0.214	0.091	0.135	0.019
Age ↔ Gender	0.011	0.032	0.019	0.738
Years in school ↔ Age	0.077	0.107	0.041	0.472
Household wealth ↔ Gender	−0.132	0.112	−0.067	0.238
Years in school ↔ Gender	−0.071	0.048	−0.084	0.141
Area of residence ↔ Gender	−0.002	0.012	−0.012	0.837
Age ↔ Area of residence	−0.011	0.026	−0.025	0.657
Years In school ↔ Household wealth	2.584	0.405	0.391	<0.001

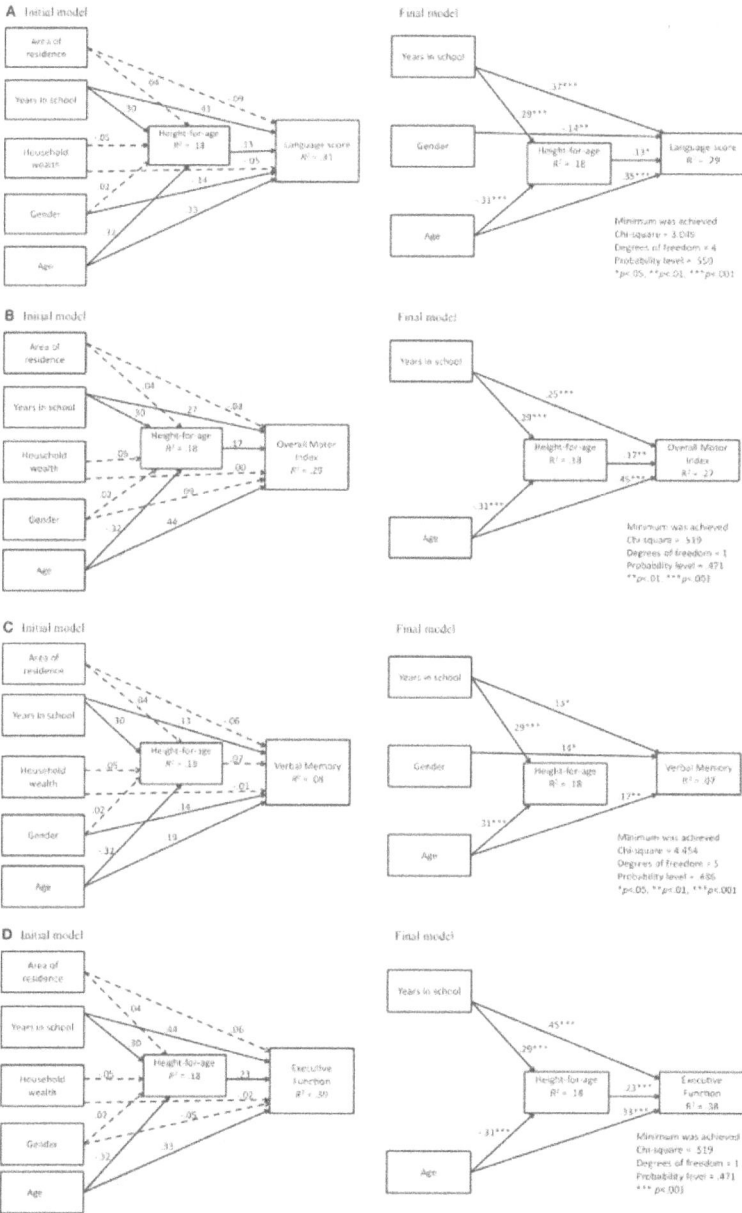

FIGURE 2: (A) Initial and final models for language score. (B) Initial and final models for motor skills. (C) Initial and final models for verbal memory score. (D) Initial and final models for executive function score.

6.3.5 LANGUAGE SKILLS

The model for language skills (Figure (Figure2A)2A) fitted well, TLI >0.99, CFI >0.99, RMSEA <0.05. School attendance and age were related directly and indirectly (through nutritional status) to language skills. While more years of being in school were associated with both better nutritional status and higher language scores, associations of nutritional status and outcomes with gender and age were less consistently observed. Younger children had better nutritional status while older children had better language outcomes. Boys had higher language scores than girls. The indirect path from gender through nutritional status was not significant. Direct paths from height-for-age Z-scores to outcome indicated associations of better nutritional status with higher scores on the language test. These results suggest that the influences of school and age (but not gender) on language scores were partially mediated through nutritional status.

6.3.6 MOTOR ABILITIES

The model for motor abilities had an excellent fit, χ^2 (1, N = 308) = 0.519, p = 0.47; TLI >0.99, CFI >0.99, RMSEA <0.05 (Figure (Figure2B).2B). Paths linking longer attendance at school and higher age with outcome suggest that these two variables were directly and indirectly associated with motor abilities. Direct paths from height-for-age Z-scores to outcome indicated associations of better nutritional status with higher scores on the motor test.

6.3.7 VERBAL MEMORY

The model for verbal memory had a good fit, χ^2 (5, N = 308) = 4.45, p = 0.49; TLI >0.99, CFI >0.99, RMSEA <0.05, but it explained very little of the variance observed (Figure (Figure2C).2C). School attendance, gender, and age had a direct effect on verbal memory. As with the other models, the association between gender and nutritional status remained nonsignificant. Gender had a small effect on outcome and this effect favored girls. The path coefficient from nutritional status to verbal memory was not significant.

6.3.8 EXECUTIVE FUNCTION

The model for executive function also had a good fit, χ^2 (1, N = 308) = 0.519, p = 0.47; TLI >0.99, CFI >0.99, RMSEA <0.05 (Figure (Figure2D).2D). School attendance and age showed strong links with executive function indicating associations of more schooling and higher age with higher scores on executive function tests. Moreover, the direct and indirect effects were significant and the path coefficient from nutritional status to executive function was higher than for all other outcomes.

6.4 DISCUSSION

Although the direct effects of poor nutritional status on child neurocognitive functioning have been well-documented in the literature, very little is known about the complexities of that relationship in a multiple risk environment. Through the use of SEM, this study has attempted to elucidate some of the pathways through which nutritional status and other contextual characteristics may influence outcome in school-age children.

The risk factors for poor nutritional status in this population included older age, rural place of residence, low household wealth levels and not attending school. That younger children had a better nutritional status than their older counterparts was not unexpected; similar findings have been reported in earlier studies among infant (Powell and Grantham-McGregor, 1985) and school-age populations (Senbanjo et al., 2011). We also found that the prevalence of stunting was higher in rural than peri-urban areas. As rural areas tend to have high concentrations of people with low education and income levels, children are more likely to suffer the effects of these deprivations, though poorer nutritional status. Fotso (2006), in an effort to compare the magnitude of inequities in child malnutrition in urban and rural areas of selected countries in sub-Saharan Africa, reported similar findings. Moreover, in the current study, children from the least wealthy households faced the greatest risk of being stunted, compared to their counterparts in the most wealthy households, corroborating earlier findings in similar resource-restricted settings (Fotso, 2006). Our finding that levels of stunting were higher among children not attending school could be explained as follows. Children from poor families are more likely to end up with poor nutritional status (Abubakar et al., 2008), and consequently, less likely to attend school (Ivanovic et al., 2012).

In turn, poor nutritional status predicted poorer outcomes on all the tests. These findings are consistent with reports from studies among infants and school-age children living in similar and different contexts (Sigman et al., 1989; Abubakar et al., 2008; Kar et al., 2008; Bangirana et al., 2009). Poor nutritional status results in a wide range of cognitive deficits linked to structural abnormalities of different parts of the brain (Kar et al., 2008). Because stunting occurs in early childhood, these results provide evidence that the effects of poor nutritional status may be long-lasting, especially if appropriate interventions are not put in place.

The data show evidence for associations between background variables and nutritional status, and between nutritional status and multiple cognitive skills. As expected, the paths linking the variables to nutritional status and children's performance differed in magnitude for each outcome. The novelty, level of familiarity with and requirements of the various tasks could perhaps explain the differences observed. Mediated influences of nutritional status, as well as the direct effects of background variables were stronger for tests with a higher degree of novelty, which were less familiar and which had more complicated task requirements. For instance, the requirement to keep a shopping list in memory is a familiar common activity for school-age children. This may be a plausible explanation for the lack of sensitivity to nutritional status influences and weak direct effects observed on verbal memory.

Noteworthy in the current study is the negative relationship between age and nutritional status. Similar patterns have been reported in earlier studies which have recorded a dramatic rise in the prevalence of stunting with age among African children (Stoltzfus et al., 1997; Hautvast et al., 2000; Senbanjo et al., 2011). Stoltzfus et al. (1997) as well as Glewwe and Jacoby (1995) have postulated that, parents probably enrol the more healthy children in school at earlier ages. As a result, a pattern of higher prevalence of poor nutritional status among children who are older emerges. The same situation may pertain to the current study context. Strong age effects were seen on motor skills, language abilities and executive function, a finding which may be attributed to the following. Children's vocabularies expand as their semantic development takes effect (Zembar and Blume, 2009) hence older children do better than younger ones on vocabulary tests. A rapid increase of muscle strength and maturation of physical abilities related to balance and coordination also takes place in middle childhood (Zembar and Blume, 2009) resulting in better performance on motor tests among older children. Also, as this is a particularly active stage of maturation of executive function, children make significant cognitive advancements during middle childhood (Brocki and Bohlin, 2004).

Associations of gender with nutritional status and with motor skills and executive function did not reach significance. The literature on gender differences in nutritional status and gender influences on child outcomes illustrates a non-uniform pattern. Studies in sub-Saharan Africa, for example, report higher levels of stunting among boys (Semproli and Gualdi-Russo, 2007; Wamani et al., 2007; Goon et al., 2011), while studies from elsewhere have recorded higher levels for girls (Chowdbury et al., 2008). Although the literature on malnutrition seems to suggest that the differences in the manner in which boys and girls are treated may help one gender overcome early adversity, this did not seem to be the case in the current study. Our study also revealed that boys achieved higher scores on the language test while the reverse was true for verbal memory. Contrasting findings have, however, been reported in other studies where girls are found to consistently outperform boys on both measures (Kramer et al., 1997; Lowe et al., 2003). Perhaps in their day to day interactions, boys had more extensive prior experience with the objects that were represented pictorially on the language test hence they had an advantage over girls in naming the items. On the other hand, superior verbal memory scores for girls may be attributed to earlier maturation of their brains.

Our index for household wealth did not have significant direct or indirect effects on any of the child outcomes. On the contrary, several studies have reported that socioeconomic status is a strong predictor of both nutritional status (Brooks-Gunn and Duncan, 1997; Ndukwu et al., 2013) and outcomes in children (Bradley and Corwyn, 2002; Santos et al., 2008).

The lack of an association between household wealth and child outcomes is not without precedence; an earlier study among infants living within the same context (Abubakar et al., 2008) has reported similar findings. We offer a couple of explanations for the non-significant direct effects of household wealth on nutritional status and child outcomes. First, we speculate that this finding may relate to the overwhelming influence of other factors, such as school attendance, among children at this age. This is evidenced by the moderate correlation seen between household wealth and school attendance. Secondly, our study was conducted within a context in which the majority of families live in economically depressed conditions. This may be the reason why, even though the indicators included in our SES measure distinguished one household from another, these differences were not significant in relation to the outcomes under study.

Although other studies have reported that children residing in rural areas have a substantially higher risk of poor nutritional status compared to their urban counterparts (Hautvast et al., 2000; Fox and Heaton, 2012), our study did not show evidence of such associations. The primary reason for this finding was that the current study was conducted within a predominantly rural context. Variations in children's area of residence may therefore have been too subtle to create any real differences in outcomes for children.

In the final trimmed models, school attendance had both direct and indirect (via nutrition) effects and was the most influential environmental predictor of nutritional status and child outcomes. The possibility that the nutrition-related benefits afforded by a school feeding program may explain this finding was negated by the fact that it was only in one school that children were offered food in school. When school attendance was taken into account, associations of nutritional status and cognitive functions with demographic factors like household wealth lost their significance; any bivariate associations washed out with the effects of going to school. This finding provides evidence that school attendance captures family resources more globally and meaningfully (such that there were no independent effects of area of residence and household wealth). Our models are also consistent with earlier studies that have demonstrated that where school attendance is not universal, even a little school exposure is associated with improved test-taking performance. In part, this may be due to increased test-taking awareness, as well as to methods of instruction, curriculum content or the types of questions that teachers ask, accelerating the development of cognitive skills over and above other factors (Holding et al., 2004; Alcock et al., 2008). Going to school thus offers opportunities for learning and practice, and also trains children to follow instructions, hence the strong associations observed with tasks of higher order functioning.

Building up on previous similar work in this area, similarities were seen in the magnitude of the associations between background variables and nutritional status. However, the relationship between SES, stunting and outcome seen among infants (Abubakar et al., 2008) within the same context was not fully replicated in the current study population. This may have been because older children are exposed to more varied environments. Furthermore, as with the infant study, the direct path between household wealth and outcome in our study was not significant. As re-iterated earlier on in this discussion, school attendance seemed to exert a greater influence than household wealth on nutritional status, and had strong direct associations with all outcomes (except verbal memory). A plausible explanation for this finding is that by the time children attain the age of going to school (around 6 years in the study context), the individual effects of socioeconomic status diminish as household wealth becomes an important determinant of whether or not a child goes to school (Mishra et al., 2007). Parents who are doing relatively well economically are able both provide more nutritious meals for their children as well as to retain their children in school. On the other hand, poor nutritional status may reflect limited economic resources. School attendance patterns of children from less wealthy households may be characterized by prolonged absenteeism or dropouts as their parents are unable to initiate and maintain their children's schooling (Mendez and Adair, 1999). Such children are thus likely to benefit less from the effects of school exposure. In light of these associations, school attendance could therefore be considered a proxy for household wealth, which in turn is strongly related to the nutritional status of the child. That there is a complex interactive relationship among the three factors is supported by the suggestion by Mukudi (2003) that the association between school attendance and nutritional status is a function of socioeconomic status. These associations could be more extensively explored through a longitudinal study.

Some of the major difficulties that emerge when comparing the effects of background variables on child development in different populations arise from the differences in environments to which they are exposed and in the outcomes tested. As noted by Goon et al. (2011), historical data such as birth weight, birth order, duration of breastfeeding and birth interval would likely provide a picture of previous states of malnutrition and provide further understanding of its aetiology within the current study population.

The estimated models demonstrated the continued importance of nutritional status as a powerful predictor of outcomes even as children grow older. Significant direct effects of the background variables on child outcomes suggest that the estimated models do not fully explain pathways through which they might influence child outcomes. The unexplained variance may be found in the home environment, an area which remains poorly investigated among rural African populations. Interventions to ameliorate the negative effects of poor nutritional status earlier on may mitigate the need for costly interventions later on, especially for those growing up in the contexts of poverty and poor nutrition.

REFERENCES

1. Abubakar A., Van de Vijver F., Van Baar A., Mbonani L., Kalu R., et al. (2008). Socioeconomic status, anthropometric status, and psychomotor development of Kenyan children from resource-limited settings: a path- analytic study. Early Hum. Dev. 84, 613–621 10.1016/j.earlhumdev.2008.02.003

2. Acham H., Kikafunda J. K., Oluka S., Malde M. K., Tylleskar T. (2008). Height, weight, body mass index and learning achievement in Kumi district, East of Uganda. Sci. Res. Essay 3, 1–8

3. Ackerman P. L., Cianciolo A. T. (2000). Cognitive, perceptual-speed, and psychomotor determinants of individual differences during skill acquisition. J. Exp. Psychol. Appl. 6, 259–290 10.1037/1076-898X.6.4.259

4. Alcock K. J., Holding P. A., Mung'ala-Odera V., Newton C. R. J. C. (2008). Constructing tests of cognitive abilities for schooled and unschooled children. J. Cross-Cultural Psych. 39, 529–551 10.1177/0022022108321176

5. Arbuckle J. (1988). AMOS: Analysis of Moment Structures User's Guide. Temple University Press

6. Badenhorst C. J., Steyn N. P., Jooste P. L., Nel J. H., Kruger M., Oelofse A., et al. (1993). Nutritional status of Pedi schoolchildren aged 6-14 years in two rural areas of Lebowa: a comprehensive nutritional survey of dietary intake, anthropometric,

biochemical, haematological and clinical measurements. South Afr. J. Food Sci. Nutr. 5, 112–119

7. Bangirana P., John C. C., Idro R., Opok R. O., Byarugaba J., Jurek A. M., et al. (2009). Socioeconomic predictors of cognition in Ugandan children: implications for community interventions. PLoS ONE 4:e7898 10.1371/journal.pone.0007898

8. Bentler P. M., Chou C. (1987). Practical issues in structural equation modeling. Soc. Methods Res. 16, 78–117 10.1177/0049124187016001004

9. Bhandari A., Ghosh B. N. (1980). A longitudinal study of fine motor-adaptive, personal-social, and language-speech developments of the children from birth to one year of age in an urban community. Indian J. Med. Res. 71, 289–302.

10. Bollen K. A. (1989). Structural Equations with Latent Variables, New York, NY: John Wiley and Sons, Inc

11. Bradley R. H., Corwyn R. F. (2002). Socioeconomic status and child development. Annu. Rev. Psychol. 53, 371–399 10.1146/annurev.psych.53.100901.135233

12. Brocki K. C., Bohlin G. (2004). Executive functions in children aged 6 to 13: a dimensional and developmental study. Dev. Neuropsychol. 26, 571–593 10.1207/s15326942dn2602_3

13. Brooks-Gunn J., Duncan G. J. (1997). The effects of poverty on children. Future Child 7, 55–71 10.2307/1602387

14. Browne M. W., Cudeck R. (1993). Alternative ways of assessing model fit, in Testing Structural Equation Models, eds Boller K. A., Long J. S., editors. (Beverly, MA: Sage;), 136–162

15. Chang-Lopez S. M. (2007). Effects of Early Childhood Stunting on Behaviour, School Achievement and Fine Motor Abilities at Age 11-12 Years. Kingston, ON: The University of the West Indies

16. Chowdbury S., Chakraborty T., Ghosh T. (2008). Prevalence of undernutrition in Santal children of Puruliya District, West Bengal. Indian Pediatr. 45, 43–46

17. de Onis M., Blössner M., Borghi E. (2012). Prevalence and trends of stunting among pre-school children, 1990-2020. Public Health Nutr. 15, 142–148 10.1017/S1368980011001315

18. Duc L. T. (2009). The Effect of Early Age Stunting on Cognitive Achievement Among Children in Vietnam. Oxford, UK: Department of International Development, University of Oxford

19. Engle P. L., Black M. M. (2008). The effect of poverty on child development and educational outcomes. Ann. N.Y. Acad. Sci. 1136, 243–256 10.1196/annals.1425.023

20. FAO Kenya. (2007). Food Security District Profiles. Nairobi: FAO

21. Fischer K. W., Bullock D. (1984). Cognitive development in school-age children: conclusions and new directions, in Development During Middle Childhood: The Years From Six to Twelve, ed Collins W. A., editor. (Washington, DC: National Academy of Sciences Press;), 70–146

22. Fotso J.-C. (2006). Child health inequities in developing countries: differences across urban and rural areas. Int. J. Equity Health 5, 9–18 10.1186/1475-9276-5-9

23. Fox K., Heaton T. B. (2012). Child nutritional status by rural/urban residence: a cross-national analysis. J. Rural Health 28, 380–391 10.1111/j.1748-0361.2012.00408.x

24. Glewwe P., Jacoby H. (1995). An economic analysis of delayed primary school enrollment in a low income country: the role of childhood nutrition. Rev. Econ. Stat. 77, 156–169 10.2307/2110001

25. Goon D. T., Toriola A. L., Shaw B. S., Amusa L. O., Monyeki M. A., Akinyemi O., et al. (2011). Anthropometrically determined nutritonal status of urban primary school-children in Makurdi, Nigeria. BMC Public Health 11:769 10.1186/1471-2458-11-769

26. Hautvast J. L. A., Tolboom J. J. M., Kafwembe E. M., Musonda R. M., Mwanakasale V., van Staveren W. A., et al. (2000). Severe linear growth retardation in rural Zambian children: the influence of biological variables. Am. J. Clin. Nutr. 71, 550–559.

27. Holding P. A., Taylor H. G., Kazungu S. D., Mkala T., Gona J., Mwamuye B., et al. (2004). Assessing cognitive outcomes in a rural African population: Development of a neuropsychological battery in Kilifi District, Kenya. J. Int. Neuropsychol. Soc.. 10, 246–260 10.1017/S1355617704102166

28. Ivanovic D. M., Olivares M. G., Castro C. G., Ivanovic R. M. (2012). Nutrition and learning in Chilean school age children: Chile's Metropolitan Region Survey 1986-1987. Nutrition 12, 321–328 10.1016/S0899-9007(96)80054-2

29. Kahuthu R., Muchoki T., Nyaga C., editors. (eds.). (2005). Kilifi District Strategic Plan 2005-2010 for Implementation of the National Population Policy for Sustainable Development. Nairobi: National Coordinating Agency for Population and Development

30. Kar B. R., Rao S. L., Chandramouli B. A. (2008). Cognitive development in children with chronic protein energy malnutrition. Behav. Brain Funct. 4, 31–42 10.1186/1744-9081-4-31

31. Kariger P. K., Stoltzfus R. J., Olney D., Sazawal S., Black R., Tielsch J. M., et al. (2005). Iron deficiency and physical growth predict attainment of walking but not crawling in poorly nourished Zanzibari infants. J. Nutr. 135, 814–819.

32. Kenya National Bureau of Statistics (KNBS) ICF Macro. (2010). Kenya Demographic and Health Survey 2008–2009. Calverton, MD: KNBS and ICF Macro

33. Kitsao-Wekulo P. K., Holding P. A., Taylor H. G., Abubakar A., Connolly K. (2012). Neuropsychological testing in a rural African school-age population: evaluating contributions to variability in test performance. Assessment. [Epub ahead of print]. 10.1177/1073191112457408

34. Kramer J. H., Delis D. C., Kaplan E., O'Donnel L., Prifitera A. (1997). Developmental sex differences in verbal learning. Neuropsychol. Rev. 11, 577–584 10.1037/0894-4105.11.4.577

35. Lowe P. A., Mayfield J. W., Reynolds C. R. (2003). Gender differences in memory test performance among children and adolescents. Arch. Clin. Neuropsychol. 18, 865–878 10.1016/S0887-6177(02)00162-2

36. Lwambo N. J., Brooker S., Siza J. E., Bundy D. A., Guyatt H. (2000). Age patterns in stunting and anaemia in African schoolchildren: a cross-sectional study in Tanzania. Eur. J. Clin. Nutr. 54, 36–40 10.1038/sj.ejcn.1600890

37. McDonald C. M., Manji K. P., Kupka R., Bellinger D. C., Spiegelman D., Kisenge R., et al. (2013). Stunting and wasting are associated with poorer psychomotor and mental development in HIV-exposed Tanzanian infants. J. Nutr. 143, 204–214 10.3945/jn.112.168682

38. Mendez M. A., Adair L. S. (1999). Severity and timing of stunting in the first two years of life affect performance on cognitive tests in late childhood. J. Nutr. 129, 1555–1562

39. Mishra V., Arnold F., Otieno F., Cross A., Hong R. (2007). Education and nutritional status of orphans and children of HIV-infected parents in Kenya. AIDS Edu. Pre. 19, 383–395 10.1521/aeap.2007.19.5.383

40. Mukudi E. (2003). Nutrition status, education participation and school achievement among Kenyan middle-school children. Nutrition 19, 612–616 10.1016/S0899-9007(03)00037-6

41. Mung'ala-Odera V., Meehan R., Njuguna P., Mturi N., Alcock K., Carter J. A., et al. (2004). Validity and reliability of the 'Ten Questions' Questionnaire for detecting moderate to severe neurological impairment in children aged 6-9 years in rural Kenya. Neuroepidemiology 23, 67–72 10.1159/000073977

42. Nabag F. O. (2011). Comparative study of nutritional status of urban and rural school girl children in Khartoum State, Sudan. J. Sci. Technol. 12, 60–68

43. Ndukwu C., Egbuonu I., Ulasi T., Ebenebe J. (2013). Determinants of undernutrition among primary school children residing in slum areas of a Nigerian city. Niger. J. Clin. Pract. 16, 178–183 10.4103/1119-3077.110142

44. Olney D. K., Kariger P. K., Stoltzfus R. J., Khalfan S. S., Ali N. S., Tielsch J. M., et al. (2009). Development of nutritionally at-risk young children is predicted by malaria, anemia, and stunting in Pemba, Zanzibar. J. Nutr. 139, 763–772 10.3945/jn.107.086231

45. Olney D. K., Pollitt E., Kariger P. K., Khalfan S. S., Ali N. S., Tielsch J. M., et al. (2007). Young Zanzibari children with iron deficiency, iron deficiency anemia, stunting, or malaria have lower motor activity scores and spend less time in locomotion. J. Nutr. 137, 2756–2762

46. Omigbodun O. O., Adediran K., Akinyemi J. O., Omigbodun A. O., Adedokun B. O., Esan O. (2010). Gender and rural-urban differences in the nutritional status of in-school adolescents in south-western Nigeria. J. Biosoc. Sci. 42, 653–676 10.1017/S0021932010000234

47. Pollitt E., Golub M., Gorman K., Grantham-McGregor S., Levitsky D., Schürch B., et al. (1996). A reconceptualization of the effects of undernutrition on children's biological, psychosocial, and behavioral development. Soc. Res. Child Dev. 10, 1–24

48. Pollitt E., Husaini M. A., Harahap H., Halati S., Nugraheni A., Sherlock A. O. (1994). Stunting and delayed motor development in rural West Java. Am. J. Hum. Biol. 6, 627–635 10.1002/ajhb.1310060511

49. Powell C. A., Grantham-McGregor S. (1985). The ecology of nutritional status and development in young children in Kingston, Jamaica. Am. J. Clin. Nutr. 41, 1322–1331

50. Santos D. N., Assis A. M., Bastos A. C., Santos L. M., Santos C. A., Strina A., et al. (2008). Determinants of cognitive function in childhood: a cohort study in a middle income context. BMC Public Health 8:202 10.1186/1471-2458-8-202

51. Semproli S., Gualdi-Russo E. (2007). Childhood malnutrition and growth in a rural area of Western Kenya. Am. J. Phys. Anthropol. 132, 463–469 10.1002/ajpa.20470

52. Senbanjo I. O., Oshikoya K. A., Odusanya O. O., Njokanma O. F. (2011). Prevalence of and risk factors for stunting among school children and adolescents in Abeokuta, Southwest Nigeria. J. Health Popul. Nutr. 29, 364–370 10.3329/jhpn.v29i4.8452

53. Sigman M., Neumann C., Jansen A. A. J., Bwibo N. (1989). Cognitive abilities of Kenyan chidren in relation to nutrition, family characteristics, and education. Child Dev. 60, 1463–1474 10.2307/1130935

54. Stoltzfus R. J., Albonico M., Tielsch J. M., Chwaya H. M., Savioli L. (1997). Linear growth retardation in Zanzibari school children. J. Nutr. 127, 1099–1105 [PubMed]

55. The Partnership for Child Development. (1998). The health and nutritional status of schoolchildren in Africa: evidence from school-based health programmes in Ghana and Tanzania. Trans. R. Soc. Trop. Med. Hyg. 92, 254–261

56. Wachs T. D. (1995). Relation of mild-to-moderate malnutrition to human development: correlational studies. J. Nutr. 125, 2245S–2254S

57. Wamani H., AstrØm A. N. Peterson S. Tumwine J. K. Tylleskär T. (2007). Boys are more stunted than girls in sub-Saharan Africa: a meta-analysis of 16 demographic and health surveys. BMC Pediatr. 7:17 10.1186/1471-2431-7-17

58. World Health Organization. (2007). Growth Reference Data for 5-19 Years. Geneva: WHO

59. Zembar M. J., Blume L. B. (2009). Middle Childhood Development: A Contextual Approach, Columbus, OH: Prentice Hall

MILD IODINE DEFICIENCY DURING PREGNANCY IS ASSOCIATED WITH REDUCED EDUCATIONAL OUTCOMES IN THE OFFSPRING: 9-YEAR FOLLOW-UP OF THE GESTATIONAL IODINE COHORT

KRISTEN L. HYNES, PETR OTAHAL, IAN HAY, AND JOHN R. BURGESS

Iodine is essential for neurodevelopment in utero and in childhood, with deficiency being a major cause of preventable intellectual impairment (1). The serious neurodevelopmental consequences of severe iodine deficiency (ID) on the fetus are well documented and include cretinism, which manifests as motor, cognitive, and auditory defects (2). ID, however, results in a spectrum of disorders with many speculating that even mild maternal ID has subtle impacts on fetal development. Recent reviews are not conclusive as to whether low maternal dietary iodine intake in areas of mild deficiency leads to measurable effects on cognition and neurodevelopment of the offspring (3, 4).

Clinical trials of iodine supplementation in pregnancy in regions of mild ID have typically focused on positive changes in maternal and fe-

Printed with permission from Kristen L. Hynes, Petr Otahal, Ian Hay, and John R. Burgess. Mild Iodine Deficiency During Pregnancy Is Associated With Reduced Educational Outcomes in the Offspring: 9-Year Follow-up of the Gestational Iodine Cohort. The Journal of Clinical Endocrinology & Metabolism *(2013),* **98***,5. DOI: http://dx.doi.org/10.1210/jc.2012-4249.*

tal thyroid function and volumes but have not examined long-term developmental consequences in the offspring. To our knowledge, there are only three studies reporting neurodevelopmental outcomes in offspring after supplementation of mothers with mild ID. Berbel et al (5) reported significantly delayed neurobehavioral performance in children (aged 18 months) if their mothers did not receive iodine supplementation by 4 to 6 weeks of gestation. Similarly, Velasco et al (6) found that children (aged 3–18 months) had higher psychomotor development scores if their mothers were given supplements from the first trimester. Both interventions provide preliminary evidence that even mild gestational ID may have an adverse impact on fetal neurodevelopment and subsequent infant functioning. In contrast, Murcia et al (7) reported that higher maternal intake of iodine-containing supplements was associated with lower scores on the Psychomotor Development Index of the Bayley Scales of Infant Development in their children (aged 1 year).

In addition to gestational studies, there is increasing evidence from observational population studies that less severe cognitive and motor impairment occurs in apparently normal individuals from areas of ID (8). Children without cretinism from iodine-deficient regions of Iran were found to have growth retardation and neurological, auditory, and psychomotor impairments (9). Boyages et al (10) reported impaired intellectual and neuromotor development in apparently normal Chinese children, with a shift in the distribution of cognitive skills to a lower level. Furthermore, randomized controlled trial data show that postgestational supplementation can lead to significantly improved mental performance of children from areas of mild (11), moderate (12), and severe ID (13).

We compared educational outcomes of children (aged 9 years) born to women assessed as being iodine deficient (urinary iodine concentration [UIC] <150 μg/L) or sufficient (UIC ≥150 μg/L) during pregnancy. Gestation occurred during 1999–2001, a documented period of mild ID (median UIC, 77.5 μg/L) in the Tasmanian population (14), with the children subsequently growing up in an environment considered to be replete (14, 15) (median UIC, 108.0 μg/L) after introduction of voluntary iodine fortification (16). We investigate whether mild gestational ID has long-term effects on educational outcomes.

7.1 MATERIALS AND METHODS

Urinary iodine (UI) samples were collected from volunteers in a study documenting the impact of advancing gestation on UIC. The methods have been published previously (17). In brief, women attending antenatal clinics at the Royal Hobart Hospital (Tasmania, Australia) consented to give between 1 and 3 random urine samples. Samples were analyzed by the Institute of Clinical Pathology and Medical Research at Westmead Hospital (Sydney, Australia), which complies with International Organization for Standardization/International Electrotechnical Commission standard 17025. UIC was determined using the modified Sandell-Kolthoff reaction (18) and is reported as micrograms of iodine per liter of urine. Gestational age at UI collection was recorded and retrospectively confirmed postdelivery. For mothers providing more than 1 sample, mean UIC and gestation age were calculated. World Health Organization (WHO) indicators of iodine nutrition during pregnancy were used to classify the women as having adequate ($\geq$150 µg/L) or insufficient iodine (<150 µg/L) (19). Birth weight and maternal date of birth were obtained from medical records. No information regarding use of iodine supplements or exposure to iodine-based antiseptics during delivery was consistently available. Offspring from singleton pregnancies are reported.

Longitudinal follow-up of 2 sources of education assessment (provided by the Tasmanian Government Department of Education) was conducted when the offspring were in Grade 3 (in 2009 and 2010) at aged 9 years. Ethics approval to link individual education data with the Gestational Iodine Cohort data was granted by the Tasmanian Health and Medical Human Research Ethics Committee (Ref. No. H11592).

7.1.1 NATIONAL ASSESSMENT PROGRAM—LITERACY AND NUMERACY (NAPLAN)

NAPLAN tests are standardized criteria-referenced measures of individual student's performance in literacy (reading, writing, and language conventions [spelling, grammar, and punctuation]) and numeracy. Testing is conducted annually by the Australian Federal Government in all schools for Grades 3, 5, 7, and 9.

7.1.2 STUDENT ASSESSMENT AND REPORTING INFORMATION SYSTEM (SARIS)

SARIS is used by Tasmanian State Government schools to record individual student's academic achievement in assessments in English-literacy and Mathematics-numeracy. The system records students' progress in speaking and listening, reading and viewing, and writing and the capacity to work mathematically, understanding numbers, algebra, function and pattern, space and measurement, and chance and data.

In contrast to the Wechsler Intelligence Scale for Children (WISC), which is a measure of students' cognitive ability and intellectual capabilities and designed to provide an individual's intelligence quotient score; the NAPLAN and SARIS are group- measures of students' school-based performance with reference to the Australian and Tasmanian literacy and numeracy curriculum.

Stata/IC12.1 was used for statistical analysis. Means (SD) are presented for continuous measures and percentages for categorical measures. UIC was skewed; thus, median and interquartile range are presented. The Pearson correlation was used to show associations (the Spearman correlation was used if data were skewed). χ^2 tests were used to show group differences for categorical data and t tests were used for continuous data. Univariable regression models between educational outcome measures at follow-up and continuous gestational UICs were examined initially. Model building of educational outcomes with categorical gestational UIC ($\geq 150/<150$ µg/L) followed, initially unadjusted and then with adjustment for biological covariates (gestational age at UI collection, maternal age, gestational length, birth weight, and sex) and with further adjustment for socioeconomic status (SES) covariates (maternal education and maternal occupation). Model covariates were only included in models for reasons of clinical importance or a demonstrated confounding effect (assessed by a 10% change in gestational UIC coefficient and association with outcome and gestational UIC).

7.2 RESULTS

From the original cohort (n = 433), 228 offspring were traced and linked to educational data. Examination of gestational measures revealed no statistical differences between those followed-up at 9 years and those lost to follow-up.

During gestation, 367 urine samples (collected between October 1999 and November 2001) were provided (123 women provided 1 sample, 71 provided 2 samples, and 34 provided 3 samples). The overall median UIC, using the mean UI value for each pregnancy (n = 228), was 81 µg/L (interquartile range, 46.5–166 µg/L), indicating mild ID. Mean gestational age at UI collection was 24.6 (SD 9.8) weeks (range, 8–41 weeks).

Using the WHO (19) cut point for adequate iodine nutrition during pregnancy, 71.1% (162 of 228) of women had UICs <150 µg/L. Table 1 details characteristics of children whose mothers had adequate UIC (≥150 µg/L) and insufficient UIC (<150 µg/L). There were no statistically significant differences (P < .05) between the 2 groups in any characteristics measured during gestation and birth or for the SES measures recorded when the children were at school. Statistically significant differences were found in NAPLAN spelling and grammar scores and in SARIS English-literacy scores; children born to mothers with insufficient iodine nutrition had poorer outcomes. The results for NAPLAN reading approached significance, but NAPLAN writing and both numeracy measures were not significantly different.

Table 2 shows the relationship between each education outcome (which showed an association with UIC in Table 1) and the biological and SES characteristics. Characteristics that were significant (P = .05 or P = .01) may indicate possible confounding of the association between educational outcomes and UIC. All four education measures (NAPLAN spelling, grammar, and reading and SARIS English-literacy) had small, but significant, positive correlations with birth weight; low-birth-weight children (data not shown) had significantly reduced scores in all outcomes. Sex was observed to be significantly related to spelling, reading, and English-literacy, with boys scoring lower than girls. Significant associations between reading and English-literacy were seen with respect to maternal occupation, but only with English-literacy for maternal education. Paternal occupation and education were significantly associated with grammar, reading, and English- literacy.

TABLE 1: Characteristics of Children by Maternal UIC During Pregnancy: Data for the Cohort of Children (Aged 9 Years) Followed-Up in 2009–2010 in Year 3 (n = 228)

	UIC ≥150 µg/L	n	UIC <150 µg/L	n	P Value[a]
Gestational measures					
Maternal age at birth of child, y	28.2 (5.8)	66	28.2 (6.1)	162	.957
Gestational length, wk[b]	38.9 (2.2)	65	39.1 (1.8)	161	.543
Preterm birth (<37 wk), %	12.3	8/65	7.5	12/161	.245
Birth weight, g[c]	3405 (501)	66	3408 (602)	159	.971
Low birth weight (≤2500 g), %	6.1	4/66	7.6	12/159	.693
Male sex, %	40.9	27/66	49.4	80/162	.245
Gestational age at time of UI collection, wk	24.2 (9.6)	66	24.7 (9.9)	162	.718
School age measures					
Maternal education (>year 10), %	65.6	42/64	68.8	108/157	.648
Maternal occupation, %[d]	20.3	12/59	22.1	33/149	.775
Paternal education (>year 10), %	73.2	41/56	68.2	92/135	.488
Paternal occupation, %[d]	37.3	19/51	26.6	33/124	.162
Indigenous statuse	11.1	7/63	13.8	22/159	.587
2009/2010 Grade 3 education measures					
NAPLAN					
Spelling score	412.0 (104.9)	62	370.9 (84.5)	155	.003
Grammar score	408.1 (103.0)	62	377.2 (97.0)	155	.038
Reading score	413.0 (97.7)	62	387.2 (87.2)	155	.058
Writing score	409.8 (73.0)	62	395.9 (70.6)	155	.197
Numeracy score	385.8 (86.1)	59	378.5 (80.6)	152	.564
SARIS					
English-literacy score	5.78 (1.12)	66	5.45 (1.03)	162	.034
Mathematics-numeracy score	5.67 (1.07)	66	5.45 (1.09)	162	.158

Data are means (SD) for continuous variables and percentages for categorical variables. [a]P values were calculated using t tests for continuous variables and χ^2 tests for categorical variables. [b]Length of gestation was unknown for 2 children. [c]Birth weight was unknown for 3 children. [d]Occupation was divided into 2 categories: unemployed/manual vs professional/ paraprofessional/managers. The percentage in the latter group is given. [e]Indigenous status: percentage shown is for those indicating Aboriginal, Torres Strait Islander, or both Aboriginal and Torres Strait Islander status.

TABLE 2: Relationship Between Education Outcomes and Possible Confounders

	NAPLAN				
	Spelling	Grammar	Reading	SARIS: English-Literacy	n^a
Gestational measures					
Maternal age at birth of child, y	0.0816	0.1023	0.1565b	0.1190	217, 228
Gestation					
Gestational age at time of UI collection, wk	−0.0022	−0.0624	−0.0075	−0.0023	217, 228
Gestational length, wk	0.0522	0.0533	0.1033	0.0111	216, 226
Birth weight, g	0.1970c	0.1696[b]	0.1529[b]	0.1426b	214, 225
Sex					
Male	367.2 (89.9)[b]	376.0 (95.8)	378.9 (97.7)[b]	5.31 (1.02)[c]	103, 107
Female	396.6 (92.9)	395.0 (102.3)	408.7 (82.1)	5.75 (1.07)	114, 121
School age measures					
Maternal education					
≤Grade 10	369.1 (88.3)	376.7 (91.6)	379.5 (75.9)	5.32 (0.92)[b]	66, 71
>Grade 10	390.1 (92.2)	391.7 (103.2)	403.3 (95.8)	5.68 (1.11)	144, 150
Maternal occupation[d]					
1	381.4 (90.5)	384.0 (96.8)	388.4 (83.7)[c]	5.49 (0.99)[c]	154, 163
2	407.3 (90.3)	414.0 (101.8)	431.5 (98.4)	6.00 (1.20)	44, 45
Paternal education					
≤Grade 10	376.0 (90.0)	364.7 (104.0)[b]	374.6 (81.7)[b]	5.30 (1.04)b	46, 58
>Grade 10	393.4 (93.2)	399.9 (98.9)	410.5 (90.6)	5.71 (1.05)	127, 133
Paternal occupation[d]					
1	386.2 (93.9)	379.5 (96.2)c	389.8 (80.3)b	5.47 (1.05)c	116, 123
2	404.8 (86.2)	423.1 (107.0)	425.5 (96.1)	5.99 (1.04)	52, 52
Indigenous					
Yes	352.1 (81.5)	353.5 (109.6)	367.8 (80.7)	5.05 (1.01)c	27, 29
No	387.3 (94.0)	390.4 (98.4)	399.4 (92.7)	5.62 (1.07)	185, 193

For continuous variables (ie, maternal age, gestational age at the time of UI collection, gestational length, and birth weight), correlation coefficients are shown. The Spearman rank correlation was used if variables were skewed. For categorical variables (ie, sex, parental education and occupation, and indigenous status), mean values (SD) are shown. t tests were used to calculate the P value. [a]The number of children with each education outcome varied. The first n is for NAPLAN outcomes, and the second is for SARIS outcomes. [b]P < .05. [c]P < .01. [d]Occupation was divided into 2 categories: 1, unemployed/manual; 2, professional/paraprofessional/managers.

TABLE 3: Differences in Educational Outcome Scores for Children of Mothers With Inadequate UIC (<150 µg/L) During Pregnancy Compared With Mothers With Adequate UIC (≥150 µg/L)

Educational Outcome	Unadjusted			Adjusted for Biological Factors[a]			Adjusted for Biological and Socioeconomic Factors[b]		
	β (95% CI)	P	n	β (95% CI)	P	n	β (95% CI)	P	n
NAPLAN									
Spelling	-41.1 (-68.0 to -14.3)	.003	217	-42.2 (-68.4 to -15.9)	.002	214	-38.6 (-65.5 to -11.6)	.005	193
Grammar	-30.9 (-60.2 to -1.7)	.038	217	-30.3 (-59.5 to -1.2)	.042	214	-29.1 (-59.9 to 1.8)	.065	193
Reading	-25.8 (-52.6 to 0.9)	.058	217	-27.7 (-54.0 to -1.4)	.039	214	-18.5 (-45.7 to 8.6)	.179	193
Writing	-13.9 (-35.0 to 7.2)	.197	217	-11.9 (-32.8 to 9.1)	.267	214	-7.9 (-30.2 to 14.2)	.487	193
Numeracy	-7.3 (-32.1 to 17.6)	.564	211	-5.0 (-29.9 to 20.0)	.697	208	+1.4 (-24.2 to 26.9)	.915	188
SARIS									
English-literacy	-0.33 (-0.63 to -0.03)	.034	228	-0.31 (-0.61 to -0.008)	.045	224	-0.30 (-0.62 to 0.01)	.059	202
Mathematics-numeracy	-0.22 (-0.54 to 0.09)	.158	228	-0.23 (-0.54 to 0.09)	.155	224	-0.25 (-0.58 to 0.08)	.140	202

[a] Adjusted for gestational age at the time of UI collection, maternal age at birth of child, gestational length at time of birth, birth weight, and sex. [b] Adjusted for all the above and for maternal education and occupation.

Univariable examination of UIC as a continuous variable showed a significant positive association with spelling (β = 0.049, P = .033). No associations were found with grammar (β = 0.026, P = .295), reading (β = 0.040, P = .080), numeracy (β = 0.044, P = .100), English-literacy (β = 0.0003, P = .198), or Mathematics-numeracy (β = 0.0002, P = .321), although writing approached significance (β = 0.034, P = .056).

Table 3 shows the associations between UIC and education outcomes using the UIC 150 µg/L cut point. In unadjusted models, spelling, grammar, and English-literacy showed significant associations with UIC and approached significance for reading. No significant associations were found for writing, numeracy, or Mathematics- numeracy. When the associations were significant, the children whose mothers had insufficient UIC had lower education outcome scores. These represent a 10.0%, a 7.6%, and a 5.7% reduction in spelling, grammar, and English-literacy scores, respectively, for the insufficient group.

Associations with spelling, grammar, and English-literacy remained significant and reading became significant after adjustment for gestational and birth factors. In the models adjusted for these biological factors, for both spelling and English-literacy, birth weight and sex were significant factors, with higher-birth-weight children and girls having better education outcomes. For grammar, none of the adjustment factors were significant; for reading, older mother, higher birth weight, and female sex had significant positive associations.

After further adjustment for possible confounding by maternal education and occupation, the association between insufficient UIC and poorer spelling remained significant. Grammar and English-literacy were borderline significant and showed little change in the coefficients. Reading was no longer significant. Further adjustment for paternal education and occupation and for indigenous status (data not shown) did not materially change the coefficients.

7.3 DISCUSSION

This study demonstrates a reduction in spelling, grammar, and general English-literacy performance in children of mothers with a gestational

UIC below the current established cut point for sufficiency (150 µg/L) (19) in comparison with performance of the offspring of mothers with adequate levels. It is well established in areas of severe ID that insufficient maternal iodine during gestation can result in severe and irreversible impairment of fetal neurocognitive development (20). Our findings add support to previous studies reporting that maternal ID in areas of mild-to-moderate deficiency can result in less severe, but measurable, long-lasting impacts (21).

Determining the severity of gestational ID is problematic. Thyroid volume measurement does not indicate recent intake; and thyroid hormone measurements are insensitive. To examine impacts on the fetus, a measure of recent maternal iodine levels is needed. UIC from a spot urine sample reflects intake of ingested iodine for the past 24 hours, although variation due to circadian rhythm influence and postmeal UIC peaks does occur (22). Whereas median UIC from spot samples is the recommended method for determining population iodine status, the large variability in iodine concentration makes it a less than ideal tool for determining individual status. König et al (23) have suggested that to be used as an individual measure, a minimum of 10 spot samples are required. Although not ideal, our study uses UIC to classify pregnant women as being sufficient (≥150 µg/L) or deficient (<150 µg/L) in iodine. For approximately half (46%) of the women, status was based on the mean of 2 or 3 samples. The effect of combining multiple UICs was to increase the overall median value of the cohort. This regression to the mean results in any misclassification of iodine status toward a higher, rather than a lower, level.

Our finding of a difference in educational outcomes using UIC ≥150 µg/L as the cut point for sufficiency lends support for this current WHO recommendation (19) for pregnant women, which is higher than the general population cut point of UIC ≥100 µg/L. Iodine utilization increases by up to 50% during pregnancy, with a concomitant increase in renal iodine clearance. Consequently, women from communities with apparently normal iodine nutrition are at risk of inadequate iodine nutrition during pregnancy (24, 25). This fact has led to recommendations for routine supplementation of pregnant women in North America and Australia with estimated adequate requirements of 160 µg of iodine/day and a Recommended Dietary Allowance of 220 µg/day (26–28).

Restoration of normal fetomaternal iodine nutrition as early as possible in gestation appears to be associated with the greatest benefits for long-term neurodevelopmental outcomes in areas of severe (3) and mild to moderate ID (5, 6). Studies have shown improvements in neurocognitive and psychomotor indices for children of mildly iodine-deficient women who receive supplementation. Previous findings from the Gestational Iodine Cohort provided evidence that supplementation throughout pregnancy is necessary because of the influence of gestational stage on UI excretion. Stilwell et al (17) reported that a range of factors resulted in decreasing iodine excretion with advancing gestation. Whereas median UICs early in pregnancy were higher than the population median, levels fell below the population level by week 16. Similar decreases in UIC from the first to the third trimester have been described by Smyth et al (29) and Brander et al (30), with both also finding that first trimester UICs were significantly higher than the UICs from mildly deficient population controls. This elevation in UIC in early pregnancy to levels of apparent sufficiency, in women from areas of mild ID, is due partly to increases in renal iodine excretion and may give a false indication of iodine adequacy for the developing fetus. Caution is therefore needed when associations between UIC and later neurodevelopmental outcomes are examined; adjustment for gestational stage at time of UI collection (as applied to Table 3 adjusted models) is required to account for UI variation. These studies provide support for current Australian and North American supplementation recommendations and suggest that maintenance of continuous adequate iodine nutrition during pregnancy is required to ensure that preventable adverse consequences do not occur.

Our study focuses on the impacts of mild deficiency during pregnancy but not during childhood. Children were born between March 2000 and December 2001, with the majority of pregnancies occurring during a time of documented mild ID in Tasmania (14, 31). In October 2001, a voluntary iodine fortification program was implemented whereby bread manufacturers substituted regular salt with iodized salt (16). Most children (82.9%) were born before October 2001, with the remaining 39 (17.1%) arriving within 6 weeks of the fortification program being implemented, having had the greater part of their gestation occur in a deficient environment. After fortification, surveys indicated that general population iodine levels had increased to be within the optimal range (median UIC, 108.0 μg/L) (14, 15). The timing of the change from population ID to sufficiency assists us in separating the impacts of mild ID on neurodevelopment during gestation from those that might occur during childhood. Unfortunately, we are unable to examine the important role of breastfeeding on early development, because data were not available. Mammary tissue is known to concentrate iodine (32) for the purpose of supplying the offspring, which necessitates an increase in maternal dietary intake for sufficiency to be assured. A review of iodine nutrition and breastfeeding (33) highlights the importance of adequate maternal iodine nutrition to ensure that breastfed neonates are not at risk of impaired neurological development. It is likely, both before and after bread fortification, that some exclusively breastfed children whose mother's diets were low in iodine may have continued developing in a suboptimal iodine environment.

Persistence, in our cohort, of reduced outcomes in areas of literacy (particularly spelling), but not reading or numeracy, suggests some gestational neurocognitive processes specific to spelling are affected and may be difficult to remediate via adequate iodine nutrition during childhood. The association with spelling, but not other outcomes, suggests there is not a general cognitive delay or confounding by SES factors. Indeed, our modeling proposes that parental education and occupation have no material impact on spelling outcomes. This finding is supported by the results of a spelling intervention of 8-year-old Australian children in which phonological awareness and oral language interventions were more important than parental education levels and family literacy practices in predicting measures of spelling (34).

The NAPLAN spelling instrument in this study required Grade 3 students to read a sentence and identify and correct errors in frequently used one-syllable words and some frequently used two-syllable words with double letters. This regimen tests both phonological (auditory pathways) and orthographical (visual pathways) capacity and involves elements of working memory and processing speed. To successfully complete the tasks, children must hold multiple ideas in their heads (ie, knowledge of sentence meaning and knowledge of the incorrect and correct words), while working quickly to complete the tasks; this necessitates high-level working memory and fast processing speed, respectively. Ormrod and Cochran (35) reported that although measures of reading and verbal ability accounted for a large proportion of the variability in spelling ability, working memory capacity was a significant predictor for learning to spell and spelling ability. Learning to spell has a large phonological component involving auditory blending of sounds (36), as well as cognitive processing and memory recall abilities to understand and recognize differences between 2 phonetically similar words (37). These results are consistent with the idea that specific spelling disability is a residual problem for individuals who have slow verbal and auditory processing speed and auditory short-term memory difficulties (38). Severe ID is known to result in deaf-mutism and mild ID in reductions in hearing thresholds (39, 40) that can be improved by supplementation (41, 42). Given that spelling is not remediated by exposure to an iodine-fortified environment in our cohort, we propose that a central auditory processing disorder influencing working memory, rather than a hearing threshold deficit, may be at work.

Support for this theory can be found in the NAPLAN numeracy testing at Grade 3. Children use one-to-one correspondence techniques requiring use of visual processing skills to identify patterns. Use of visual processing skills for numeracy tasks and combined use of visual (orthographical) and auditory (phonological) processing skills for spelling tasks provide possible evidence that visual pathways are either not affected by ID during gestation or that any impact may be improved by childhood supplementation, whereas auditory pathways affected during gestation do not recover with subsequent supplementation.

Further support for a hypothesis involving deficits in processing and working memory can be found in populations with mild ID, in whom childhood supplementation has resulted in improvements in some, but not all, areas of cognition and motor performance. Gordon et al (11) reported that supplementation of mildly deficient New Zealand 10- to 13-year-olds resulted in improvements in 2 cognitive subtests (picture concepts and matrix reasoning) from the WISC, but no improvements in subtests for letter-number sequencing or symbol search. The picture concepts and matrix reasoning tests assess perceptual reasoning, whereas the letter-number sequencing and the symbol search tests assess working memory and processing speed. The WISC picture concepts and matrix reasoning tests require visual processing skills similar to those tested in the NAPLAN numeracy test. Improvements in perceptual reasoning but not in working memory have similarly been shown after supplementation of moderate to severely iodine-deficient 10- to 12-year-old Albanian children (12) using the Raven's Colored Progressive Matrices test and WISC Digit Span (Forwards and Backwards) test, respectively. Results for processing speed, however, varied with no associations found using the WISC Coding test, but improvement in the supplemented group using the WISC Symbol Search, the Rapid Object Naming, and Rapid Target Marking tests.

The Generation R Study from The Netherlands, which examined executive functioning in children (aged 4 years) using the Behavior Rating Inventory of Executive Function provides further evidence that working memory is affected by mild gestational ID (43). Children whose mothers were in the lowest decile of UIC during pregnancy had higher problems scores on 2 of the 5 scales (inhibition and working memory) compared with those of children of mothers in the highest decile; no significant differences were reported for other 3 scales.

Although the evidence is not conclusive, it suggests that working memory and processing speed are affected by ID during gestation and are resistant to supplementation during childhood. It is not possible from the data available to determine definitively whether a central auditory processing disorder, as opposed to a more pervasive neurodevelopmental defect, is responsible for the observed association. Although our study is not a random sample, it does suggest that despite restitution of adequate iodine nutrition in early childhood, ID during embryonic and fetal development has a demonstrable long-term impact on educational performance. Findings from this study and others provide support for the theory that even mild ID at critical periods of fetal development can lead to deficits that are extremely resistant to restoration by later iodine sufficiency or even irreversible.

Further research on the long-term impacts of mild ID during pregnancy on offspring and studies to determine the prevalence of iodine supplementation during pregnancy and lactation appear warranted. Despite introduction of mandatory iodine fortification in Australia in 2009, awareness among women of the role of iodine nutrition is low (44), and the impact of a recent recommendation from the Australian National Health and Medical Research Council that pregnant and breastfeeding women take a daily iodine supplement (45) is unknown. Whereas our study was able to demonstrate that the 150 μg/L cut point enables us to distinguish between sufficiency and deficiency with respect to educational outcomes, it also adds weight to the call for reexamination of current recommendations to ensure that it is truly sufficient for avoiding fetal brain damage in regions of mild ID. As highlighted by the review of Zimmermann and Andersson (46), use of the median UIC of school-aged children cannot be considered a good proxy for the general population and is inappropriate for pregnant and lactating women. Their suggestion that UIC be extrapolated using iodine intake and then interpreted using the estimated adequate requirements cut point method would provide for more robust estimations of population sufficiency. It seems vital that a prospective iodine supplementation intervention of pregnant and breastfeeding women at risk of mild ID, with longitudinal follow-up of their offspring, be conducted to determine appropriate recommendations for supplementation. Although mandatory fortification in Australia may have led to sufficiency in the general population (based on UIC surveys of children), pregnant women are still at risk of deficiency, which may result in long-term irreversible, but preventable, consequences for their offspring.

REFERENCES

1. Delange F. Iodine deficiency as a cause of brain damage. Postgrad Med J. 2001;77:217–220.
2. Zimmermann MB. Iodine deficiency. Endocr Rev. 2009;30:376–408.
3. Zimmermann MB. Iodine deficiency in pregnancy and the effects of maternal iodine supplementation on the offspring: a review. Am J Clin Nutr. 2009;89:668S–672S. .
4. Skeaff SA. Iodine deficiency in pregnancy: the effect on neurodevelopment in the child. Nutrients. 2011;3:265–273.
5. Berbel P , Mestre JL , Santamariá A , et al.. Delayed neurobehavioral development in children born to pregnant women with mild hypothyroxinemia during the first month of gestation: the importance of early iodine supplementation. Thyroid. 2009;19:511–519.
6. Velasco I , Carreira M , Santiago P , et al.. Effect of iodine prophylaxis during pregnancy on neurocognitive development of children during the first two years of life. J Clin Endocrinol Metab. 2009;94:3234–3241.
7. Murcia M , Rebagliato M , Iñiguez C , et al.. Effect of iodine supplementation during pregnancy on infant neurodevelopment at 1 year of age. Am J Epidemiol. 2011;173:804–812.
8. Bleichrodt N , Born MP. A metaanalysis of research on iodine and its relationship to cognitive development. In: , Stanbury JB, ed. The Damaged Brain of Iodine De-

ficiency: Cognitive, Behavioral, Neuromotor, and Educative Aspects. New York: Cognizant Communication Corporation; 1994:195–200.

9. Azizi F , Kalani H , Kimiagar M , et al.. Physical, neuromotor and intellectual impairment in non-cretinous schoolchildren with iodine deficiency. Int J Vitam Nutr Res. 1995;65:199–205.

10. Boyages SC , Collins JK , Maberly GF , Jupp JJ , Morris J , Eastman CJ. Iodine deficiency impairs intellectual and neuromotor development in apparently-normal persons. A study of rural inhabitants of north-central China. Med J Aust. 1989;150:676–682.

11. Gordon RC , Rose MC , Skeaff SA , Gray AR , Morgan KM , Ruffman T. Iodine supplementation improves cognition in mildly iodine-deficient children. Am J Clin Nutr. 2009;90:1264–1271.

12. Zimmermann MB , Connolly K , Bozo M , Bridson J , Rohner F , Grimci L. Iodine supplementation improves cognition in iodine-deficient schoolchildren in Albania: a randomized, controlled, double-blind study. Am J Clin Nutr. 2006;83:108–114.

13. van den Briel T , West CE , Bleichrodt N , van de Vijver FJ , Ategbo EA , Hautvast JG. Improved iodine status is associated with improved mental performance of schoolchildren in Benin. Am J Clin Nutr. 2000;72:1179–1185.

14. Hynes KL , Blizzard CL , Otahal P , et al.. History of iodine deficiency in school children in Tasmania, Australia. In: , Preedy VR , Burrow GN , Watson RR, eds. Comprehensive Handbook on Iodine: Nutritional, Biochemical, Pathological and Therapeutic Aspects. New York: Elsevier; 2009:1235–1251.

15. Seal JA , Doyle Z , Burgess JR , Taylor R , Cameron AR. Iodine status of Tasmanians following voluntary fortification of bread with iodine. Med J Aust. 2007;186:69–71.

16. Seal JA , Johnson EM , Doyle Z , Shaw K. Tasmania: doing its wee bit for iodine nutrition. Med J Aust. 2003;179:451–452.

17. Stilwell G , Reynolds PJ , Parameswaran V , Blizzard L , Greenaway TM , Burgess JR. The influence of gestational stage on urinary iodine excretion in pregnancy. J Clin Endocrinol Metab. 2008;93:1737–1742.

18. Dunn JT , Crutchfield HE , Gutekunst R , Dunn AD. Two simple methods for measuring iodine in urine. Thyroid. 1993;3:119–123.

19. Andersson M , de Benoist B , Delange F , Zupan J. Prevention and control of iodine deficiency in pregnant and lactating women and in children less than 2-years-old: conclusions and recommendations of the Technical Consultation. Public Health Nutr. 2007;10:1606–1611.

20. Hetzel BS. Iodine deficiency and fetal brain damage. N Engl J Med. 1994;331:1770–1771.

21. de Escobar GM , Obregón MJ , Del Rey FE. Iodine deficiency and brain development in the first half of pregnancy. Public Health Nutr. 2007;10:1154–1570.

22. Als C , Helbling A , Peter K , Haldimann M , Zimmerli B , Gerber H. Urinary iodine concentration follows a circadian rhythm: a study with 3023 spot urine samples in adults and children. J Clin Endocrinol Metab. 2000;85:1367–1369.

23. König F , Andersson M , Hotz K , Aeberli I , Zimmermann MB. Ten repeat collections for urinary iodine from spot samples or 24-hour samples are needed to reliably estimate individual iodine status in women. J Nutr. 2011;141:2049–2054.

24. Gowachirapant S , Winichagoon P , Wyss L , et al.. Urinary iodine concentrations indicate iodine deficiency in pregnant Thai women but iodine sufficiency in their school-aged children. J Nutr. 2009;139:1169–1172.

25. Burgess JR , Seal JA , Stilwell GM , Reynolds PJ , Taylor ER , Parameswaran V. A case for universal salt iodisation to correct iodine deficiency in pregnancy: another salutary lesson from Tasmania. Med J Aust. 2007;186:574–576.

26. National Health and Medical Research Council. Nutrient Reference Values for Australia and New Zealand Including Recommended Dietary Intakes. Canberra, Australia: National Health and Medical Research Council; 2006.

27. Stagnaro-Green A , Abalovich M , Alexander E , et al.. Guidelines of the American Thyroid Association for the diagnosis and management of thyroid disease during pregnancy and postpartum. Thyroid. 2011;21:1081–1125.

28. De Groot L , Abalovich M , Alexander EK , et al.. Management of thyroid dysfunction during pregnancy and postpartum: an Endocrine Society clinical practice guideline. J Clin Endocrinol Metab. 2012;97:2543–2565.

29. Smyth PP , Hetherton AM , Smith DF , Radcliff M , O'Herlihy C. Maternal iodine status and thyroid volume during pregnancy: correlation with neonatal iodine intake. J Clin Endocrinol Metab. 1997;82:2840–2843.

30. Brander L , Als C , Buess H , et al.. Urinary iodine concentration during pregnancy in an area of unstable dietary iodine intake in Switzerland. J Endocrinol Invest. 2003;26:389–396.

31. Hynes K. Urinary Iodine Status of Tasmanian Primary School Children. Pilot Study 1996, Phase I 1998–99, Phase II 2000–01. Final Project Report for the Tasmanian State Government Department of Health and Human Services. Hobart, Tasmania: Menzies Centre for Population Health Research; 2001.

32. Brown-Grant K. The iodide concentrating mechanism of the mammary gland. J Physiol (Lond). 1957;135:644–654.

33. Azizi F , Smyth P. Breastfeeding and maternal and infant iodine nutrition. Clin Endocrinol (Oxf). 2009;70:803–809.

34. Fielding-Barnsley R , Hay I. Comparative effectiveness of phonological awareness and oral language intervention for children with low emergent literacy skills. Aust J Lang Literacy. 2012;35:271–286.

35. Ormrod JE , Cochran KF. Relationship of verbal ability and working memory to spelling achievement and learning to spell. Read Res Instruct. 1988;28:33–43.

36. Marshall CM , Snowling MJ , Bailey BJ. Rapid auditory processing and phonological ability in normal readers and readers with dyslexia. J Speech Lang Hear Res. 2001;44:925–940.

37. Ehri LC. Learning to read and learning to spell are on and the same, almost. In: , Perfetti CA , Rieben L , Fayol M, eds. Learning to Spell: Research, Theory, and Practice Across Languages. Mahwah, NJ: Lawrence Erlbaum Associates, 1997:237–270.

38. Newman S , Fields H , Wright S. A developmental study of specific spelling disability. Br J Educ Psychol. 1993;63:287–296.

39. van den Briel T , West CE , Hautvast JG , Ategbo EA. Mild iodine deficiency is associated with elevated hearing thresholds in children in Benin. Eur J Clin Nutr. 2001;55:763–768.

40. Soriguer F , Millón MC , Munoz R , et al.. The auditory threshold in a school-age population is related to iodine intake and thyroid function. Thyroid. 2000;10:991–999.

41. Wang YY , Yang SH. Improvement in hearing among otherwise normal schoolchildren in iodine-deficient areas of Guizhou, China, following use of iodized salt. Lancet. 1985;2:518–520.

42. Azizi F , Mirmiran P , Hedayati M , Salarkia N , Noohi S , Rostamian D. Effect of 10 yr of the iodine supplementation on the hearing threshold of iodine deficient schoolchildren. J Endocrinol Invest. 2005;28:595–598.

43. van Mil NH , Tiemeier H , Bongers-Schokking JJ , et al.. Low urinary iodine excretion during early pregnancy is associated with alterations in executive functioning in children. J Nutr. 2012;142:2167–2174.

44. Charlton K , Yeatman H , Lucas C , et al.. Poor knowledge and practices related to iodine nutrition during pregnancy and lactation in Australian women: pre- and post-iodine fortification. Nutrients. 2012;4:1317–1327.

45. National Health and Medical Research Council. Iodine Supplementation for Pregnant and Breastfeeding Women. Canberra, Australia: National Health and Medical Research Council; 2010.

46. Zimmermann MB , Andersson M. Assessment of iodine nutrition in populations: past, present, and future. Nutr Rev. 2012;70:553–570.

PART II

NUTRITION AND CHILDREN WITH SPECIAL NEEDS

CHAPTER 8

DIETARY PATTERNS IN CHILDREN WITH ATTENTION DEFICIT/ HYPERACTIVITY DISORDER (ADHD)

HAE DONG WOO, DONG WOO KIM, YOUNG-SEOUB HONG, YU-MI KIM, JU-HEE SEO, BYEONG MOO CHOE, JAE HONG PARK, JE-WOOK KANG, JAE-HO YOO, HEE WON CHUEH, JUNG HYUN LEE, MIN JUNG KWAK, AND JEONGSEON KIM

8.1 INTRODUCTION

Attention deficit hyperactivity disorder (ADHD) is one of the most commonly diagnosed neurobehavioral disorders in childhood, and it often lasts into adulthood [1]. ADHD prevalence rates vary by age, gender, and ethnicity [2,3]. Boys are more likely to have ADHD than girls, and higher rates of ADHD in younger age groups have been observed in studies of children and adolescents [4]. Worldwide, the overall prevalence of ADHD/ hyperkinetic disorder (HD) was found to be 5.29% in a pooled analysis [2]. The prevalence of ADHD is 8.7% in US children aged eight to 15 years [5] and 9.7% in Iranian school-aged children [6]. In Korea, the prevalence of ADHD is 7.6% in elementary school children with a mean age of 9.4

Dietary Patterns in Children with Attention Deficit/Hyperactivity Disorder (ADHD). © Woo HD, Kim DW, Hong Y-S, Kim Y-M, Seo J-H, Choe BM, Park JH, Kang J-W, Yoo J-H, Chueh HW, Lee JH, Kwak MJ, and Kim J. Nutrients 6,4 (2014); doi:10.3390/nu6041539. Licensed under a Creative Commons Attribution 3.0 Unported License, http://creativecommons.org/licenses/by/3.0/.

years [7] and upper-grade elementary school children with a mean age of 11.6 years [8]. The etiology of ADHD is multifactorial, and both genetic and environmental factors may be involved in ADHD [9]. Family and twin studies have shown that genes play an important role in the development of ADHD. Genome-wide association studies are inconclusive, but candidate gene studies suggest the involvement of genes related to the receptors and transporters of dopamine and serotonin [10,11]. Proposed ADHD environmental risk factors include heavy metal and chemical exposures such as lead, mercury, organochlorine, organophosphates, and phthalates, as well as nutritional and lifestyle/psychosocial factors [5].

The effect of diet and dietary supplements is unclear, but considerable evidence suggests that dietary factors are associated with childhood behavioral disorders such as ADHD [12,13]. Low levels of copper, iron, zinc, magnesium, and omega-3 fatty acids have been reported in children with ADHD, and sugar, artificial food colorings, and preservatives are associated with an increased risk of ADHD [12,13]. Recently, the association between dietary pattern and ADHD has been examined in several studies [6,20,21]. As nutrients are consumed in combination and because nutrients are highly interrelated, the study of dietary patterns is useful to further understand the overall role of diet in ADHD. Thus, the purpose of this study was to determine the association between various dietary patterns and ADHD among Korean school-aged children.

8.2 EXPERIMENTAL SECTION

8.2.1 STUDY POPULATION

We conducted a hospital-based case-control study using elementary school students who visited several university hospitals in Busan, Korea, from April to September, 2013. ADHD cases were recruited from two university hospitals (Dong-A and Inje University). ADHD was diagnosed by psychiatrists based on the *Diagnostic and Statistical Manual of Mental Disorders*-Fourth Edition (DSM-IV). Some children with ADHD have concurrent condition such as tic disorder (motor type), anxiety disorder, oppositional defiant disorder, Tourette's disorder, depression, and learning disability. A total of 117 cases, which consented to participate in research, were recruited, and age- and sex-matched controls were recruited from three university hospitals (Dong-A, Pusan, and Kosin University). Controls who did not have severe chronic diseases, a history of ADHD diagnosis and any related disease, such as mental disorder and tic disorder were recruited. Additional test using ADHD Rating Scale (ARS) for controls was performed to exclude ADHD cases. After excluding seven participants who did not complete the questionnaire, a total of 202 controls were recruited. To exclude the seasonal variation in dietary intake, the dietary survey season was also matched in the analysis. Frequency matching by grade (two years), sex, and season (three months) was conducted. A total of 192 elementary school students aged seven to 12 years (96 students with ADHD and 96 healthy controls) were finally selected. Each participant and their legal guardian were provided with an informed consent form according to the procedures approved by the Institutional Review Board of the National Cancer Center.

8.2.2 DATA COLLECTION

The legal guardians of the participants were asked to complete a self-administered questionnaire, which was used to gather information on demographics, lifestyle, and the medical histories of the participants and their parents. A trained interviewer facilitated the 24-h recalls (24HR) interviews face-to-face, and another two non-consecutive 24HR interviews were conducted by telephone between April and September 2013. Individual food intake was calculated using CAN-PRO 4.0 (Computer Aided Nutritional Analysis Program, The Korean Nutrition Society, Seoul, Korea). Mercury and lead exposure from food was calculated using dietary consumption data and their concentrations in 118 core food items. Consumption of omega-3 fatty acids was estimated as the sum of eicosapentaenoic acid (EPA) and docosahexaenoic acid (DHA).

TABLE 1: General characteristics of study population 1.

Characteristics	Controls (n = 96)	Cases (n = 96)	P
Age (year)	9.1 ± 1.8	9.0 ± 1.7	
Sex, male (%)	65 (67.7)	65 (67.7)	
Total energy intake (kcal)	2027.3 ± 381.7	1879.2 ± 380.7	0.008
Weight (kg)	34.3 ± 9.6	33.1 ± 10.4	0.427
Body mass index (cm/m2)	18.2 ± 2.9	17.5 ± 3.2	0.122
Gestation age (week)	39.0 ± 1.7	39.0 ± 1.7	0.787
Birth weight (kg)	3.3 ± 0.5	3.2 ± 0.5	0.099
Breastfeeding, yes (%)	80 (83.3)	70 (72.9)	0.081
Mother's age (year)	38.6 ± 3.7	39.5 ± 4.1	0.133
Birth order	1.5 ± 0.7	1.4 ± 1.1	0.651
Father's education, n (%)			
<High school	22 (22.9)	45 (47.9)	<0.001
College	53 (55.2)	41 (43.6)	
Graduate school	21 (21.9)	8 (8.5)	
Father's occupation, n (%)			
Professional	26 (27.1)	15 (15.6)	0.001
Office/service worker	44 (45.8)	28 (29.2)	
Manual worker	13 (13.5)	28 (29.2)	
Other	13 (13.5)	25 (26.0)	
Father's smoking status, n (%)			
Seldom or Never	37 (39.0)	24 (26.4)	0.188
Current	42 (44.2)	49 (53.9)	
Former	16 (16.8)	18 (19.8)	

1 All analyses were performed with the data matched for age, sex, and dietary survey season.

8.2.3 STATISTICAL ANALYSIS

Principal-components analysis (PROC FACTOR) was used to extract the participants' dietary patterns using 32 predefined food groups. We used a varimax rotation to enhance the interpretability of the analyzed factors.

We determined how many factors to retain after evaluating the eigenvalue, scree test, and interpretability. The dietary patterns were named according to the factors with the highest scores among the defined food groups for each dietary factor. Each dietary pattern's factor score was categorized by tertile for further analysis. Using a Student t-test for continuous variables and a chi-square test for categorical variables, we compared the general characteristics between students with ADHD and controls. The trend test was performed to analyze the associations between each of the dietary patterns and ADHD using a generalized linear model with adjustments for total energy intake. Odds ratios (ORs) and 95% confidence intervals (CIs) for ADHD were calculated across the tertiles of dietary pattern scores using logistic regression models. The lowest tertile of each dietary pattern was used as the reference. To assess the trend across the tertiles, we assigned median values to each tertile of the dietary pattern scores as a continuous variable. We performed the statistical analysis using SAS version 9.2 (SAS Institute Inc., Cary, NC, USA). All P values were two-tailed (α = 0.05).

8.3 RESULTS

The general characteristics of the study population are presented in Table 1. The mean ages of the controls and students with ADHD were 9.1 and 9.0 years, respectively. The total energy intake was higher in controls than in students with ADHD ($p = 0.008$). Father's educational background and occupation significantly differed between ADHD students and controls ($p < 0.001$ and $p = 0.001$, respectively).

PCA identified four major dietary patterns among the 32 food groups, and the associated factor loading scores with absolute values ≥ 0.20 are shown in Table 2. The "traditional" dietary pattern was characterized by high intakes of condiments, vegetables, tofu/soymilk, and mushrooms. The "seaweed-egg" dietary pattern included high intakes of seaweeds, fats/oils, sweets, and eggs. The "traditional-healthy" dietary pattern included high intakes of kimchi, grains, bonefish, and low intakes of fast foods and beverages. The "snack" dietary pattern was characterized by high intakes of snacks and processed meat and a low intake of noodles. Lean fish, other seafood, and yogurt were not listed due to their low factor loadings in all examined dietary patterns. Each dietary pattern explained 8.0%, 6.0%, 5.6%, and 5.4% of the variation in food intake, respectively.

The distribution of characteristics by dietary pattern score tertiles is presented in Table 3. Increasing scores in the traditional and traditional-healthy patterns were correlated with a decreased percent energy from fat (P for trend = 0.001; P for trend <0.001, respectively), whereas the percent energy from carbohydrate increased as the score of the traditional-healthy pattern increased (P for trend <0.001). Fatty acids were significantly associated with dietary pattern scores. The traditional pattern score was associated with a high intake of total fatty acids; the seaweed-egg and traditional-healthy pattern scores were associated with high intakes of PUFAs and omega-3 fatty acids, whereas the snack pattern score was negatively associated with the intakes of total fatty acids, PUFAs, and MUFAs. Regarding mineral intake, calcium intake was positively associated with the scores of the traditional, traditional-healthy, and snack patterns, and iron was positively associated with the scores of the traditional and traditional-healthy patterns. Heavy metal exposure via food consumption was also assessed, and mercury was positively associated with the traditional, traditional-healthy, and snack patterns; lead was positively associated with the traditional and snack patterns.

The ORs and 95% CIs of ADHD were analyzed across the tertiles of dietary pattern scores (Table 4). The OR (95% CI) in the highest tertiles of the traditional dietary pattern compared to those in the lowest tertiles in crude model was 0.29 (0.13–0.64), but a significant association was not observed in multivariate model 2 (OR: 0.76, 95% CI: 0.26–2.24). The seaweed-egg pattern was not significantly associated with ADHD in any of the models. The snack pattern score was positively associated with the risk of ADHD, but a significant association was observed only in the second tertile in crude model and multivariate model 1. Students in the highest tertile of the traditional-healthy pattern score had an increased risk of ADHD in the multivariate-adjusted models when compared with those in the lowest tertile (OR (95% CI): 0.32 (0.13–0.82) in multivariate model 1; 0.31 (0.12–0.79) in multivariate model 2).

TABLE 2: Factor loadings for the four major dietary patterns derived from principal components analysis with orthogonal rotation.

Foods/Food Groups	Traditional	Seaweed-Egg	Traditional-Healthy	Snack
Condiments	0.75			
Vegetables	0.56		0.20	
Tofu, Soymilk	0.53			
Mushrooms	0.49			
Salted fermented seafood	0.34			
Fruits	0.32	−0.22		−0.31
Seaweeds		0.69		
Fats, Oils	0.29	0.68		
Sweets	0.27	0.43		0.33
Egg		0.41		
Potatoes	0.22	0.35		
Processed fruit products		0.33		
Legumes		0.29		
Kimchi			0.58	−0.23
Grains	0.23		0.56	
Bonefish	0.28		0.52	0.26
Fatty fish	0.29		0.23	−0.38
Snack				0.49
Processed meats				0.44
Bread				0.43
Milk				0.30
Shellfish			−0.22	
Beverages		0.22	−0.44	
Fast foods			−0.49	
Rice cake		−0.36		
Seeds	0.23			
Dairy products			−0.23	−0.23
Meats			−0.31	−0.31
Noodles		0.24		−0.49
Variance of explained (%)	8.0	6.0	5.6	5.4

Factor loadings with absolute values ≥0.20 were listed in the table among 32 food groups.

TABLE 3. Distribution of characteristics by the tertiles of dietary pattern scores.

Characteristics	Traditional				Seaweed-Egg			
	T1	T2	T3	P Trend	T1	T2	T3	P Trend
Age (year)	8.7 (1.8)	9.1 (1.7)	9.5 (1.6)	0.014	8.9 (1.6)	9.0 (1.8)	9.2 (1.8)	0.270
Sex, female (%)	32 (43.2)	19 (25.7)	11 (25.0)	0.023	28 (40.6)	22 (33.9)	12 (20.7)	0.018
BMI (kg/m2)	17.9 (3.3)	17.6 (3.0)	18.3 (2.7)	0.533	17.6 (2.5)	17.7 (3.1)	18.4 (3.6)	0.171
Education, ≥college (%)	41 (56.9)	51 (68.9)	31 (70.5)	0.109	41 (59.4)	40 (63.5)	42 (72.4)	0.132
Total energy intake (kcal)	1757.7 (353)	2005.6 (325)	2194.2 (383)	<0.001	1898.9 (418)	1897.2 (362)	2080.8 (352)	0.008
Carbohydrate (g)	248.6 (44.7)	284.5 (49.5)	315.4 (59.2)	0.013	273.0 (61.6)	272.3 (51.4)	289.5 (53.9)	0.216
Carbohydrate (% energy)	56.6 (6.5)	56.5 (6.2)	57.0 (4.9)	0.057	57.4 (6.3)	57.1 (6.0)	55.3 (5.5)	0.173
Protein (g)	67.1 (22.3)	78.2 (14.4)	86.0 (15.2)	0.198	71.0 (18.7)	74.0 (21.6)	83.2 (15.3)	0.016
Protein (% energy)	15.0 (3.0)	15.6 (2.2)	15.6 (1.7)	0.075	14.9 (2.2)	15.4 (2.8)	16.0 (2.2)	0.005
Fat (g)	56.9 (19.1)	63.3 (18.4)	68.1 (18.4)	<0.001	59.7 (20.6)	59.4 (18.2)	67.3 (17.4)	0.951
Fat (% energy)	28.3 (5.1)	27.9 (5.1)	27.4 (4.4)	0.001	27.7 (5.3)	27.6 (4.9)	28.7 (4.6)	0.792
Total fatty acids (g)	29.2 (12.8)	33.1 (14.2)	33.2 (12.6)	0.031	28.9 (13.9)	30.9 (12.7)	35.7 (12.7)	0.080
PUFAs (g)	6.9 (2.5)	8.7 (3.4)	8.5 (2.7)	0.798	6.4 (2.6)	7.8 (2.1)	10.1 (3.2)	<0.001
MUFAs (g)	10.9 (5.7)	12.2 (5.9)	12.4 (5.3)	0.057	10.8 (5.9)	11.5 (5.4)	13.1 (5.5)	0.245
Omega-3 fatty acids (g)	0.10 (0.26)	0.23 (0.48)	0.34 (0.62)	0.134	0.25 (0.57)	0.20 (0.38)	0.15 (0.38)	0.059
Calcium (mg)	491.5 (222)	587.7 (171)	730.0 (224)	0.002	565.1 (225)	558.1 (230)	632.8 (206)	0.755
Iron (mg)	10.4 (2.3)	13.5 (4.8)	16.6 (8.4)	<0.001	12.2 (7.3)	12.8 (5.3)	14.1 (3.4)	0.447
Zinc (mg)	8.2 (2.1)	9.8 (2.0)	10.5 (1.9)	0.112	8.9 (2.2)	9.1 (2.3)	10.2 (1.9)	0.063
Mercury (μg/kg bw)	0.19 (0.05)	0.22 (0.06)	0.22 (0.07)	0.027	0.20 (0.06)	0.21 (0.06)	0.21 (0.06)	0.965
Lead (μg/kg bw)	0.43 (0.14)	0.50 (0.14)	0.53 (0.17)	0.022	0.48 (0.17)	0.47 (0.13)	0.49 (0.16)	0.954

Characteristics	Traditional-Healthy				Snack			
	T1	T2	T3	P Trend	T1	T2	T3	P Trend
Age (year)	9.2 (1.7)	8.8 (1.8)	9.1 (1.7)	0.746	9.8 (1.7)	8.8 (1.7)	8.8 (1.7)	0.002
Sex, female (%)	31 (41.9)	18 (29.0)	13 (23.2)	0.022	13 (25.0)	34 (42.5)	15 (25.0)	0.906
BMI (kg/m2)	17.8 (3.1)	17.8 (3.0)	18.0 (3.3)	0.644	19.5 (3.7)	17.4 (2.3)	17.0 (2.8)	<0.001
Education, ≥college (%)	47 (63.5)	41 (67.2)	35 (63.6)	0.956	32 (61.5)	52 (66.7)	39 (65.0)	0.719
Total energy intake (kcal)	1946.2 (411)	1893.1 (391)	2029.3 (343)	0.225	2088.5 (361)	1812.7 (362)	2023.5 (387)	0.354
Carbohydrate (g)	266.5 (56.5)	272.8 (52.1)	298.1 (55.8)	<0.001	292.7 (58.3)	260.5 (53.4)	287.7 (52.8)	0.566

TABLE 3: *Cont.*

Characteristics	Traditional				Seaweed-Egg			
	T1	T2	T3	P Trend 2	T1	T2	T3	P Trend
Carbohydrate (% energy)	54.6 (6.0)	57.7 (5.9)	58.3 (5.5)	<0.001	55.6 (6.1)	57.2 (6.3)	56.9 (5.5)	0.326
Protein (g)	77.4 (23.4)	71.8 (17.3)	77.9 (15.2)	0.294	82.6 (15.6)	71.2 (21.4)	75.8 (18.1)	0.079
Protein (% energy)	15.7 (3.1)	15.1 (1.9)	15.2 (1.9)	0.293	15.7 (2.4)	15.5 (2.8)	14.8 (1.9)	0.047
Fat (g)	65.7 (20.5)	58.5 (19.2)	60.6 (16.3)	<0.001	67.7 (18.0)	56.0 (17.9)	64.7 (19.8)	0.872
Fat (% energy)	29.7 (4.6)	27.2 (5.0)	26.5 (4.6)	<0.001	28.7 (5.1)	27.3 (5.0)	28.2 (4.6)	0.843
Total fatty acids (g)	30.4 (12.9)	30.6 (12.1)	34.3 (15.1)	0.244	38.3 (16.9)	28.3 (10.0)	30.3 (11.9)	0.001
PUFAs (g)	7.6 (3.1)	7.7 (2.8)	8.8 (3.0)	0.046	9.1 (3.2)	7.5 (2.5)	7.7 (3.3)	0.018
MUFAs (g)	11.3 (5.5)	11.4 (5.2)	12.8 (6.4)	0.300	14.8 (7.5)	10.4 (4.0)	10.9 (4.7)	<0.001
Omega-3 fatty acids (g)	0.13 (0.34)	0.18 (0.36)	0.33 (0.63)	0.024	0.29 (0.66)	0.19 (0.38)	0.14 (0.31)	0.124
Calcium (mg)	553.3 (227)	551.3 (195)	658.0 (231)	0.016	555.1 (221)	541.2 (206)	663.5 (227)	<0.001
Iron (mg)	12.0 (4.1)	12.8 (5.0)	14.6 (7.6)	0.026	13.8 (3.8)	12.0 (4.6)	13.7 (7.8)	0.669
Zinc (mg)	9.3 (2.5)	9.2 (2.1)	9.7 (2.0)	0.909	10.1 (2.1)	8.7 (2.1)	9.6 (2.3)	0.293
Mercury (µg/kg bw)	0.19 (0.05)	0.21 (0.06)	0.23 (0.06)	0.003	0.19 (0.06)	0.21 (0.06)	0.22 (0.06)	0.001
Lead (µg/kg bw)	0.45 (0.13)	0.49 (0.15)	0.50 (0.18)	0.125	0.44 (0.16)	0.47 (0.14)	0.51 (0.16)	0.006

1 Tertiles of dietary pattern scores; 2 P trend was calculated using generalized linear models for continuous variables and using Mantel–Haenszel chi-squared tests for categorical variables; P trend of nutrient and metal consumption was adjusted for total energy intake; PUFAs: Polyunsaturated fatty acids, MUFAs: Monounsaturated fatty acids.

TABLE 4: Distribution of characteristics by the tertiles of dietary pattern scores 1.

Dietary Pattern		N Control/ Case	Crude Model	Multivariate Model[1][2]	Multivariate Model[2][3]
Traditional	T1[4]	32/42	1	1	1
	T2	32/42	1.00 (0.52–1.92)	1.32 (0.61–2.84)	1.88 (0.80–4.42)
	T3	32/12	0.29 (0.13–0.64)	0.43 (0.18–1.04)	0.76 (0.26–2.24)
	P trend[5]		0.003	0.072	0.615
Seaweed-egg	T1	32/37	1	1	1
	T2	32/33	0.89 (0.45–1.76)	0.66 (0.30–1.44)	0.70 (0.31–1.55)
	T3	32/26	0.70 (0.35–1.42)	0.64 (0.29–1.41)	0.84 (0.36–1.94)
	P trend		0.321	0.271	0.682
Traditional-healthy	T1	32/42	1	1	1
	T2	32/30	0.71 (0.36–1.41)	0.60 (0.27–1.32)	0.57 (0.25–1.29)
	T3	32/24	0.57 (0.28–1.15)	0.32 (0.13–0.77)	0.31 (0.12–0.79)
	P trend		0.113	0.011	0.014
Snack	T1	32/20	1	1	1
	T2	32/48	2.40 (1.17–4.91)	2.93 (1.22–7.05)	2.34 (0.95–5.79)
	T3	32/28	1.40 (0.66–2.98)	1.69 (0.70–4.07)	1.59 (0.65–3.91)
	P trend		0.571	0.451	0.505

1 All analyses were performed with the data matched for age, sex, and dietary survey season; 2 Adjusted for gestation age, birth weight, mother's age, birth order, father's education, and father's occupation; 3 Model 2 + additional adjustment for total energy intake, omega-3 fatty acids, lead, and mercury consumption; 4 Tertiles of dietary pattern scores; 5 Tests for trend were conducted by assigning the median value to each tertile of heavy metal intake as a continuous variable.

8.4 DISCUSSION

The present study identified four dietary patterns. The traditional-healthy dietary pattern, characterized by high intakes of kimchi, grains, and bonefish, and low intakes of fast foods and beverages, was associated with lower odds having ADHD. Although the present study focused on dietary factors, significant associations with ADHD were found in father's education and occupation. Socioeconomic status of children is generally related to household income, and parent's educational background and occupation. Children from lower socioeconomic status are more likely diagnosed with ADHD than children from higher socioeconomic status in previous studies [14,15,16,17]. Family income [14,15], parent's education [15,16,17] and occupation [15,16] were significantly associated with ADHD. Education status of mother was highly correlated with that of fathers in this study, and occupation of mother did not vary compared to that of father's. Thus, fathers' educational background and occupation were used as surrogate of socioeconomic status. As those variables were high associated with ADHD, we adjusted them for the analysis.

The role of diet in the behavior of children has been controversial, but associations between several nutritional factors and child behavior such as ADHD have been continually suggested [12,13]. Food additives, sugar, and aspartame are considered negative factors in the development of ADHD, and thus, dietary intervention studies with special diets, including additive-free and sugar elimination diets, have been conducted. A meta-analysis has reported that artificial food coloring is associated with childhood hyperactivity [18]. However, in a sugar elimination intervention study, there was no evidence that refined sugar affected child behavior [19,20,21,22,23,24].

The role of polyunsaturated fatty acids (PUFAs), particularly omega-3 fatty acids, in relation to neurodevelopmental disorders has been studied because omega-3 fatty acids play a critical role in brain development and function [25]. Children with ADHD have lower levels of omega-3 fatty acids, and the supplementation of omega-3 fatty acids can reduce the symptoms of ADHD in school-aged children and adolescents [26,27]. However, there was no clear evidence of improvement in ADHD symptoms with omega-3 supplementation in randomized controlled trials, but these findings could be the result of methodological problems [28,29]. The association between dietary pattern score and fatty acid intake was investigated in this study. The traditional, seaweed-egg, and traditional-healthy pattern scores were negatively associated with ADHD, although only the traditional-healthy pattern had a statistically significant association; moreover, they were positively associated with fatty acid intake. By contrast, the snack pattern score showed a positive association with ADHD and was negatively associated with the intake of total fatty acids, PUFAs, and MUFAs. However, additional adjustment for omega-3 fatty acid intake did not change the statistically significant association between the traditional-healthy dietary pattern and ADHD. Thus, the factors associated with the beneficial effects of a healthy dietary pattern might be complex.

Regarding mineral intake, calcium was positively associated with the scores of the traditional, traditional-healthy, and snack patterns, and iron was positively associated with the scores of the traditional and traditional-healthy patterns. Zinc was not associated with any of the four pattern scores. Iron deficiency may be associated with ADHD [30] because iron stores in the brain can influence dopamine-dependent functions [31,32]. A case-control study in India reported that the serum ferritin level was lower in children with ADHD [33], while another study found that ADHD symptoms in children with low serum ferritin levels were alleviated following iron supplementation [34]. In a 19-year follow-up study, the iron status of Costa Rican children was found to be associated with behavioral problems in adolescents [35]. The role of zinc nutrition in ADHD is not clear, but evidence suggests that zinc is beneficial in the treatment of children with ADHD [36,37]. Zinc deficiency is involved in dopamine transporter dysfunction [38], and intervention studies have found that zinc supplementation can reduce ADHD symptoms in children with low zinc levels [39,40,41]. Both, low iron and zinc levels have been associated with dopamine metabolism, and low levels of iron and zinc are involved in impaired dopamine transmission in subjects with ADHD [42,43,44,45].

Heavy metal exposure via food consumption was also investigated. Mercury was positively associated with the traditional, traditional-healthy, and snack patterns, and lead was positively associated with the traditional and snack patterns. The association between lead exposure and ADHD has been widely studied, and a meta-analysis has reported that lead exposure is positively associated with ADHD symptoms [46]. In a study with school-aged children living in two Romanian cities near a metal-processing plant, an association with ADHD was observed only for lead exposure, not aluminum or mercury exposure [47]. An association between the blood mercury level and ADHD in Chinese children in Hong Kong has been observed [48], but a significant association was not found in a cross-sectional study of Romanian children [47] or in a Children's Health and Environment Research (CHEER) study that surveyed elementary schools in six South Korean cities [49,50]. A more clear association with ADHD has been observed for lead exposure, even at low concentrations [49,50]. Prenatal mercury exposure is associated with an increased risk of neurobehavioral disorders, and lead exposure in childhood has been associated with ADHD [51]. In this study, lead and mercury consumption was positively correlated with the traditional-healthy dietary pattern, but it did not alter the beneficial effects of the traditional-healthy dietary pattern on ADHD.

Recently, associations between dietary patterns and ADHD have been examined in several cross-sectional studies [6,20,21]. One study, which included a population-based cohort of adolescents, reported that a Western-style dietary pattern, characterized by high intakes of fat, refined sugars, and sodium and low intakes of fiber, folate, and omega-3 fatty acids, was associated with increased odds of an ADHD diagnosis, whereas a healthy dietary pattern, with high intakes of fiber, folate, and omega-3 fatty acids, was not correlated with the diagnosis of ADHD [20]. In a study of adolescents in China, three major dietary patterns were identified, and dietary patterns characterized by a high intake of snacks or animal-derived foods were associated with higher odds for psychological symptoms [21]. In Iranian school-aged children, four major dietary patterns were identified. The higher scores of the dietary patterns associated with a high intake of sweets and fast food were associated with greater odds for having ADHD, but no significant association was observed for the healthy or Western dietary patterns [6]. In this study, traditional-healthy dietary pattern was positively associated with dietary factors, such as PUFAs and minerals that are known for beneficial effects on ADHD. Another beneficial effect of the traditional-healthy dietary pattern might be associated with the low fast food intake. Junk foods are generally high in fat, sugar, additives, artificial food colorings, and preservatives, which may negatively affect ADHD symptoms [52]. Overall, the traditional-healthy dietary pattern was associated with many dietary factors that affect childhood behavioral disorders, such as ADHD.

The present study has several limitations. As this was a case-control study, it is possible that dietary intake was affected by an individual's health status and social background. Thus, causal inference cannot be determined. Results could differ by ADHD types, but information about ADHD type was not gathered for subgroup analysis due to small sample size. However, such pattern analyses are useful to further understand the diet of ADHD children as a whole rather than classifying it by a single nutrient or food group.

8.5 CONCLUSIONS

The traditional-healthy dietary pattern, which is characterized by high intakes of kimchi, grains, and bonefish, and low consumption of fast foods and beverages, appears to be negatively associated with ADHD in school-aged Korean children.

REFERENCES

1. Wilens, T.E.; Biederman, J.; Spencer, T.J. Attention deficit/hyperactivity disorder across the lifespan. Annu. Rev. Med. 2002, 53, 113–131, doi:10.1146/annurev. med.53.082901.103945.
2. Polanczyk, G.; de Lima, M.; Horta, B.; Biederman, J.; Rohde, L. The worldwide prevalence of ADHD: A systematic review and metaregression analysis. Am. J. Psychiatry 2007, 164, 942–948, doi:10.1176/appi.ajp.164.6.942.
3. Cuffe, S.P.; Moore, C.G.; McKeown, R.E. Prevalence and correlates of ADHD symptoms in the national health interview survey. J. Atten. Disord. 2005, 9, 392–401, doi:10.1177/1087054705280413.
4. Boyle, C.A.; Boulet, S.; Schieve, L.A.; Cohen, R.A.; Blumberg, S.J.; Yeargin-Allsopp, M.; Visser, S.; Kogan, M.D. Trends in the prevalence of developmental disabilities in US children, 1997–2008. Pediatrics 2011, 127, 1034–1042, doi:10.1542/peds.2010-2989.
5. Froehlich, T.E.; Anixt, J.S.; Loe, I.M.; Chirdkiatgumchai, V.; Kuan, L.; Gilman, R.C. Update on environmental risk factors for attention-deficit/hyperactivity disorder. Curr. Psychiatry Rep. 2011, 13, 333–344, doi:10.1007/s11920-011-0221-3.
6. Azadbakht, L.; Esmaillzadeh, A. Dietary patterns and attention deficit hyperactivity disorder among Iranian children. Nutrition 2012, 28, 242–249, doi:10.1016/j.nut.2011.05.018.
7. Kim, E.; Kwon, H.; Ha, M.; Lim, M.; Oh, S.; Kim, J.; Yoo, S.; Paik, K. Relationship among attention-deficit hyperactivity disorder, dietary behaviours and obesity. Child Care Health Dev. 2014, doi:10.1111/cch.12129.

8. Jang, C.-B.; Kim, H.-Y. The relationship between attention deficit hyperactivity disorder, dietary habit and caffeine intake in upper-grade elementary school children. Korean J. Nutr. 2012, 45, 522–530, doi:10.4163/kjn.2012.45.6.522.

9. Biederman, J. Attention-deficit/hyperactivity disorder: A selective overview. Biol. Psychiatry 2005, 57, 1215–1220, doi:10.1016/j.biopsych.2004.10.020.

10. Bobb, A.J.; Castellanos, F.X.; Addington, A.M.; Rapoport, J.L. Molecular genetic studies of ADHD: 1991 to 2004. Am. J. Med. Genet. 2006, 141, 551–565.

11. Faraone, S.V.; Khan, S.A. Candidate gene studies of attention-deficit/hyperactivity disorder. J. Clin. Psychiatry 2005, 67, 13–20.

12. Millichap, J.G.; Yee, M.M. The diet factor in attention-deficit/hyperactivity disorder. Pediatrics 2012, 129, 330–337, doi:10.1542/peds.2011-2199.

13. Cormier, E.; Elder, J.H. Diet and child behavior problems: Fact or fiction? Pediatr. Nurs. 2007, 33, 138–143.

14. Saadi, H.R.; Shamsuddin, K.; Sutan, R.; Alshaham, S.A. Socio-maternal risk factors of ADHD among Iraqi children: A case-control study. Open J. Prev. Med. 2013, 3, 251–257, doi:10.4236/ojpm.2013.32034.

15. Al Hamed, J.; Taha, A.; Sabra, A.; Bella, H. Attention deficit hyperactivity disorder (ADHD): Is it a health problem among male primary school children. Bahrain Med. Bull. 2008, 30, 1–9.

16. Kalff, A.; Kroes, M.; Vles, J.; Bosma, H.; Feron, F.; Hendriksen, J.; Steyaert, J.; van Zeben, T.; Crolla, I.; Jolles, J. Factors affecting the relation between parental education as well as occupation and problem behaviour in Dutch 5-to 6-year-old children. Soc. Psychiatry Psychiatr. Epidemiol. 2001, 36, 324–331, doi:10.1007/s001270170036.

17. Khamis, V. Family environment and parenting as predictors of attention-deficit and hyperactivity among Palestinian children. J. Soc. Serv. Res. 2006, 32, 99–116, doi:10.1300/J079v32n04_06.

18. Schab, D.W.; Trinh, N.H.T. Do artificial food colors promote hyperactivity in children with hyperactive syndromes? A meta-analysis of double-blind placebo-controlled trials. J. Dev. Behav. Pediatr. 2004, 25, 423–434, doi:10.1097/00004703-200412000-00007.

19. Wolraich, M.L.; Wilson, D.B.; White, J.W. The effect of sugar on behavior or cognition in children. JAMA 1995, 274, 1617–1621, doi:10.1001/jama.1995.03530200053037.

20. Howard, A.L.; Robinson, M.; Smith, G.J.; Ambrosini, G.L.; Piek, J.P.; Oddy, W.H. ADHD is associated with a "Western" dietary pattern in adolescents. J. Atten. Disord. 2011, 15, 403–411, doi:10.1177/1087054710365990.

21. Weng, T.T.; Hao, J.H.; Qian, Q.W.; Cao, H.; Fu, J.L.; Sun, Y.; Huang, L.; Tao, F.B. Is there any relationship between dietary patterns and depression and anxiety in Chinese adolescents? Public Health Nutr. 2012, 15, 673–682, doi:10.1017/S1368980011003077.

22. Sinha, S.R.; Kossoff, E.H. The ketogenic diet. Neurologist 2005, 11, 161–170, doi:10.1097/01.nrl.0000160818.58821.d2.

23. Murphy, P.; Likhodii, S.S.; Hatamian, M.; Burnham, W.M. Effect of the ketogenic diet on the activity level of Wistar rats. Pediatr. Res. 2005, 57, 353–357, doi:10.1203/01.PDR.0000150804.18038.79.

24. Murphy, P.; Burnham, W. The ketogenic diet causes a reversible decrease in activity level in Long-Evans rats. Exp. Neurol. 2006, 201, 84–89, doi:10.1016/j.expneurol.2006.03.024.

25. Horrocks, L.A.; Farooqui, A.A. Docosahexaenoic acid in the diet: Its importance in maintenance and restoration of neural membrane function. Prostaglandins Leukot. Essent. Fatty Acids 2004, 70, 361–372, doi:10.1016/j.plefa.2003.12.011.

26. Kirby, A.; Woodward, A.; Jackson, S.; Wang, Y.; Crawford, M. Childrens' learning and behaviour and the association with cheek cell polyunsaturated fatty acid levels. Res. Dev. Disabil. 2010, 31, 731–742, doi:10.1016/j.ridd.2010.01.015.

27. Colter, A.L.; Cutler, C.; Meckling, K.A. Fatty acid status and behavioural symptoms of attention deficit hyperactivity disorder in adolescents: A case-control study. Nutr. J. 2008, 7, 79–85.

28. Raz, R.; Gabis, L. Essential fatty acids and attention/deficit-hyperactivity disorder: A systematic review. Dev. Med. Child Neurol. 2009, 51, 580–592, doi:10.1111/j.1469-8749.2009.03351.x.

29. Richardson, A.J. Omega-3 fatty acids in ADHD and related neurodevelopmental disorders. Int. Rev. Psychiatry 2006, 18, 155–172, doi:10.1080/09540260600583031.

30. Konofal, E.; Lecendreux, M.; Arnulf, I.; Mouren, M.-C. Iron deficiency in children with attention-deficit/hyperactivity disorder. Arch. Pediatr. Adolesc. Med. 2004, 158, 1113–1115, doi:10.1001/archpedi.158.12.1113.

31. Solanto, M.V. Dopamine dysfunction in AD/HD: Integrating clinical and basic neuroscience research. Behav. Brain Res. 2002, 130, 65–71, doi:10.1016/S0166-4328(01)00431-4.

32. Erikson, K.M.; Jones, B.C.; Hess, E.J.; Zhang, Q.; Beard, J.L. Iron deficiency decreases dopamine D1 and D2 receptors in rat brain. Pharmacol. Biochem. Behav. 2001, 69, 409–418, doi:10.1016/S0091-3057(01)00563-9.

33. Juneja, M.; Jain, R.; Singh, V.; Mallika, V. Iron deficiency in Indian children with attention deficit hyperactivity disorder. Indian Pediatr. 2010, 47, 955–958, doi:10.1007/s13312-010-0160-9.

34. Konofal, E.; Lecendreux, M.; Deron, J.; Marchand, M.; Cortese, S.; Zaïm, M.; Mouren, M.C.; Arnulf, I. Effects of iron supplementation on attention deficit hyperactivity disorder in children. Pediatr. Neurol. 2008, 38, 20–26, doi:10.1016/j.pediatrneurol.2007.08.014.

35. Corapci, F.; Calatroni, A.; Kaciroti, N.; Jimenez, E.; Lozoff, B. Longitudinal evaluation of externalizing and internalizing behavior problems following iron deficiency in infancy. J. Pediatr. Psychol. 2010, 35, 296–305, doi:10.1093/jpepsy/jsp065.

36. Arnold, L.E.; DiSilvestro, R.A. Zinc in attention-deficit/hyperactivity disorder. J. Child Adolesc. Psychopharmacol. 2005, 15, 619–627, doi:10.1089/cap.2005.15.619.

37. Sinn, N. Nutritional and dietary influences on attention deficit hyperactivity disorder. Nutr. Rev. 2008, 66, 558–568, doi:10.1111/j.1753-4887.2008.00107.x.

38. Lepping, P.; Huber, M. Role of Zinc in the Pathogenesis of Attention-Deficit Hyperactivity Disorder. CNS Drugs 2010, 24, 721–728.

39. Bilici, M.; Yıldırım, F.; Kandil, S.; Bekaroğlu, M.; Yıldırmış, S.; Değer, O.; Ülgen, M.; Yıldıran, A.; Aksu, H. Double-blind, placebo-controlled study of zinc sulfate in the treatment of attention deficit hyperactivity disorder. Prog. Neuropsychopharmacol. Biol. Psychiatry 2004, 28, 181–190, doi:10.1016/j.pnpbp.2003.09.034.

40. Akhondzadeh, S.; Mohammadi, M.-R.; Khademi, M. Zinc sulfate as an adjunct to methylphenidate for the treatment of attention deficit hyperactivity disorder in children: A double blind and randomized trial [ISRCTN64132371]. BMC Psychiatry 2004, 4, doi:10.1186/1471-244X-4-9.

41. Arnold, L.E.; DiSilvestro, R.A.; Bozzolo, D.; Bozzolo, H.; Crowl, L.; Fernandez, S.; Ramadan, Y.; Thompson, S.; Mo, X.; Abdel-Rasoul, M. Zinc for attention-deficit/hyperactivity disorder: Placebo-controlled double-blind pilot trial alone and combined with amphetamine. J. Child Adolesc. Psychopharmacol. 2011, 21, 1–19, doi:10.1089/cap.2010.0073.

42. Oner, O.; Oner, P.; Bozkurt, O.H.; Odabas, E.; Keser, N.; Karadag, H.; Kızılgün, M. Effects of zinc and ferritin levels on parent and teacher reported symptom scores in attention deficit hyperactivity disorder. Child Psychiatry Hum. Dev. 2010, 41, 441–447, doi:10.1007/s10578-010-0178-1.

43. Kozielec, T.; Starobrat-Hermelin, B. Assessment of magnesium levels in children with attention deficit hyperactivity disorder (ADHD). Magnes. Res. 1997, 10, 143–148.

44. Starobrat-Hermelin, B.; Kozielec, T. The effects of magnesium physiological supplementation on hyperactivity in children with attention deficit hyperactivity disorder (ADHD). Positive response to magnesium oral loading test. Magnes. Res. 1997, 10, 149–156.

45. Mousain-Bosc, M.; Roche, M.; Rapin, J.; Bali, J.P. Magnesium VitB6 intake reduces central nervous system hyperexcitability in children. J. Am. Coll. Nutr. 2004, 23, 545S–548S, doi:10.1080/07315724.2004.10719400.

46. Goodlad, J.K.; Marcus, D.K.; Fulton, J.J. Lead and attention-deficit/hyperactivity disorder (ADHD) symptoms: A meta-analysis. Clin. Psychol. Rev. 2013, 33, 417–425, doi:10.1016/j.cpr.2013.01.009.

47. Nicolescu, R.; Petcu, C.; Cordeanu, A.; Fabritius, K.; Schlumpf, M.; Krebs, R.; Krämer, U.; Winneke, G. Environmental exposure to lead, but not other neurotoxic metals, relates to core elements of ADHD in Romanian children: Performance and questionnaire data. Environ. Res. 2010, 110, 476–483, doi:10.1016/j.envres.2010.04.002.

48. Wong, V. Attention-deficit hyperactivity disorder and blood mercury level: A case-control study in Chinese children. Neuropediatrics 2006, 37, 234–240, doi:10.1055/s-2006-924577.

49. Ha, M.; Kwon, H.J.; Lim, M.H.; Jee, Y.K.; Hong, Y.C.; Leem, J.H.; Sakong, J.; Bae, J.M.; Hong, S.J.; Roh, Y.M. Low blood levels of lead and mercury and symptoms of attention deficit hyperactivity in children: A report of the children's health and environment research (CHEER). Neurotoxicology 2009, 30, 31–36, doi:10.1016/j.neuro.2008.11.011.

50. Kim, S.; Arora, M.; Fernandez, C.; Landero, J.; Caruso, J.; Chen, A. Lead, mercury, and cadmium exposure and attention deficit hyperactivity disorder in children. Environ. Res. 2013, 126, 105–110, doi:10.1016/j.envres.2013.08.008.

51. Boucher, O.; Jacobson, S.W.; Plusquellec, P.; Dewailly, É.; Ayotte, P.; Forget-Dubois, N.; Jacobson, J.L.; Muckle, G. Prenatal methylmercury, postnatal lead exposure, and evidence of attention deficit/hyperactivity disorder among inuit children

in Arctic Québec. Environ. Health Perspect. 2012, 120, 1456–1461, doi:10.1289/ehp.1204976.

52. Wiles, N.J.; Northstone, K.; Emmett, P.; Lewis, G. "Junk food" diet and childhood behavioural problems: Results from the ALSPAC cohort. Eur. J. Clin. Nutr. 2007, 63, 491–498.

CHAPTER 9

DIETARY INTAKE AND PLASMA LEVELS OF CHOLINE AND BETAINE IN CHILDREN WITH AUTISM SPECTRUM DISORDERS

JOANNA C. HAMLIN, MARGARET PAULY, STEPAN MELNYK, OLEKSANDRA PAVLIV, WILLIAM STARRETT, TINA A. CROOK, AND S. JILL JAMES

9.1 INTRODUCTION

Autism is a complex, behaviorally-defined neurodevelopmental disorder characterized by significant impairments in social interaction, verbal and nonverbal communication, and by restrictive, repetitive, and stereotypic patterns of behavior. The Centers for Disease Control estimates that the current prevalence of autism spectrum disorders (ASD) in the United States is 1 in 110 children* [1]. Nutritional screening and assessment of children with ASDs is an important clinical consideration for several reasons. First, these children often exhibit nutrition-related medical issues

---

*As of August 2014, CDC most recently estimates that about 1 in 68 children has been identified with autism spectrum disorder (ASD). (http://www.cdc.gov/ncbddd/autism/facts.html)

including gastrointestinal discomfort, bowel inflammation, diarrhea, constipation, and acid reflux [1]. Abnormal sensory processing can affect taste and texture perception leading to food avoidance and restricted food intake in many children with ASD. "Insistence on sameness" and compulsive repetitive behaviors reinforce rigid dietary preferences and lead to a limited food repertoire [2]. Finally, accumulating research indicates that nutrient metabolism and requirements may be altered in some children with ASDs compared to typically developing children [3–5]. Thus, children with ASDs have multiple risk factors that may increase the prevalence of nutrient deficiencies in this population.

Metabolic abnormalities reported in children with ASDs have primarily involved folate-dependent one-carbon metabolism. Paşca et al. reported hyperhomocysteinemia and abnormal methionine metabolite levels in children with AD and PDD-NOS [6]. They also noted an increased prevalence of the C677T MTHFR polymorphism in children with AD. Polymorphisms in this pathway limit folate availability and increase the need for other interdependent metabolites including choline and betaine [7]. In addition, James et al. found that children with ASDs had significantly lower plasma concentrations of methionine, S-adenosylmethionine (SAM), cystathionine, cysteine, and total glutathione (GSH) and significantly higher concentrations of S-adenosylhomocysteine (SAH), adenosine, and oxidized glutathione (GSSG) when compared to age-matched control children [8–10]. These metabolic abnormalities can lead to compromised methylation (SAM/SAH) and antioxidant/detoxification capacity (GSH/GSSG). In one study, low plasma SAM/SAH was associated with DNA hypomethylation and low plasma GSH/GSSG was associated with biomarkers of protein oxidative damage (3-nitrotyrosine, 3-chlorotyrosine) and DNA oxidative damage (8-oxode-oxyguanine) [10]. Rose et al. found a similar decrease in GSH/GSSG and oxidative damage in postmortem brain samples from individuals with autism suggesting that oxidative stress and damage may be a systemic issue in some children with autism [11].

Choline, betaine, and folate are interchangeable sources of one-carbon units. As shown in Figure 1, the metabolism of choline intersects with folate-dependent one-carbon metabolism as an alternate pathway for methionine synthesis, especially when folate availability is limited. Choline is the precursor for betaine and methyl groups derived from betaine which are used for SAM-dependent methylation reactions including the synthesis of membrane phosphatidylcholine (PC). In this way, choline indirectly serves as a precursor for the synthesis of membrane phospholipids that are essential for normal membrane fluidity, signal transduction, membrane transport and integrity [12, 13]. Choline is also a precursor for the synthesis of acetylcholine (ACh), an important neurotransmitter in both the central and autonomic nervous systems. In the central nervous system, ACh is an important neuromodulator of sensory perceptions and inducer of REM sleep and is important for sustaining attention [14]. Finally, as a methyl donor for SAM synthesis, choline deficiency has been shown in animal models to contribute to global DNA hypomethylation and epigenetic abnormalities [15]. Low plasma SAM levels and DNA hypomethylation have also been shown to be present in children with autism [10].

Choline was recognized by the Institute of Medicine (IOM) as an essential nutrient in 1998 [16]. Good dietary sources of choline include eggs, liver, beef, chicken, fish, milk, cruciferous vegetables, beans, and peanuts, whereas betaine is primarily obtained from wheat bran, wheat germ, and spinach [9, 10]. Notably, betaine intake has been negatively associated with the Western diet high in meat, sugar, and fat [11]. Zeisel [17] observed the following symptoms when healthy individuals consumed a choline deficient diet: (1) hepatic steatosis, (2) muscle damage, (3) DNA damage, and (4) changes in lymphocyte gene expression. In addition, low plasma choline levels have been associated with increased anxiety [18].

Although choline and its metabolites are important contributors to normal folate-dependent one-carbon metabolism, dietary intake and plasma levels of these nutrients have not been investigated in the ASD population. Therefore, the purpose of the study was to determine whether age-specific dietary intake of these nutrients was within the adequate range by national standards and whether dietary intake was correlated with plasma levels in a subset of these children.

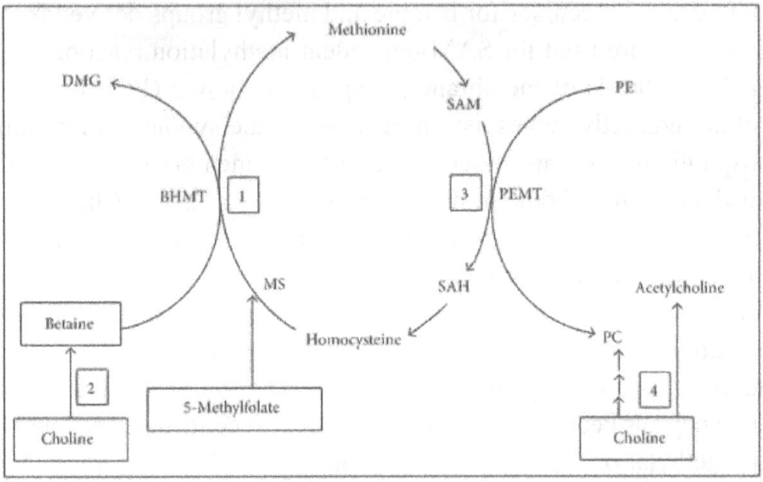

FIGURE 1: Interrelated and interdependent pathways of (1) folate- and betaine-dependent methionine resynthesis from homocysteine utilizing folate-dependent methionine synthase (MS) and betaine-dependent betaine:homocysteine methyltransferase (BHMT); (2) choline-dependent betaine synthesis; (3) phosphtidylethanoloamine methyltransferasse (PEMT) conversion of phosphatidylethanolamine (PE) to phosphatidylcholine (PC); and (4) choline-dependent synthesis of PC and acetylcholine.

9.2 SUBJECTS AND METHODS

9.2.1 STUDY PARTICIPANTS

Nutritional data on choline and betaine intake from food was obtained from 288 children with ASDs who participated in the Autism Intervention Research Network for Physical Health (AIR-P) Study on Diet and Nutrition in Children with Autism and they were recruited from four national sites including Pittsburg, Pennsylvania, Little Rock, Arkansas, Rochester, New York, and Denver, Colorado. A subgroup of 35 of the 288 ASD participants and 32 control participants whose parents consented to a blood draw participated in an ancillary study in which plasma choline metabolites were measured and compared between groups. Inclusion criteria for the ASD group included children 2–11 years of age with clinical diagnoses of an ASD based on the Diagnostic and Statistical Manual IV criteria and the Autism Diagnostic Observation Schedule (ADOS). Control participants were 3–10 years of age and had no medical history of behavioral or neurological abnormalities, as determined by parent report, and were control participants in an ongoing NICHD-sponsored study of children with autism (SJJ: R011HD051873). Control children were age and sex-matched to the case children for the plasma analysis and were limited to parents who agreed to have their child's blood drawn. The study protocols and informed consents were approved by the Institutional Review Boards at each site where data were collected.

9.2.2 DIETARY DATA

Three-day food records were collected from caregivers of the participants in the ASD group (n = 288). Trained personnel used a standardized method to instruct caregivers on recording all foods, beverages, and supplements consumed by the participants for three consecutive days, including one weekend day. Completed records were returned to each site for review and caregivers were contacted if information was missing or unclear. Records from each site were sent to Rochester, New York for analysis using the Nutrition Data System for Research (NDSR) software versions 2009 and 2010, developed by the Nutrition Coordinating Center (University of Minnesota, Minneapolis, MN). Individual food intake results were based on the mean intake from all three days of data collection.

9.2.3 PLASMA DATA

Plasma concentrations of choline and betaine were obtained from 67 participants (35 with ASD and 32 controls) whose parents consented to the blood draw. Participants were instructed to fast 12 hours prior to the blood draw. The maximum blood drawn was 25 mL per participant. The blood sample was obtained within two weeks of the completion of the 3-day food record. After samples were obtained and deidentified, they were sent to the Autism Treatment Network/Intellectual & Developmental Disabilities Research Center (ATN/IDDRC) Biorespository in Denver, Colorado for storage. A 250 uL aliquot was sent to the Autism Genomics Laboratory in Little Rock, Arkansas for analysis. Choline and betaine concentrations were measured using a Dionex High Performance Liquid Chromatography-Ultraviolet System coupled to an electrospray ionization (ESI) tandem mass spectrometer using Thermo-Finnagen LCQ. Samples of 30 μL were deprotenized with three volumes of acetonitrile and further analyzed using normal phase chromatography on silica gel column. It was equilibrated with a mixture of 15 mmol/L ammonium formate and acetonitrile in a ratio of 25 : 75 by volume. It was eluted with a linear gradient of increasing proportions of ammonium formate, as described in greater detail in Holm et al. [19].

9.2.4 STATISTICAL ANALYSIS

Statistical analyses were conducted using SPSS (version 21.0) and Excel software (Microsoft Office 2007; Microsoft Corp., Redmond, WA). Descriptive statistics were used to describe the study participants' demographic characteristics. Means, standard deviations, and ranges were used to describe the dietary intake of the ASD group. Pearson's product-moment correlation coefficients were used to test the relationships between dietary intake and plasma levels of choline and betaine in the ASD group. Student's t-tests were used to determine if differences existed in plasma concentrations between groups. Statistical significance was set at 0.0.

9.3 RESULTS

9.3.1 PARTICIPANT CHARACTERISTICS

Among the 288 ASD participants, 86.1% were male, 25.7% (74) were in the 1–3-year-age category, 61.5% (177) were in the 4–8-year-age category, and 12.8% (37) were in the 9–11-year-age category. Greater than 90% of the participants were Caucasian. Within the subgroup of children evaluated for plasma and dietary intake of choline and betaine, 11 of the 35 children (32%) were 1–3 years old, 19 children (54%) were 4–8 years old, and 5 children (14%) were 8–11 years of age. Anthropometric data from the ASD subgroup (n = 35) and control group (n = 32) indicated that 27% of children in the ASD group were in the overweight and obese categories compared to 23% in the control group. Additionally, fewer children in the ASD group were classified as underweight compared to the control group (6% versus 10%, resp.).

TABLE 1: Mean dietary intake of choline and betaine in children with ASD (n = 288).

Age	Choline intake (mg) (mean ± SE)	AI[a] for choline (mg)	Choline intake less than AI[a] (% children)	Betaine intake[b] (mg/kg) (mean ± SE)	Betaine intake less than 3.5 mg/kg (% children)
1–3 y (n = 72)	176 ± 10	200	68.7%	4.6 ± 0.18	30%
4–8 y (n = 178)	182 ± 5	250	84%	4.7 ± 0.47	23%
9–11 y (n = 38)	238 ± 14	375	93.2%	4.6 ± 0.20	18%

Note: [a]AI: adequate intake; [b]average adult betaine intake = ~5 mg/kg [14, 15].

9.3.2 DIETARY INTAKE OF PARTICIPANTS WITH ASD

Dietary intake data is based on three-day food records of the 288 ASD participants analyzed at the time of paper preparation. As shown in Table 1, choline intake was below the AI for more than 69% in all age categories. The proportion of children with intake below the AI increased progressively with age (range 69–93%). No dietary reference intake levels have been established for betaine; however, the average US adult betaine intake has been estimated to be ~5 mg/kg/day [20, 21]. The mean betaine intake in the children with autism was ~4.6 mg/kg/day across all age groups. However, the percent of children whose intake was less than 3.5 mg/Kg/day was 30% in the 1–3 yr age group, 23% in the 4–8 yr age group, and 18% in the 9–11 yr age group.

9.3.3 RELATIONSHIPS BETWEEN DIETARY INTAKE AND PLASMA CONCENTRATIONS OF CHOLINE AND BETAINE IN ASD GROUP

Relationships between dietary intake and plasma concentrations of choline and betaine in the ASD cohort (n = 35) were investigated using Pearson's product-moment correlation coefficients. There was a strong, positive correlation between dietary intake and plasma choline concentrations: r = 0.86, n = 35, and P < 0.001, with low intake associated with low plasma choline concentrations (Figure 2). Similarly, dietary intake and plasma betaine concentrations showed a strong, positive correlation: r = 0.67, n = 35, and P < 0.001, with low dietary intake associated with low plasma betaine concentrations (Figure 3).

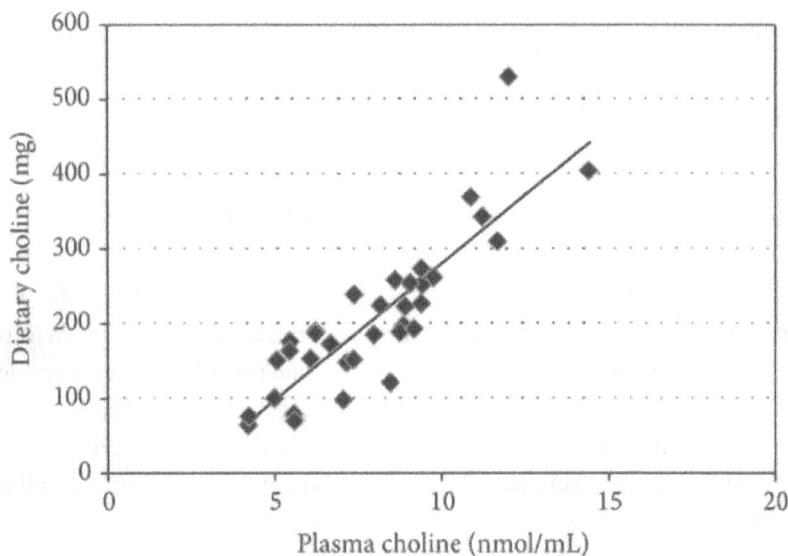

FIGURE 2: Correlation between dietary intake and plasma choline concentrations in children with ASD (n = 35). r = 0.86 and P ≤ 0.001 using Pearson's product-moment correlation coefficient. ASD: autism spectrum disorder.

9.3.4 COMPARISON OF PLASMA METABOLITE CONCENTRATIONS IN ASD AND CONTROL GROUPS

A comparison of plasma concentrations of choline and betaine was made between the ASD cohort (n = 35) and the control group (n = 32) and is presented in Figure 4. Student's t-test demonstrated that participants in the ASD group had significantly lower plasma concentrations of choline and betaine compared to the control group (P < 0.001) as well as a significant decrease in the betaine : choline ratio.

9.4 DISCUSSION

The results of the AIR-P study of diet and nutrition in children with autism demonstrate for the first time that the majority of children with ASDs be-

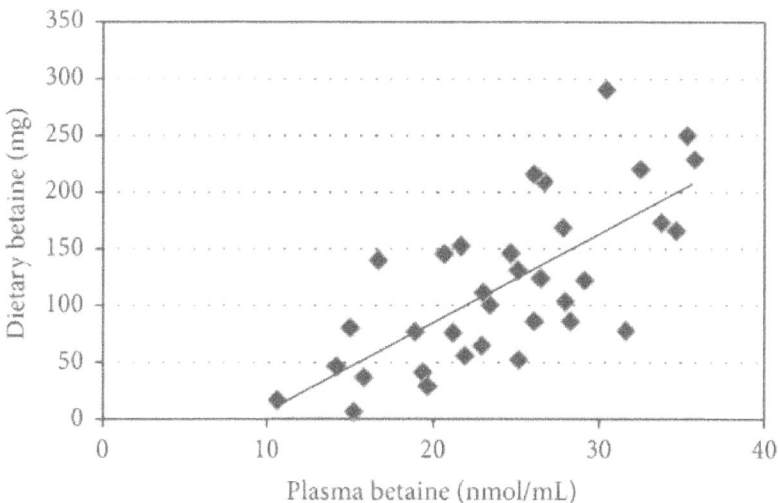

FIGURE 3: Correlation between dietary intake and plasma betaine concentrations in children with ASD (n = 35). r = 0.67 and P ≤ 0.001 using Pearson's product-moment correlation coefficient. ASD: autism spectrum disorder.

tween 3 and 11 years of age consume inadequate amounts of dietary choline. A strong correlation between choline and betaine dietary intake and
plasma levels was observed in a subset of these children suggesting that
the choline-betaine-homocysteine pathway for methionine synthesis may
be compromised. The significant decrease in choline:betaine intake ratio
presented in Figure 4 is consistent with this possibility. Research studies
have shown that insufficient dietary folate increases requirement for choline and betaine-derived methyl groups and conversely, choline and betaine deficiency increases the requirement for folate-derived methyl groups
[17]. Thus, dietary deficits in both pathways for methionine synthesis may
be compromised in children with ASDs and additively contribute to the
low methionine and SAM levels previously reported in these children
[8–10]. Importantly, reduced synthesis of SAM, the major intracellular
methyl donor, can lead to DNA hypomethylation and epigenetic abnormalities associated with abnormal gene expression, genomic imprinting,
and genomic instability [22]. Significant decreases in plasma methioinine
and SAM associated with DNA hypomethylation have been reported in
children with ASDs relative to age-matched control children [10].

It is not known whether supplemental choline or betaine would increase methionine and SAM synthesis in children with autism. However,
works by Atkinson et al. [23] and Innis et al. [24] support the positive effects of choline and betaine in other studies. Atkinson et al. conducted a
randomized crossover study in healthy males (n = 8) that measured betaine
and homocysteine concentrations after consuming meals or supplements
containing choline or betaine. They found that betaine from meals and
supplements acutely increased plasma betaine. Additionally, both betaine
and choline helped alleviate the rise in homocysteine concentrations following a postmethionine load. Innis et al. found that a choline supplement
in children with cystic fibrosis resulted in significant increased methionine, SAM, the SAM/SAH methylation ratio, and the GSH/GSSG redox
ratio. Because the metabolic profile of children with ASDs is similar to
that observed in children with cystic fibrosis, it is possible that choline
supplementation may similarly improve methylation status in children
with ASDs.

Consistent with low choline status, El-Ansary et al. [25] found that
phosphatidylethanolamine, phosphatidylserine, and phosphatidylcholine

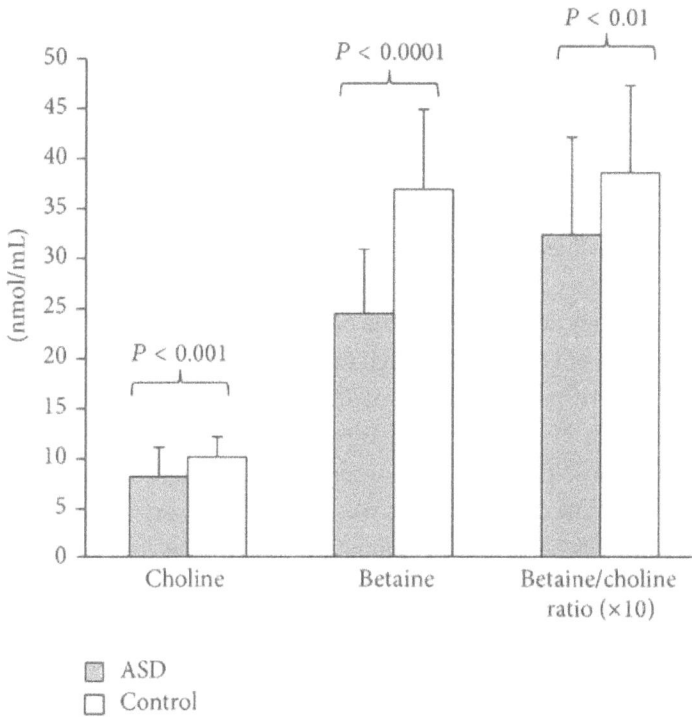

FIGURE 4: Plasma levels of choline, betaine, and the betaine/choline ratio in children with autism compared to age-matched controls.

were significantly lower in a group of Saudi Arabian children with ASDs (n = 25) compared to a control group (n = 16). They suggested that the lower levels of these phospholipids could be related to oxidative stress and inflammation. Similarly, James et al. found decreased plasma levels of cysteine, glutathione, and the ratio of reduced to oxidized glutathione (GSH/GSSG) in children with ASDs compared to a control group, indicating that some children with ASDs have reduced antioxidant capacity and evidence of oxidative stress [8]. Other researchers have reported higher homocysteine levels in children with ASDs [6] which is important to consider since choline and betaine have been shown to reduce these levels, especially when given in addition to methionine. In addition to inadequate intake of choline and betaine, the AIR-P study of diet and nutrition in children with autism reported that calcium, vitamin E, vitamin D, and fiber intake are also inadequate when compared to NHANES normative data [2].

A final consideration is the role of choline deficiency in brain development, memory, and anxiety. In rodent models, multiple studies have shown that choline deficiency and supplementation affect neurodevelopment. The offspring of choline-supplemented pregnant rodents have improved visuospatial and auditory memory and perform better in behavioral tests, whereas choline deficiency seems to have the opposite effect [26, 27]. Fewer studies have been done in humans, although the elderly and patients with Alzheimer's disease have reduced levels of free choline and phosphatidylcholine in the brain [28, 29]. A recent large population based study of 5,918 men and women participating in the Hordaland [18] Health Study, found that low plasma choline concentrations were significantly associated with higher anxiety levels. Behavioral alterations associated with low plasma choline levels in children with ASDs warrant further research consideration.

The present study had several possible limitations. First, it is possible that parents who consented to participate may have been more concerned about nutrition and feeding behaviors in their children such that their dietary patterns might be different from the general population of children with ASD. We were unable to make comparisons regarding the diets of the unaffected control children since food records were only collected for children with ASDs. Also, it is unclear if the differences observed in plasma concentrations between case and control groups are reflective of their dietary intake or abnormal metabolism or both. While the adequacy of choline intake was determined using the standard AI levels, a component of the dietary reference intakes that is intended for healthy individuals, it is uncertain if these standards can be applied to children with ASDs, especially since abnormalities in nutrient metabolism have been found in these children.

9.5 CONCLUSIONS

In summary, choline plays an essential role as a methyl-group donor in the synthesis of the membrane phospholipid components of cell membranes as well as in the synthesis of the neurotransmitter acetylcholine. The data in the AIR-P diet and nutrition study indicate that 69 to 93% of children with ASDs consumed diets that were inadequate in choline. Importantly, low choline and betaine intake were associated with low plasma levels of these nutrients suggesting that there could be functional consequences related to folate and phospholipid metabolism. Future research should consider whether these metabolic imbalances can be corrected with dietary counseling or supplement interventions and whether metabolic improvement is associated with improvement in some behavioral symptoms.

REFERENCES

1. T. Buie, D. B. Campbell, G. J. Fuchs 3rd, et al., "Evaluation, diagnosis, and treatment of gastrointestinal disorders in individuals with ASDs: a consensus report," Pediatrics, vol. 125, supplement 1, pp. S1–18, 2010.
2. S. L. Hyman, P. A. Stewart, B. Schmidt, et al., "Nutrient intake from food in children with autism," Pediatrics, vol. 130, supplement 2, pp. S145–S153, 2012.
3. D. A. Rossignol and R. E. Frye, "A review of research trends in physiological abnormalities in autism spectrum disorders: immune dysregulation, inflammation, oxidative stress, mitochondrial dysfunction and environmental toxicant exposures," Molecular Psychiatry, vol. 17, no. 4, pp. 389–401, 2012.
4. R. E. Frye, L. C. Huffman, and G. R. Elliott, "Tetrahydrobiopterin as a novel therapeutic intervention for autism," Neurotherapeutics, vol. 7, no. 3, pp. 241–249, 2010.
5. S. J. James, S. Melnyk, G. Fuchs et al., "Efficacy of methylcobalamin and folinic acid treatment on glutathione redox status in children with autism," American Journal of Clinical Nutrition, vol. 89, no. 1, pp. 425–430, 2009.
6. S. P. Paşca, E. Dronca, T. Kaucsár et al., "One carbon metabolism disturbances and the C677T MTHFR gene polymorphism in children with autism spectrum disorders," Journal of Cellular and Molecular Medicine, vol. 13, no. 10, pp. 4229–4238, 2009.
7. K.-A. Da Costa, O. G. Kozyreva, J. Song, J. A. Galanko, L. M. Fischer, and S. H. Zeisel, "Common genetic polymorphisms affect the human requirement for the nutrient choline," The FASEB Journal, vol. 20, no. 9, pp. 1336–1344, 2006.
8. S. J. James, P. Cutler, S. Melnyk et al., "Metabolic biomarkers of increased oxidative stress and impaired methylation capacity in children with autism," American Journal of Clinical Nutrition, vol. 80, no. 6, pp. 1611–1617, 2004.
9. S. J. James, S. Melnyk, S. Jernigan et al., "Metabolic endophenotype and related genotypes are associated with oxidative stress in children with autism," American Journal of Medical Genetics B, vol. 141, no. 8, pp. 947–956, 2006.
10. S. Melnyk, G. J. Fuchs, E. Schulz, et al., "Metabolic imbalance associated with methylation dysregulation and oxidative damage in children with autism," Journal of Autism and Developmental Disorders, vol. 42, no. 3, pp. 367–377, 2012.

11. S. Rose, S. Melnyk, O. Pavliv, et al., "Evidence of oxidative damage and inflammation associated with low glutathione redox status in the autism brain," Translational Psychiatry, vol. 2, article e134, 2012.

12. D. E. Vance, "Physiological roles of phosphatidylethanolamine N-methyltransferase," Biochimica et Biophysica Acta, vol. 1831, no. 3, pp. 626–632, 2013.

13. S. H. Zeisel, "Choline phospholipids: Signal transduction and carcinogenesis," The FASEB Journal, vol. 7, no. 6, pp. 551–557, 1993.

14. F. Kimura, "Cholinergic modulation of cortical function: a hypothetical role in shifting the dynamics in cortical network," Neuroscience Research, vol. 38, no. 1, pp. 19–26, 2000.

15. M. D. Niculescu, C. N. Craciunescu, and S. H. Zeisel, "Dietary choline deficiency alters global and gene-specific DNA methylation in the developing hippocampus of mouse fetal brains," The FASEB Journal, vol. 20, no. 1, pp. 43–49, 2006.

16. L. M. Sanders and S. H. Zeisel, "Choline: dietary requirements and role in brain development," Nutrition Today, vol. 42, no. 4, pp. 181–186, 2007.

17. S. H. Zeisel, "Choline: clinical nutrigenetic/nutrigenomic approaches for identification of functions and dietary requirements," Journal of Nutrigenetics and Nutrigenomics, vol. 3, no. 4-6, pp. 209–219, 2010.

18. I. Bjelland, G. S. Tell, S. E. Vollset, S. Konstantinova, and P. M. Ueland, "Choline in anxiety and depression: The Hordaland Health Study," American Journal of Clinical Nutrition, vol. 90, no. 4, pp. 1056–1060, 2009.

19. P. I. Holm, P. M. Ueland, G. Kvalheim, and E. A. Lien, "Determination of choline, betaine, and dimethylglycine in plasma by a high-throughput method based on normal-phase chromatography-tandem mass spectrometry," Clinical Chemistry, vol. 49, no. 2, pp. 286–294, 2003.

20. E. Cho, S. H. Zeisel, P. Jacques et al., "Dietary choline and betaine assessed by food-frequency questionnaire in relation to plasma total homocysteine concentration in the Framingham Offspring Study," American Journal of Clinical Nutrition, vol. 83, no. 4, pp. 905–911, 2006.

21. A. Bidulescu, L. E. Chambless, A. M. Siega-Riz, S. H. Zeisel, and G. Heiss, "Usual choline and betaine dietary intake and incident coronary heart disease: The Atherosclerosis Risk in Communities (ARIC) Study," BMC Cardiovascular Disorders, vol. 7, article 20, 2007.

22. M. A. Caudill, J. C. Wang, S. Melnyk et al., "Intracellular S-adenosylhomocysteine concentrations predict global DNA hypomethylation in tissues of methyl-deficient cystathionine β-synthase heterozygous mice," Journal of Nutrition, vol. 131, no. 11, pp. 2811–2818, 2001.

23. W. Atkinson, J. Elmslie, M. Lever, S. T. Chambers, and P. M. George, "Dietary and supplementary betaine: acute effects on plasma betaine and homocysteine concentrations under standard and postmethionine load conditions in healthy male subjects," American Journal of Clinical Nutrition, vol. 87, no. 3, pp. 577–585, 2008.

24. S. M. Innis, A. G. F. Davidson, S. Melynk, and S. J. James, "Choline-related supplements improve abnormal plasma methioninehomocysteine metabolites and glutathione status in children with cystic fibrosis," American Journal of Clinical Nutrition, vol. 85, no. 3, pp. 702–708, 2007.

25. A. K. El-Ansary, A. G. Ben Bacha, and L. Y. Al- Ayahdi, "Impaired plasma phospholipids and relative amounts of essential polyunsaturated fatty acids in autistic patients from Saudi Arabia," Lipids in Health and Disease, vol. 10, article 63, 2011.
26. S. H. Zeisel, "Choline: critical role during fetal development and dietary requirements in adults," Annual Review of Nutrition, vol. 26, pp. 229–250, 2006.
27. S. H. Zeisel, "The fetal origins of memory: the role of dietary choline in optimal brain development," Journal of Pediatrics, vol. 149, supplement 5, pp. S131–S136, 2006.
28. R. M. Nitsch, J. K. Blusztajn, A. G. Pittas, B. E. Slack, J. H. Growdon, and R. J. Wurtman, "Evidence for a membrane defect in Alzheimer disease brain," Proceedings of the National Academy of Sciences of the United States of America, vol. 89, no. 5, pp. 1671–1675, 1992.
29. B. M. Cohen, P. F. Renshaw, A. L. Stoll, R. J. Wurtman, D. Yurgelun-Todd, and S. M. Babb, "Decreased brain choline uptake in older adults: an in vivo proton magnetic resonance spectroscopy study," Journal of the American Medical Association, vol. 274, no. 11, pp. 902–907, 1995.

CHAPTER 10

ASSOCIATION BETWEEN PSYCHIATRIC DISORDERS AND IRON DEFICIENCY ANEMIA AMONG CHILDREN AND ADOLESCENTS: A NATIONWIDE POPULATION-BASED STUDY

MU-HONG CHEN, TUNG-PING SU, YING-SHEUE CHEN, JU-WEI HSU, KAI-LIN HUANG, WEN-HAN CHANG, TZENG-JI CHEN, AND YA-MEI BAI

10.1 BACKGROUND

According to the World Health Organization, iron deficiency (ID) is the most prevalent nutritional deficiency. A 30% prevalence of iron deficiency anemia (IDA), at a minimum, has been noted among children, adolescents, and women in non-industrialized countries, and ID is also the most prevalent nutritional deficiency in industrialized countries [1-4]. ID, defined by two or more abnormal measurements (serum ferritin, transferrin satura-

Association between Psychiatric Disorders and Iron Deficiency Anemia among Children and Adolescents: A Nationwide Population-Based Study. © Chen M-H, Su T-P, Chen Y-S, Hsu J-W, Huang K-L, Chang W-H, Chen T-J, and Bai Y-M. BMC Psychiatry *13,161 (2013); doi:10.1186/1471-244X-13-161.*

tion, erythrocyte protoporphyrin), is insidious and uneasily detected by patients themselves and may not develop significant clinical symptoms [1-4]. IDA is characterized by a defect in hemoglobin synthesis owing to significant ID, resulting in the reduced capacity of the red blood cells to deliver oxygen to body cells and tissues, and many clinical symptoms, such as pale conjunctiva, shortness of breath, dizziness, and lethargy [1-4]. The main risk factors for IDA and ID include a low intake of iron, poor absorption of iron from diets, chronic loss of iron (i.e., ulcer, metrorrhagia), and some specific periods of life when iron requirements are especially high, such as growth and pregnancy [1-4].

Iron is an essential component of hemoglobin, myoglobin, and many enzymes in cellular metabolism and DNA replication and repair. It also plays a crucial role in the development of the central neurological system [5-8], autoimmune system [9-11], endocrine system [12-15], and cardiovascular system [16,17]. In the development of the brain, iron accounted for the myelination of white matter [18,19] and the development and functioning of the different neurotransmitter systems, including the dopamine, norepinephrine, and serotonin systems [20-22]. In vivo microdialysis studies using post-weaning iron-deficient rats and mice demonstrated that they exhibited deficits in intracellular dopamine concentrations and in the density of dopamine and dopamine transporter receptors, with variable amounts of loss by brain region [23-26]. Anderson et al. showed that decreased iron significantly reduced extracellular concentrations of norepinephrine in the caudate putamen, and altered levels of norepinephrine due to reduced iron levels may be the result of changes in the expression of norepinephrine transport and norepinephrine receptor proteins in the locus ceruleus and basal ganglia [27,28]. A reduction in serotonin transporter binding was noted in the nucleus accumbens and olfactory tubercle in iron-deficient rats [21], and the serotonin concentration in the brain was significantly correlated with the non-heme iron level [29].

In summary, IDA and ID were significantly associated with an alteration of monoamine neurotransmitters and the abnormal myelination of white matter, and is probably related to childhood/adolescence-onset psychiatric disorders. There is well documented evidence in the literature that IDA has a significant influence on cognitive development, intelligence, and developmental delay [30,31]. However, the association between IDA and other childhood/adolescence-onset psychiatric disorders is still limited. Some clinical studies supposed that brain ID involved in the pathophysiology of attention deficit hyperactivity disorder (ADHD) [32] and ferritin level was related to behavioral symptoms in ADHD patients [33]. But, Millichap et al. disclosed no significant difference in severity of ADHD symptoms between children with ADHD who had the lower serum ferritin levels (<20 ng/mL) and those who had the higher levels (>60 ng/mL) [34]. And a high prevalence, up to 30%, of IDA was observed in children with autism spectrum disorder (ASD), which was supposed to potentially compromise their communication and behavior [35,36]. As for schizophrenia, bipolar disorder (BD), unipolar depressive disorder, and anxiety disorder, the data are quite limited. This study, using a nationwide population-based insurance database with a case–control method and the largest sample size, attempted to clarify the association between IDA and various psychiatric disorders among children and adolescents with IDA. We hypothesized that children and adolescents with ADHD exhibited the higher risk of having a psychiatric disorder.

10.2 METHODS

10.2.1 DATA SOURCE

The National Health Insurance (NHI) program was implemented in Taiwan in 1995. Since 2001, Taiwan's NHI has covered 96.9% of all 23,000,000 residents of Taiwan. The completeness and accuracy of the NHI claims database has been audited by the Department of Health and the Bureau of NHI. The database provides demographic and medical information on insured residents, including age, gender, prescription drugs, prescription date, and the prescription and diagnosis using the International Classification of Diseases, 9th Revision, Clinical Modification (ICD-9-CM). The NHI Research Database (NHIRD) has been used extensively in many epidemiologic studies in Taiwan [37-39]. Our study was approved by Institutional Review Board of Taipei Veterans General Hospital (2012-04-012BC).

10.2.2 INCLUSION CRITERIA FOR IDA AND PSYCHIATRIC DISORDERS

In this study, 1,000,000 subjects, approximately 4.3% of the population of Taiwan, were randomly selected from the NHIRD. The study comprised all children and adolescents (aged younger than 18) who were identified by the diagnostic code of "iron deficiency anemia" (ICD-9-CM: 280) between January 1, 1996 and December 31, 2008. Diagnosis was given by board-certificated pediatricians and physicians. Coexistent psychiatric disorders were investigated by specific diagnostic codes, and included schizophrenia (ICD-9-CM code: 295), BD (ICD-9-CM code: 296 except 296.2 and 296.3), unipolar depressive disorder (ICD-9-CM codes: 296.2, 296.3, 300.4, and 311 for major depressive disorder, dysthymic disorder, depressive disorder, not specified), obsessive-compulsive disorder (OCD) (ICD-9-CM code: 300.3), anxiety disorder (ICD-9-CM code: 300 except 300.3 and 300.4), ASD (ICD-9-CM code: 299), ADHD (ICD-9-CM code: 314), tic disorder (ICD-9-CM: 307.2), delayed development (ICD-9-CM code: 315), and mental retardation (ICD-9-CM code: 317~319). Finally, gastrointestinal ulcer (ICD-9-CM code: 531~534), metrorrhagia (ICD-9-CM code: 626.2 and 626.6), and premenopausal menorrhea (ICD-9-CM code: 627.0) were used as covariates. All psychiatric diagnoses were given by board-certified psychiatrists. The diagnoses of delayed development and mental retardation were given by board-certificated psychiatrists, rehabilitation specialists, and pediatricians.

10.2.3 CONTROL GROUP

The age and gender-matched control group (4 for every patient in the study cohort) was randomly identified from subjects who had no major physical illnesses, including cancer (ICD-9-CM code: 140~239), hematological disease (ICD-9-CM code: 280~289), chronic liver disease (ICD-9-CM code: 570~573), chronic renal disease (ICD-9-CM code: 585, 586), chronic inflammatory disease (ICD-9-CM code: 710 for diffuse diseases of connective tissue, 714 for rheumatoid arthritis and other inflammatory polyarthropathies, 720 for ankylosing spondylitis and other inflammatory spondylopathies, 555 for Crohn's disease, 556 for idiopathic proctocolitis), chronic infectious disease (ICD-9-CM code: 010~018 for tuberculosis, 042~044 for human immunodeficiency virus, 070 for viral hepatitis, 090~099 for syphilis, 390~392 for rheumatic fever, 730 for osteomyelitis), endocrine disease (ICD-9-CM code: 240~246 for thyroid disease, 249~250 for diabetes mellitus, 252 for parathyroid disease, 253 for pituitary disease, 255 for adrenal gland disease), and nutritional deficiency (ICD-9-CM code: 260~269).

10.2.4 STATISTICAL ANALYSIS

For between-group comparisons, the independent t test was used for continuous variables and Pearson's X^2 test or Fisher's exact test was applied for nominal variables, where appropriate. Multiple logistic regressions were performed to calculate the OR with 95% confidence intervals (CI) after adjusting for ulcer, metrorrhagia, and premenopausal menorrhea (because ulcer and metrorrhagia were two important risks causing IDA of children and adolescents). A two-tailed P-value of less than 0.05 was considered statistically significant. All data processing and statistical analyses were performed with Statistical Package for Social Science (SPSS) version 17 software (SPSS Inc) and Statistical Analysis Software (SAS) version 9.1 (SAS Institute, Cary, NC).

10.3 RESULTS

10.3.1 DEMOGRAPHIC CHARACTERISTICS OF THE IDA PATIENTS AND CONTROL GROUP

A total of 2957 children and adolescents (1060 males and 1897 females) were identified as having IDA from the 1,000,000-person sample population between January 1, 1996 and December 31, 2008. The mean age was 10.59 ± 6.02 years and male patients were significantly younger than the females (7.46±5.68 vs. 12.34±5.46, p<0.001). Male IDA patients exhibited a significantly higher prevalence of ASD (1.6% vs. 0.4%, p<0.001), ADHD (6.0% vs. 1.1%, p<0.001), tic disorder (1.3% vs. 0.5%, p=0.027), delayed development (8.5% vs. 3.4%, p<0.001), and mental retardation (4.4% vs. 1.5%, p<0.001) than the females (Table 1). In comparing the difference between the IDA patients and the control group, the IDA patients had a significantly increased prevalence of psychiatric comorbidities, including unipolar depressive disorder (1.6% vs. 0.6%, p<0.001), BD (0.4% vs. 0.1%, p<0.001), anxiety disorder (1.5% vs. 0.7%, p<0.001), ASD (0.8% vs. 0.3%, p<0.001), ADHD (2.8% vs. 1.8%, p<0.001), tic disorder (0.8% vs. 0.5%, p=0.044), delayed development (5.2% vs. 2.4%, p<0.001), and mental retardation (2.5% vs. 1.0%, p<0.001) (Table 2).

TABLE 1: Characteristics of patients with iron deficiency anemia (IDA)

Characteristics of IDA	Male	Female	p-value	All
No.	1060	1897		
Age (years)	7.46±5.68	12.34±5.46	<0.001	10.59±6.02
Associated diseases, N (%)				
Schizophrenia	2 (0.2)	6 (0.3)	0.719	8 (0.3)
Unipolar depressive disorder	12 (1.1)	36 (1.9)	0.104	48 (1.6)
Bipolar disorder	2 (0.2)	11 (0.6)	0.154	13 (0.4)
OCD	1 (0.1)	3 (0.2)	>0.999	4 (0.1)
Anxiety disorder	21 (2.0)	24 (1.3)	0.158	45 (1.5)
ASD	17 (1.6)	7 (0.4)	0.001	24 (0.8)
ADHD	64 (6.0)	20 (1.1)	<0.001	84 (2.8)
Tic disorder	14 (1.3)	9 (0.5)	0.027	23 (0.8)
Delayed development	90 (8.5)	64 (3.4)	<0.001	154 (5.2)
Mental retardation	47 (4.4)	28 (1.5)	<0.001	75 (2.5)

OCD obsessive-compulsive disorder, ASD autistic spectrum disorder, ADHD attention-deficit hyperactivity disorder.

TABLE 2: Characteristics of patients with iron deficiency anemia (IDA) and control subjects

Characteristics	IDA	Control	p-value
No.	2957	11828	
Age (years)	10.59±6.02	10.59±6.02	
Sex, N (%)			
Male	1060 (35.8)	4240 (35.8)	
Female	1897 (64.2)	7588 (64.2)	
Associated diseases, N (%)			
Schizophrenia	8 (0.3)	14 (0.1)	0.063
Unipolar depressive disorder	48 (1.6)	66 (0.6)	<0.001
Bipolar disorder	13 (0.4)	7 (0.1)	<0.001
OCD	4 (0.1)	8 (0.1)	0.274
Anxiety disorder	45 (1.5)	80 (0.7)	<0.001
ASD	24 (0.8)	32 (0.3)	<0.001
ADHD	84 (2.8)	207 (1.8)	<0.001
Tic disorder	23 (0.8)	56 (0.5)	0.044
Delayed development	154 (5.2)	278 (2.4)	<0.001
Mental retardation	75 (2.5)	114 (1.0)	<0.001

IDA iron deficiency anemia, OCD obsessive-compulsive disorder, ASD autistic spectrum disorder, ADHD attention-deficit and hyperactivity disorder.

10.3.2 ODDS RATIO OF PSYCHIATRIC DISORDERS

In examining the association between IDA and childhood/adolescence-onset psychiatric disorders, multiple logistic regression analysis was used to evaluate the OR of psychiatric comorbidity among those with IDA, after adjusting for age, gender, ulcer, metrorrhagia, and premenopausal menorrhea. Patients with IDA were prone to having a significantly higher chance of being associated with unipolar depressive disorder (OR=2.34, 95% CI=1.59~3.46), BD (OR=5.80, 95% CI=2.24~15.05), anxiety disorder (OR=2.17, 95% CI=1.49~3.16), ASD (OR=3.08, 95% CI=1.79~5.28), ADHD (OR=1.67, 95% CI=1.29~2.17), tic disorder

(OR = 1.70, 95% CI = 1.03 ~ 2.78), delayed development (OR = 2.45, 95% CI = 2.00 ~ 3.00), and mental retardation (OR = 2.70, 95% CI = 2.00 ~ 3.65) (Table 3). We also investigated the gender effect on IDA and associated psychiatric comorbidities (Table 3). A significantly increased risk of unipolar depressive disorder (OR = 2.36, 95% CI = 1.10 ~ 5.10), anxiety disorder (OR = 1.73, 95% CI = 1.02 ~ 2.94), ASD (OR = 2.66, 95% CI = 1.41 ~ 5.00), ADHD (OR = 1.51, 95% CI = 1.12 ~ 2.04), delayed development (OR = 1.95, 95% CI = 1.50 ~ 2.53), and mental retardation (OR = 3.09, 95% CI = 2.08 ~ 4.61) were observed in male IDA patients in comparison with females, while a significantly higher risk of unipolar depressive disorder (OR = 2.37, 95% CI = 1.51 ~ 3.73), BD (OR = 5.56, 95% CI = 1.98 ~ 15.70), anxiety disorder (OR = 2.69, 95% CI = 1.57 ~ 4.62), ASD (OR = 4.07, 95% CI = 1.39 ~ 11.90), ADHD (OR = 2.00, 95% CI = 1.14 ~ 3.49), tic disorder (OR = 2.95, 95% CI = 1.27 ~ 6.86), delayed development (OR = 3.48, 95% CI = 2.48 ~ 4.88), and mental retardation (OR = 2.13, 95% CI = 1.34 ~ 3.40) were noted in female IDA patients compared with males (Table 3).

10.3.3 ODDS RATIO OF PSYCHIATRIC DISORDER STRATIFIED BY AGE

We performed adjusted multiple logistic regression stratified by age to elucidate the association between IDA and various psychiatric comorbidities, focusing on children and adolescents with IDA, respectively (Table 3). Children were defined as those younger than 13 and adolescents as those aged 13 ~ 18. Children with IDA exhibited a significantly higher risk of ASD (OR = 3.00, 95% CI = 1.70 ~ 5.27), ADHD (OR = 1.50, 95% CI = 1.12 ~ 1.99), delayed development (OR = 2.23, 95% CI = 1.79 ~ 2.78), and mental retardation (OR = 3.01, 95% CI = 2.09 ~ 4.32) (Table 3). Adolescents with IDA were significantly associated with unipolar depressive disorder (OR = 2.89, 95% CI = 1.84 ~ 4.54), BD (OR = 6.05, 95% CI = 1.97 ~ 18.58), anxiety disorder (OR = 3.71, 95% CI = 2.16 ~ 6.37), ADHD (OR = 2.54, 95% CI = 1.31 ~ 4.95), tic disorder (OR = 3.73, 95% CI = 1.12 ~ 12.48), delayed development (OR = 3.88, 95% CI = 2.17 ~ 6.95), and mental retardation (OR = 2.08, 95% CI = 1.22 ~ 3.57) (Table 3).

TABLE 3: Association between iron deficiency anemia (IDA) and psychiatric disorders

OR (95% CI)	Male	Female	Children (Age <13)	Adolescent (Age≥13)	All
Schizophrenia	2.20 (0.40, 12.02)	2.15 (0.76, 6.10)	4.35 (0.27, 69.56)	2.04 (0.79, 5.28)	2.11 (0.86, 5.15)
Unipolar depressive disorder	**2.36 (1.10, 5.10)**	**2.37 (1.51, 3.73)**	1.33 (0.58, 3.04)	**2.89 (1.84, 4.54)**	**2.34 (1.59, 3.46)**
Bipolar disorder	8.80 (0.80, 97.14)	**5.56 (1.98, 15.70)**	5.20 (0.83, 32.71)	**6.05 (1.97, 18.58)**	**5.80 (2.24, 15.05)**
OCD	0.78 (0.08, 7.48)	3.07 (0.67, 14.13)	--	3.01 (0.77, 11.77)	1.87 (0.55, 6.40)
Anxiety disorder	**1.73 (1.02, 2.94)**	**2.69 (1.57, 4.62)**	1.29 (0.74, 2.26)	**3.71 (2.16, 6.37)**	**2.17 (1.49, 3.16)**
ASD	**2.66 (1.41, 5.00)**	**4.07 (1.39, 11.90)**	**3.00 (1.70, 5.27)**	2.55 (0.40, 16.24)	**3.08 (1.79, 5.28)**
ADHD	**1.51 (1.12, 2.04)**	**2.00 (1.14, 3.49)**	**1.50 (1.12, 1.99)**	**2.54 (1.31, 4.95)**	**1.67 (1.29, 2.17)**
Tic disorder	1.23 (0.66, 2.30)	**2.95 (1.27, 6.86)**	1.41 (0.81, 2.43)	**3.73 (1.12, 12.48)**	**1.70 (1.03, 2.78)**
Delay in development	**1.95 (1.50, 2.53)**	**3.48 (2.48, 4.88)**	**2.23 (1.79, 2.78)**	**3.88 (2.17, 6.95)**	**2.45 (2.00, 3.00)**
Mental retardation	**3.09 (2.08, 4.61)**	**2.13 (1.34, 3.40)**	**3.01 (2.09, 4.32)**	**2.08 (1.22, 3.57)**	**2.70 (2.00, 3.65)**

OCD obsessive-compulsive disorder, ASD autistic spectrum disorder, ADHD attention-deficit hyperactivity disorder. Bold type denotes statistically significant odds ratio (OR).

10.4 DISCUSSION

The results of our clinical epidemiological study supported previous findings that IDA is significantly associated with increased risks of unipolar depressive disorder, BD, anxiety disorder, ASD, ADHD, delayed development, and mental retardation among children and adolescents.

10.4.1 MENTAL RETARDATION AND DELAYED DEVELOPMENT

Our results showed a higher prevalence of mental retardation and delayed development among subjects with IDA, which was consistent with previous findings [31,40,41]. Beltrán-Navarro et al. used the Bayley Scales of Infant Development, preschool language scales and an environmental sound perception task to assess the effect of IDA on multifaceted development in infancy (at 6 and 14 to 18 months) and showed that infants with chronic IDA did show significantly lower scores on language, environmental sound perception, and motor measures, when compared with infants with a normal iron nutritional status [42]. Studying the long-term developmental outcome of infants with IDA, Lozoff et al. found lower scores on tests of mental (i.e., intelligence) and motor functioning at age of 5 and 12 among those with IDA in infancy [31,40]. Furthermore, IDA can impair cognitive performance at all stages of life. Halterman et al. assessed 5398 children and adolescents aged 6 to 16 and demonstrated that subjects with IDA had more than twice the risk of scoring below average in scholastic achievement than the children with a normal iron status [43].

10.4.2 ATTENTION DEFICIT HYPERACTIVITY DISORDER (ADHD)

Previous studies on iron and the pathophysiology of ADHD have had inconsistent results. In a small cohort study comprising 52 ADHD children, Oner et al. found that lower ferritin levels were associated with higher hyperactivity scores in ADHD children, but did not have a significant influence on cognitive measures [33]. Using magnetic resonance imaging (MRI) to investigate the association of ADHD and brain iron levels in the putamen, pallidum, caudate, and thalamus, Cortese et al. demonstrated children with ADHD showed significantly lower brain iron levels in the right and left thalamus compared to healthy controls [32]. Other studies, however, did not find this association between ADHD and the ferritin level [34,44]. In our study, an increased risk of ADHD was noted among those with IDA, which was compatible with a recent meta-analysis result [45]. With regard to the current pathophysiology of ADHD as involving a dysfunction of the neurotransmitter systems, IDA significantly disturbed the development and functioning of norepinephrine and dopamine neurotransmitter systems.

10.4.3 AUTISM SPECTRUM DISORDER (ASD)

Previous studies have revealed that iron was associated with socio-cognitive and socio-emotional development and functioning [46-48]. A disorder in this area is one of the core symptoms of ASD. Assessing the prevalence of ID and IDA among 116 children between 3 and 16 years old with a diagnosis of ASD, Hergüner et al. revealed that 24% of patients with ASD had ID, and 15% had IDA [35]. Latif et al. analyzed the serum ferritin measurements of 96 children with ASD and suggested there was a high prevalence, up to 30 percent, of ID in children with ASD [36]. Our result showed an increased risk of ASD among children and adolescents with IDA, suggesting a possible reciprocal effect between ASD and IDA. For example, inappropriate eating habit in those subjects may be related to IDA and many children with ASD are picky eaters, which could contribute to IDA. Furthermore, diffusion-tensor MRI found impaired white matter integrity and a myelination developmental abnormality in ASD patients compared to normal subjects [49-51]. Iron was regarded as an essential component in myelination and oligodendrogenesis. Myelin synthesis was limited and altered by ID. Further study would be needed to clarify the comorbidity or causality between ASD and IDA.

10.4.4 UNIPOLAR DEPRESSIVE DISORDER

Numerous studies have reported that IDA was associated with unipolar depressive disorder, possibly through an alteration of the monoamine neurotransmitters by ID [52-54]. Lower serum ferritin concentrations were significantly correlated with depressive symptoms [53,54]. Using a longitudinal cohort study of 191 participants to evaluate the association between IDA in infancy and affective and developmental outcomes in adolescence, Lozoff et al. revealed that those with IDA in infancy exhibited more anxiety, depression, social problems, and attentional problems in later life [40]. Vahdat Shariatpanaahi et al. studied 192 female medical students and found the mean ferritin level of students with depression was significantly lower than that of healthy students [53]. Similar results were observed in a Japanese male population. In a study of 312 men, those with lower serum ferritin concentration levels had a higher prevalence of depressive symptoms [54]. Our result, showing an increased risk of unipolar depressive disorder among those with IDA, was compatible with that of previous studies, and reconfirmed the pathophysiological association of IDA with unipolar depressive disorder.

10.4.5 BIPOLAR DISORDER (BD)

Emotional dysregulation has been deemed as one of the core neuropsychopathologies of BD [55-57]. It has been well documented that iron is associated with socio-emotional development and that ID may disturb the development of emotional regulation [40,46,47,58], although clinical studies on the association between IDA and BD are few. Our results showed a higher prevalence of BD among IDA subjects. Structural and functional changes related to emotional dysregulation such as in the dorsal and ventral prefrontal cortices and the prefrontal-subcortical and associated limbic circuitry have been considered as a neuropathology of BD [56,57]. ID has been related to perturbations in myelin formation, alterations of monoamine neurotransmitter systems, particularly in the striatum, and deficits in energy metabolism, particularly in the hippocampus and prefrontal cortex [59,60]. The effect of IDA on BD is still unclear and further study is needed to investigate the possible causality between IDA and BD. Furthermore, a significantly increased OR of BD was noted only among females with IDA after controlling gastrointestinal ulcer, metrorrhagia, and premenopausal menorrhea. Clarifying this gender effect between IDA and BD may be needed in future studies.

10.4.6 ANXIETY DISORDER

Clinical studies on the association between IDA and anxiety disorder are few. Lozoff et al. found that children with severe, chronic ID in infancy had a greater prevalence of anxiety, depression, and attention problems [40]. Some animal studies have shown an association between IDA and alterations in serotonin, norepinephrine, and gamma-aminobutyric acid (GABA) neurotransmission [21,61]. In assessing weanling rats with either an iron deficient diet or a control diet for 6 weeks, Beard et al. found reduced activity and increased anxiety-like behaviors among the iron deficient rats with significant decrements in brain iron content in the corpus striatum, prefrontal cortex, and midbrain [62]. Emotional dysregulation due to ID may be a possible mechanism explaining the association between anxiety and IDA [63-65]. In our study, both males and females with IDA had a significantly higher risk of anxiety disorder. However, establishing causality between IDA and anxiety disorder will require further study in the future.

Regarding emotional and cognitive problems, current neuroanatomical imaging studies have proven that brain development is a continuous process from infancy to late adolescence or early adulthood [66,67]. A deficiency of essential components will greatly impair the normal trajectory of brain development. Iron is regarded as one of the essential nutritional elements related to cognitive and socio-emotional development and functioning. A significantly higher risk of anxiety disorder, ASD, ADHD, delayed development, and mental retardation was noted among children (below age 13) with IDA. After entering adolescence (age 13~18), those with IDA had an increased risk of unipolar depressive disorder, BD, anxiety disorder, ADHD, delayed development, and mental retardation. These results may indicate that ID, whether in childhood or adolescence, does have a great impact on psychiatric comorbidities. Moreover, iron deletion in childhood has immediate and chronic effects on brain development, in that children with IDA exhibited an increased risk of delayed development and mental retardation with persistent sequelae of cognitive impairment and emotional problems during adolescence.

10.4.7 TIC DISORDER

We found a significantly increased risk of tic disorder among females with IDA. The association between IDA and tic disorder is unclear and rarely reported in the literature. Cortese et al. mentioned a possible iron hypothesis in a possible spectrum disorder of ADHD, restless leg syndrome, and tic disorder, because these 3 disorders were sometimes comorbid and shared a pathogenesis similar to monoamine neurotransmitter dysfunction [68]. Exploring the associations of ferritin levels with regional brain volumes among patients with Tourette's syndrome, Gorman et al. demonstrated ferritin and serum iron levels were significantly lower in the Tourette's syndrome subjects and that ferritin correlated positively with putamen volume [69]. Combining these results with ours may inspire further study to clarify the effect of iron on tic disorder or other movement disorders, especially in female populations.

Some limitations in our study should be mentioned here. First, the prevalence of psychiatric disorders was deemed underestimated because our results were derived from insurance registry-based data. Only those individuals who used the medical resource to seek psychiatric help were identified. However, patients included in our study were given a diagnosis by board-certified physicians and the diagnoses were more reliable than self-reported ones. Second, those subjects who were not diagnosed as having IDA ever but had iron deficiency problem cannot be detected in our study. The clinical study would be required to elucidate the possible association between psychiatric disorders and iron deficiency or subthreshold IDA. Third, ID may be due to inappropriate eating habits in some cases but the association among IDA, eating disorder, and episodic mood disorder with changed eating pattern is still unclear. In our study, we focused on the risks of psychiatric comorbidities in patients with IDA and the further study is required to analyze the effect of inappropriate eating pattern of specific psychiatric disorder on the risk of IDA. Fourth, we had no personal information that could contribute to an understanding of the risk of psychiatric disorders in patients, such as environmental factors (i.e. long-term life stress, traumatic experience), and family history of psychiatric disorder. Forth, the causality between IDA and psychiatric disorders cannot be proved in our study, even though our results did indicate a significant association between IDA and psychiatric disorders.

10.5 CONCLUSIONS

In conclusion, patients with IDA did have a higher risk of psychiatric disorders, including unipolar depressive disorder, BD, anxiety disorder, ASD, ADHD, delayed development, and mental retardation. When encountering patients with IDA in clinical practice, prompt iron supplementation should be considered to prevent possible psychiatric sequelae, because ID does impair the development of emotional regulation and cognition. And vice versa, psychiatrists should check the iron level in those children and adolescents with psychiatric disorders. Finally, further well-designed cohort studies are needed to elucidate the causality or comorbid effect between IDA and psychiatric disorders.

REFERENCES

1. DeMaeyer E, Adiels-Tegman M: The prevalence of anaemia in the world. World Health Stat Q 1985, 38(3):302-316.
2. Joint World Health Organization/Centers for Disease Control and Prevention Technical Consultation on the Assessment of Iron Status at the Population Level (2004: Geneva Switzerland), World Health Organization: Assessing the iron status of populations: report of a joint world health organization/centers for disease control and prevention technical consultation on the assessment of iron status at the population level. Geneva, Switzerland: Geneva: World Health Organization; 2005.
3. World Health Organization: Worldwide prevalence of anaemia 1993–2005: WHO global database on anaemia. Geneva: World Health Organization; 2008.
4. World Health Organization: Iron deficiency anaemia: assessment, prevention and control: a guide for programme managers. Geneva: World Health Organization; 2001.
5. Pollitt E: Effects of a diet deficient in iron on the growth and development of preschool and school-age children. Food Nutr Bull 1991, 13:110-118.
6. Krebs NF: Dietary zinc and iron sources, physical growth and cognitive development of breastfed infants. J Nutr 2000, 130(2S Suppl):358S-360S.
7. Lind T, Lonnerdal B, Stenlund H, Gamayanti IL, Ismail D, Seswandhana R, Persson LA: A community-based randomized controlled trial of iron and zinc supplementation in Indonesian infants: effects on growth and development. Am J Clin Nutr 2004, 80(3):729-736.
8. Webb TE, Oski FA: Iron deficiency anemia and scholastic achievement in young adolescents. J Pediatr 1973, 82(5):827-830.

9.   Gershwin ME, Keen CL, Mareschi JP, Fletcher MP: Trace metal nutrition and the immune response. Compr Ther 1991, 17(3):27-34.
10. Joynson DH, Walker DM, Jacobs A, Dolby AE: Defect of cell-mediated immunity in patients with iron-deficiency anaemia. Lancet 1972, 2(7786):1058-1059.
11. Srikantia SG, Prasad JS, Bhaskaram C, Krishnamachari KA: Anaemia and immune response. Lancet 1976, 1(7973):1307-1309.
12. Beard JL, Borel MJ, Derr J: Impaired thermoregulation and thyroid function in iron-deficiency anemia. Am J Clin Nutr 1990, 52(5):813-819.
13. Eftekhari MH, Eshraghian MR, Mozaffari-Khosravi H, Saadat N, Shidfar F: Effect of iron repletion and correction of iron deficiency on thyroid function in iron-deficient Iranian adolescent girls. Pak J Biol Sci 2007, 10(2):255-260.
14. Isguven P, Arslanoglu I, Erol M, Yildiz M, Adal E, Erguven M: Serum levels of ghrelin, leptin, IGF-I, IGFBP-3, insulin, thyroid hormones and cortisol in prepubertal children with iron deficiency. Endocr J 2007, 54(6):985-990.
15. Zimmermann MB: The influence of iron status on iodine utilization and thyroid function. Annu Rev Nutr 2006, 26:367-389.
16. Andersen HS, Gambling L, Holtrop G, McArdle HJ: Maternal iron deficiency identifies critical windows for growth and cardiovascular development in the rat postimplantation embryo. J Nutr 2006, 136(5):1171-1177.
17. Toxqui L, De Piero A, Courtois V, Bastida S, Sanchez-Muniz FJ, Vaquero MP: Iron deficiency and overload. Implications in oxidative stress and cardiovascular health. Nutr Hosp 2010, 25(3):350-365.
18. Beard JL: Why iron deficiency is important in infant development. J Nutr 2008, 138(12):2534-2536.
19. Beard JL, Wiesinger JA, Connor JR: Pre- and postweaning iron deficiency alters myelination in Sprague–Dawley rats. Dev Neurosci 2003, 25(5):308-315.
20. Beard J: Iron deficiency alters brain development and functioning. J Nutr 2003, 133(5 Suppl 1):1468S-1472S.
21. Burhans MS, Dailey C, Beard Z, Wiesinger J, Murray-Kolb L, Jones BC, Beard JL: Iron deficiency: differential effects on monoamine transporters. Nutr Neurosci 2005, 8(1):31-38.
22. Parks YA, Wharton BA: Iron deficiency and the brain. Acta Paediatr Scand Suppl 1989, 361:71-77.
23. Beard JL, Unger EL, Bianco LE, Paul T, Rundle SE, Jones BC: Early postnatal iron repletion overcomes lasting effects of gestational iron deficiency in rats. J Nutr 2007, 137(5):1176-1182.
24. Erikson KM, Jones BC, Beard JL: Iron deficiency alters dopamine transporter functioning in rat striatum. J Nutr 2000, 130(11):2831-2837.
25. Erikson KM, Jones BC, Hess EJ, Zhang Q, Beard JL: Iron deficiency decreases dopamine D1 and D2 receptors in rat brain. Pharmacol Biochem Behav 2001, 69(3–4):409-418.
26. Pinero DJ, Li NQ, Connor JR, Beard JL: Variations in dietary iron alter brain iron metabolism in developing rats. J Nutr 2000, 130(2):254-263.
27. Anderson JG, Fordahl SC, Cooney PT, Weaver TL, Colyer CL, Erikson KM: Extracellular norepinephrine, norepinephrine receptor and transporter protein and mRNA

levels are differentially altered in the developing rat brain due to dietary iron deficiency and manganese exposure. Brain Res 2009, 1281:1-14.

28. Erikson KM, Syversen T, Steinnes E, Aschner M: Globus pallidus: a target brain region for divalent metal accumulation associated with dietary iron deficiency. J Nutr Biochem 2004, 15(6):335-341.

29. Shukla A, Agarwal KN, Chansuria JP, Taneja V: Effect of latent iron deficiency on 5-hydroxytryptamine metabolism in rat brain. J Neurochem 1989, 52(3):730-735.

30. Grantham-McGregor S, Ani C: A review of studies on the effect of iron deficiency on cognitive development in children. J Nutr 2001, 131(2S-2):649S-666S.

31. Lozoff B, Jimenez E, Wolf AW: Long-term developmental outcome of infants with iron deficiency. N Engl J Med 1991, 325(10):687-694.

32. Cortese S, Azoulay R, Castellanos FX, Chalard F, Lecendreux M, Chechin D, Delorme R, Sebag G, Sbarbati A, Mouren MC: Brain iron levels in attention-deficit/hyperactivity disorder: A pilot MRI study. World J Biol Psychiatry 2012, 13(3):223-231.

33. Oner O, Alkar OY, Oner P: Relation of ferritin levels with symptom ratings and cognitive performance in children with attention deficit-hyperactivity disorder. Pediatr Int 2008, 50(1):40-44.

34. Millichap JG, Yee MM, Davidson SI: Serum ferritin in children with attention-deficit hyperactivity disorder. Pediatr Neurol 2006, 34(3):200-203.

35. Herguner S, Kelesoglu FM, Tanidir C, Copur M: Ferritin and iron levels in children with autistic disorder. Eur J Pediatr 2012, 171(1):143-146.

36. Latif A, Heinz P, Cook R: Iron deficiency in autism and Asperger syndrome. Autism 2002, 6(1):103-114.

37. Chen MH, Su TP, Chen YS, Hsu JW, Huang KL, Chang WH, Bai YM: Attention deficit hyperactivity disorder, tic disorder, and allergy: Is there a link? A nationwide population-based study. J Child Psychol Psychiatry 2013, 54(5):545-551.

38. Chen MH, Su TP, Chen YS, Hsu JW, Huang KL, Chang WH, Bai YM: Allergic rhinitis in adolescence increases the risk of depression in later life: a nationwide population-based prospective cohort study. J Affect Disord 2013, 145(1):49-53.

39. Li CT, Bai YM, Huang YL, Chen YS, Chen TJ, Cheng JY, Su TP: Association between antidepressant resistance in unipolar depression and subsequent bipolar disorder: cohort study. Br J Psychiatry 2012, 200(1):45-51.

40. Lozoff B, Jimenez E, Hagen J, Mollen E, Wolf AW: Poorer behavioral and developmental outcome more than 10 years after treatment for iron deficiency in infancy. Pediatrics 2000, 105(4):E51.

41. Pollitt E: Early iron deficiency anemia and later mental retardation. Am J Clin Nutr 1999, 69(1):4-5.

42. Beltran-Navarro B, Matute E, Vasquez-Garibay E, Zarabozo D: Effect of chronic iron deficiency on neuropsychological domains in infants. J Child Neurol 2012, 27(3):297-303.

43. Halterman JS, Kaczorowski JM, Aligne CA, Auinger P, Szilagyi PG: Iron deficiency and cognitive achievement among school-aged children and adolescents in the United States. Pediatrics 2001, 107(6):1381-1386.

44. Menegassi M, Mello ED, Guimaraes LR, Matte BC, Driemeier F, Pedroso GL, Rohde LA, Schmitz M: Food intake and serum levels of iron in children and ado-

lescents with attention-deficit/hyperactivity disorder. Rev Bras Psiquiatr 2010, 32(2):132-138.

45. Tan LN, Wei HY, Zhang YD, Lu AL, Li Y: Relationship between serum ferritin levels and susceptibility to attention deficit hyperactivity disorder in children: a Meta analysis. Zhongguo Dang Dai Er Ke Za Zhi 2011, 13(9):722-724.

46. Lozoff B: Iron deficiency and child development. Food Nutr Bull 2007, 28(4 Suppl):S560-571.

47. Lozoff B, Corapci F, Burden MJ, Kaciroti N, Angulo-Barroso R, Sazawal S, Black M: Preschool-aged children with iron deficiency anemia show altered affect and behavior. J Nutr 2007, 137(3):683-689.

48. Lozoff B, Georgieff MK: Iron deficiency and brain development. Semin Pediatr Neurol 2006, 13(3):158-165.

49. Carmody DP, Lewis M: Regional white matter development in children with autism spectrum disorders. Dev Psychobiol 2010, 52(8):755-763.

50. Conturo TE, Williams DL, Smith CD, Gultepe E, Akbudak E, Minshew NJ: Neuronal fiber pathway abnormalities in autism: an initial MRI diffusion tensor tracking study of hippocampo-fusiform and amygdalo-fusiform pathways. J Int Neuropsychol Soc 2008, 14(6):933-946.

51. Weinstein M, Ben-Sira L, Levy Y, Zachor DA, Ben Itzhak E, Artzi M, Tarrasch R, Eksteine PM, Hendler T, Ben Bashat D: Abnormal white matter integrity in young children with autism. Hum Brain Mapp 2011, 32(4):534-543.

52. Bodnar LM, Wisner KL: Nutrition and depression: implications for improving mental health among childbearing-aged women. Biol Psychiatry 2005, 58(9):679-685.

53. Vahdat Shariatpanaahi M, Vahdat Shariatpanaahi Z, Moshtaaghi M, Shahbaazi SH, Abadi A: The relationship between depression and serum ferritin level. Eur J Clin Nutr 2007, 61(4):532-535.

54. Yi S, Nanri A, Poudel-Tandukar K, Nonaka D, Matsushita Y, Hori A, Mizoue T: Association between serum ferritin concentrations and depressive symptoms in Japanese municipal employees. Psychiatry Res 2011, 189(3):368-372.

55. Leibenluft E: Severe mood dysregulation, irritability, and the diagnostic boundaries of bipolar disorder in youths. Am J Psychiatry 2011, 168(2):129-142.

56. Phillips ML: The neural basis of mood dysregulation in bipolar disorder. Cogn Neuropsychiatry 2006, 11(3):233-249.

57. Stein DJ, Horn N, Ramesar R, Savitz J: Bipolar disorder: emotional dysregulation and neuronal vulnerability. CNS Spectr 2009, 14(3):122-126.

58. Chang S, Wang L, Wang Y, Brouwer ID, Kok FJ, Lozoff B, Chen C: Iron-deficiency anemia in infancy and social emotional development in preschool-aged Chinese children. Pediatrics 2011, 127(4):e927-933.

59. Lozoff B: Early iron deficiency has brain and behavior effects consistent with dopaminergic dysfunction. J Nutr 2011, 141(4):740S-746S.

60. Schmidt AT, Ladwig EK, Wobken JD, Grove WM, Georgieff MK: Delayed alternation performance in rats following recovery from early iron deficiency. Physiol Behav 2010, 101(4):503-508.

61. Shukla A, Agarwal KN, Shukla GS: Latent iron deficiency alters gamma-aminobutyric acid and glutamate metabolism in rat brain. Experientia 1989, 45(4):343-345.

62. Beard JL, Erikson KM, Jones BC: Neurobehavioral analysis of developmental iron deficiency in rats. Behav Brain Res 2002, 134(1–2):517-524.
63. Suveg C, Morelen D, Brewer GA, Thomassin K: The emotion dysregulation model of anxiety: a preliminary path analytic examination. J Anxiety Disord 2010, 24(8):924-930.
64. Weems CF, Silverman WK: An integrative model of control: implications for understanding emotion regulation and dysregulation in childhood anxiety. J Affect Disord 2006, 91(2–3):113-124.
65. Mennin DS, Heimberg RG, Turk CL, Fresco DM: Preliminary evidence for an emotion dysregulation model of generalized anxiety disorder. Behav Res Ther 2005, 43(10):1281-1310.
66. Giedd JN, Rapoport JL: Structural MRI of pediatric brain development: what have we learned and where are we going? Neuron 2010, 67(5):728-734.
67. Toga AW, Thompson PM, Sowell ER: Mapping brain maturation. Trends Neurosci 2006, 29(3):148-159.
68. Cortese S, Lecendreux M, Bernardina BD, Mouren MC, Sbarbati A, Konofal E: Attention-deficit/hyperactivity disorder, Tourette's syndrome, and restless legs syndrome: the iron hypothesis. Med Hypotheses 2008, 70(6):1128-1132.
69. Gorman DA, Zhu H, Anderson GM, Davies M, Peterson BS: Ferritin levels and their association with regional brain volumes in Tourette's syndrome. Am J Psychiatry 2006, 163(7):1264-1272.

CHAPTER 11

VITAMIN D DEFICIENCY AND PSYCHOTIC FEATURES IN MENTALLY ILL ADOLESCENTS: A CROSS-SECTIONAL STUDY

BARBARA L. GRACIOUS, TERESA L. FINUCANE,
MERIEL FRIEDMAN-CAMPBELL, SUSAN MESSING,
AND MELISSA N PARKHURST

11.1 BACKGROUND

Vitamin D deficiency is endemic across the life span and in diverse populations throughout the world [1]. Contributing factors are lack of exposure to sunlight and insufficient dietary intake; individuals with darker skin are at higher risk due to low cutaneous synthesis and dairy-poor diets. In a study of healthy Northeastern US adolescents, more than 90% of African American teens and 55% of all teens had low vitamin D [2]. The National Health and Nutritional Examination Survey (NHANES 2001–2004) found an overall US prevalence of vitamin D insufficiency in adolescents of 61%, with 9% deficient [3].

Vitamin D Deficiency and Psychotic Features in Mentally Ill Adolescents: A Cross-Sectional Study. ©
Gracious BL, Finucane TL, Friedman-Campbell M, Messing S, and Parkhurst MN. BMC Psychiatry
12, 38 (2012); doi:10.1186/1471-244X-12-38. Licensed under Creative Commons Attribution 2.0 Generic License, http://creativecommons.org/licenses/by/2.0.

Vitamin D is well recognized as essential for intestinal calcium absorption, serum calcium homeostasis, optimal skeletal development, and the prevention of rickets and osteoporosis [4]. The importance of vitamin D to the CNS in both healthy and psychiatric populations is less well-appreciated and is vastly understudied compared to its known impact on bone health. Vitamin D receptors are present throughout the brain, and D-deficiency is associated with negative CNS effects in animal studies [5]. Vitamin D receptors and activating enzymes are particularly prominent in the hypothalamus and substantia nigra, and are involved in glucocorticoid signaling in hippocampal cells. Depletion models show maternal offspring with abnormal brain shape, cell number, and reduced neurotropic factors and receptors. Vitamin D receptor animal knock-out models show increased anxiety, decreased activity, and muscular and motor impairments, resembling phenotypic models of depression. Vitamin D is neuroprotective to hippocampal cells, through regulating calcium ion channels and activating PKC and mapPK pathways.

Clinical studies reinforce the significance of this basic work. A Finnish cohort supplemented with prenatal and infant vitamin D demonstrated reduced adult risk for schizophrenia [6]. Low vitamin D levels were found to correlate with major depression [7] and premenstrual mood symptoms in women [8], and mood disorders and cognitive impairment in older adults [9]. Two randomized controlled trials (RCT) have shown that raising vitamin D levels improved depression. The first study examined phototherapy vs. vitamin D supplementation for seasonal affective disorder, and found a positive effect for vitamin D via either supplementation or phototherapy within one month [10]. Another RCT of overweight and obese subjects, at greater risk for low vitamin D than those of normal weight, found higher levels of depression with low vitamin D; supplementation resulted in significant improvement in depressive symptoms after one year [11]. To the best of our knowledge, there have been no published studies examining vitamin D deficiency and the presence of psychosis in adolescents.

We hypothesized that, in severely mentally ill adolescents, defined as adolescents requiring either inpatient or partial hospitalization, 1) rates of vitamin D insufficiency and deficiency would be greater than those documented in general US populations, and 2) lower vitamin D levels would be associated with mental illness severity, defined as presence of psychotic features.

11.2 METHODS AND MATERIALS

11.2.1 ETHICS

The University of Rochester Research Subject Review Board approved the retrospective chart review study.

11.2.2 PARTICIPANTS

The study population included 75 females and 29 males aged 12 to 18 years admitted to the Strong Behavioral Health Child and Adolescent Acute Inpatient Service or Partial Hospitalization Service (CAPHS), Department of Psychiatry, University of Rochester, NY, between October 2008-February 2010 who had serum 25-OH vitamin D levels collected on routine admission laboratory testing as part of a quality improvement initiative.

11.2.3 DATA COLLECTION

Charts were identified by a clinical admission database of the service. Diagnostic evaluations and symptom reports from parents/legal guardians and adolescents were extracted from medical records for the period of clinical care.

11.2.4 CLINICAL DIAGNOSES

Clinical DSM-IV diagnoses were predominantly affective disorders (bipolar disorders, N=37; depressive disorders, N=36; mood disorder NOS, N=15; psychotic disorders, N=8; anxiety disorders, N=4; and ADHD/ODD N=1).

11.2.5 PATIENT-REPORTED PSYCHOSIS AND POTENTIALLY RELATED VARIABLES

Psychotic symptoms, defined as hallucinations, paranoia, or delusions, were documented on standardized admission assessment forms by the emergency room psychiatrist and the admitting attending. They were categorized dichotomously as yes/no by the second author (TLF), who was blinded to both the purpose of the study and to vitamin D levels until after record extraction was completed. Other variables examined included: race, month of admission/vitamin D level, insurance status, urban/suburban/rural residence, inpatient/partial hospital outpatient, clinical DSM-IV diagnosis, smoking status, age of onset of mental illness, admitting medications, past medications, and immediate and extended family psychiatric and medical history.

11.2.6 VITAMIN D LABORATORY ANALYSIS AND CATEGORICAL DEFINITIONS

Vitamin D 25-OH (25OHD) levels were analyzed by chemiluminescent immunoassay at ARUP laboratories, SLC, Utah, and recorded as normal if >30 ng/ml, insufficient if 20–30 ng/ml, and deficient if <20 ng/ml, as per expert guidelines [12].

11.2.7 STATISTICAL ANALYSES

Continuous data were graphically inspected for distributional assumptions; comparisons between the normal, insufficient, and deficient vitamin D groups were evaluated by ANOVAs (with t-tests subsequent to the overall analysis), Wilcoxon rank sum test, χ^2, or Fisher's exact test, as appropriate to the data. The relationship of vitamin D levels and psychosis was assessed with an ANOVA type design and the association of psychosis with vitamin D level groups with logistic regression models, assessing race as well as vitamin D level groups in a multivariate model. All analyses were carried out using SAS 9.2 on a Windows 7 platform.

TABLE 1: Patient Characteristics by 25-OH Vitamin D Levels

Variable	All N=104 X (1SD) or n (%)	Deficient (<20 ng/ ml) N=35 X (1SD) or n (%)	Not Deficient N=69 X (1SD) or n (%)	p-value*
Demographics				
Age	15.38±1.6	15.28± 1.63	15.43± 1.60	0.66
Sex (M/F) (%Male)	29/75 (27.9)	11/24 (31.4)	18/51 (27.9)	0.57
Race (White/Black/Hispanic/ Asian/ Biracial) (%White)	76/15/1/5/7 (73.1)	17/9/0/5/4 (50.0)	59/6/1/0/3 (67.0)	0.0003
Residence (Urban/ Suburban or Rural) (%Urban)	10/94 (9.6)	3/32 (8.6)	7/62 (6.7)	0.80
Insurance (Private/ Medicaid) (%Private)	65/39 (62.5)	19/16 (54.3)	46/23 (66.7)	0.22
Smoking Status (Yes/No) (%Yes)	18/67 (21.2)	9/20 (31)	9/47 (16.1)	0.11
Inpatient or Outpatient Status (Inpatient/ Outpatient) (% Inpatient)	34/70 (32.7)	14/21 (40)	20/49 (29.0)	0.26
Metabolic Variables				
Body Mass Index (BMI)	25.2±7.6	26.1±8.4	24.7±7.2	0.39
Glucose	93.9±18.1	91.7±13.8	94.9±19.7	0.42
Cholesterol, total	167.4±34.4	167.6±30.8	167.3+36.7	0.98
High Density Lipoprotein (HDL)	53.1±13.9	54.3±13.5	52.4±14.3	0.63
Low Density Lipoprotein (LDL)	94.0±25.0	95.7±21.9	93.0±26.8	0.71
Triglycerides	96.0±69.3	87.6±57.6	100.5±75.2	0.52
Pulse	79.6±15.6	78.4±12.4	80.3±16.7	0.57
Diastolic Blood Pressure	67.6±9.0	69.1±9.3	66.7±8.7	0.20
Systolic Blood Pressure	115.3±12.7	116.9±14.3	114.5±11.9	0.39
Illness Features and Family History				
Psychosis N, (%)	25 (24.0)	14 (40.0)	11 (15.9)	0.007
Immediate Family Psychosis N, (%)	10 (9.6)	4 (11.4)	6 (8.7)	0.66
Extended Family Psychosis N, (%)	10 (9.6)	5 (14.3)	5 (7.3)	0.25
Illness Age of Onset (Prepubertal/ Adolescent) (% Prepubertal)	45/55 (45)	14 (41.2)	31 (47.0)	0.69
DSM-IV diagnoses, N (%)				
Bipolar Disorders	37 (36)	13 (37)	24 (34.8)	0.81
Unipolar Depressive	36 (35)	9 (25.7)	27 (39.1)	0.17
Mood Disorder NOS	15 (14)	6 (17.1)	9 (13.0)	0.57
Anxiety Disorder NOS	5 (5)	2 (5.7)	3 (4.3)	0.76
Psychotic Disorder NOS	8 (7.7)	5 (14.3)	3 (4.3)	0.07

TABLE 1: *Cont.*

Variable	All N=104 X (1SD) or n (%)	Deficient (<20 ng/ ml) N=35 X (1SD) or n (%)	Not Deficient N=69 X (1SD) or n (%)	p-value*
Other (Yes/No) (%Yes)	3 (1.3)	0 (0.0)	3 (4.3)	0.21
Current Medication Exposure, N (%)				
Stimulants N, (%)	6 (5.8)	2(5.7)	4 (5.8)	0.99
Antidepressants N, (%)	44 (42.3)	11 (31.4)	33 (47.8)	0.11
Antipsychotics N, (%)	35 (33.7)	12 (34.3)	23 (66.7)	0.92
Anticonvulsants N, (%)	18 (17.3)	5 (14.9))	13 (18.8)	0.56
Benzodiazepines N, (%)	6 (5.8)	3 (8.6)	3 (4.35)	0.38
Other medications	31 (29.8)	8 (22.9)	23 (33.3)	0.27
Past Medication Exposure, N (%)				
Stimulants N, (%)	18 (17.3)	7 (20.0)	11 (15.9)	0.60
Antidepressants N, (%)	42 (40.4)	12 (34.3)	30 (56.5)	0.37
Antipsychotics N, (%)	21 (20.2)	6 (17.1)	15 (21.7)	0.58
Anticonvulsants N, (%)	20 (19.2)	4 (11.4)	16 (23.2)	0.15
Benzodiazepines N, (%)	3 (2.88)	0 (0.0)	3 (4.35)	0.21
Other medications	9 (8.7)	2 (5.7)	7 (10.1)	0.4

*Evaluated by ANOVA, Wilcoxon rank sum test, χ^2, or Fisher's exact test. Missing data were present for the following (N): BMI, 4;, glucose 5; cholesterol and HDL 50; LDL 49; TG 49, pulse 4, DBP and SBP 5; calcium 6; height 4; waist circumference 50; weight 3.

11.3 RESULTS

11.3.1 VITAMIN D DEFICIENCY PREVALENCE AND ASSOCIATION WITH PSYCHOSIS

Thirty-five (33.7%) adolescents were vitamin D deficient (<20 ng/ml), and an additional 40 (38.4%) were vitamin D insufficient (20–30 ng/ml). Of those with vitamin D deficiency, 40% had psychotic features compared to only 16% of the sample who were not vitamin D deficient (p<0.007). Those with D deficiency were 3½ times more likely to have psychotic features (OR 3.52, CI 1.38-8.95, 1df). Of those with normal vitamin D status, 79% (N=23/29) did not have psychotic features.

11.3.2 DEMOGRAPHIC AND OTHER RELATED VARIABLE DIFFERENCES

A comparison of demographic variables between adolescents with insufficient, deficient, and normal 25-OH D levels is presented in Table 1.

11.3.3 RACIAL DIFFERENCES

Those who were deficient were more likely to be black or Asian (Figure 1) and have psychotic features (Figure 2). Figure 3 displays the association of 25-OH vitamin D and the interaction of race and psychosis. All groups showed lower 25-OH D levels in the presence of psychosis including Asians who were all deficient. Asian (N=5) and biracial (N=7) categories were combined into the "Other" category and Hispanic/Latino ethnicity (N=1) was combined with Caucasian in the linear modeling that was conducted. Odds ratio comparisons for presence of psychosis with vitamin D deficiency as well as potential covariates, including race and medication exposure, are depicted in Table 2. Psychosis was independently related to race for the "other" group (Asian and biracial individuals) vs. white group, but not for black vs. white groups, nor significantly associated for other vs. blacks. The association of psychosis and vitamin D level was significant overall in the univariate and multivariable analyses. Of added interest was the association of psychosis with Vitamin D levels and race (Table 3). While race and vitamin D levels were associated, race and psychosis were not associated adjusting for vitamin D levels.

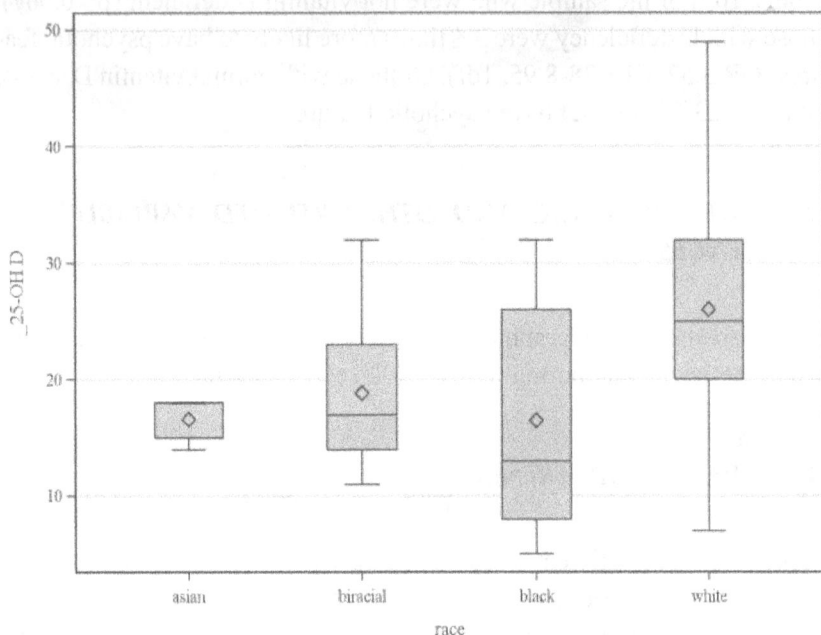

FIGURE 1: Box-Whisker plot of vitamin D levels by race.

11.3.4 FAMILY HISTORY, MEDICATION EXPOSURE, AND SEASONAL DIFFERENCES

Immediate family history of psychosis and current antidepressant exposure were also independently related to psychosis. Rates of vitamin D insufficiency and deficiency rose from December through March, peaking in March, as would be expected. No seasonal effects, however, were statistically detected (p=0.14), possibly due to both latitude and high rates of overall deficiency and insufficiency.

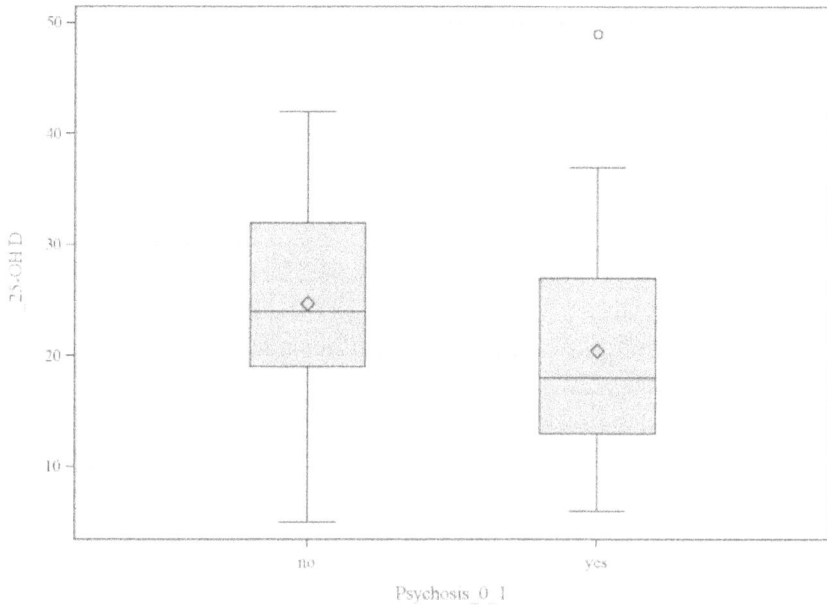

FIGURE 2: Box-Whisker plot of vitamin D levels by psychosis.

11.4 DISCUSSION

This is the first report of an association between vitamin D deficiency in adolescents and severity of mental illness, defined as presence of psychotic features. These findings are similar to a cross-sectional study also linking vitamin D deficiency and adult psychosis [13]. In a study of over 1,000 adults from combined cohorts of a longitudinal evaluation of severe mental illness and a population-based sample from the Oslo Health Study, vitamin D levels and presence of psychosis were compared between native Norwegians and dark-complexion immigrants to Norway. Prevalence of vitamin D deficiency and insufficiency in immigrants with psychosis was 80%, similar to the 72% in our sample of severely mentally ill adolescents.

Additionally, 43% of the Oslo community population with psychosis met criteria for vitamin D deficiency, also similar to the 40% of this teen sample with psychosis. In the adult epidemiologic sample, disorientation on the PANSS, weight loss, and lack of physical energy correlated with lower 25-OH D levels after controlling for major depression. Demographics, level of functioning, lifestyle habits, and BMI were not associated with vitamin D levels.

Our findings also agree with an unpublished 2011 report of a child and adolescent psychiatric population residing in the Pacific Northwest. Using the same definitions of deficiency, insufficiency, and normal ranges as in the current study, 21% of 67 youth with severe psychiatric symptoms residing in 2 Oregon residential treatment programs had vitamin D defi-

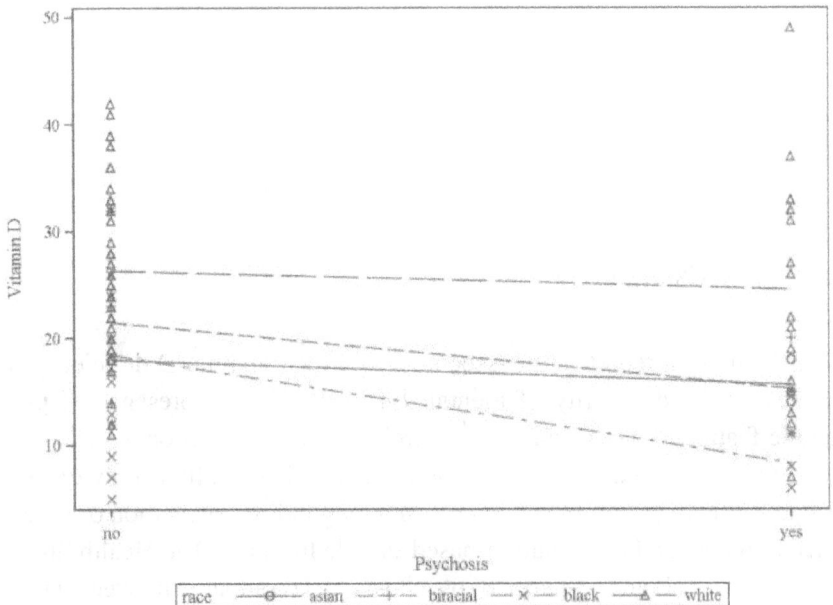

FIGURE 3: Association of psychosis, race, and interaction of psychosis and race on vitamin D level expressed as continuous data. Y-axis displays 25OH-D levels in ng/mL; left vs. right side of figure denotes mean 25OHD levels without and with psychosis by race.

ciency, vs. 14% of a comparable NHANES sample. For the children with psychotic disorders, the prevalence of vitamin D deficiency was 43% [14]. The overall mean 25-OH D level was 28.9 ng/mL, with 2/3 of the patients falling below the normal range; mean 25-OHD in the youth with psychotic disorders was 26.47 ng/mL (SD 12.42). Another group of psychiatric inpatient Parisian adolescents (N = 136) were also found to be largely vitamin D-deficient (72.4%), with the mean 25-OHD value 15–16 ng/mL, lower in blacks and North Africans [15]. No differences in mean levels were found between those taking or not taking antipsychotics, indicating that antipsychotics may not lower vitamin D absorption.

The prevalence of vitamin D deficiency in our sample of acutely mentally ill adolescents is also greater than the high rates observed in U.S. community adolescent populations (34% vs. NHANES 9%)[3] and in Australian adult private psychiatric inpatients (vitamin D deficiency 11%, defined as <25 nmol/L, or 10 ng/mL) [16]. The latter study found a 29% difference between mean levels in patients vs. controls. Our higher prevalence rates of deficiency and insufficiency may be in part due to the latitude of Rochester, NY, 43.145 degrees N. Paris, France is 48.51 N, and Geelong, Australia 38.10 S. Except during summer months, skin makes negligible vitamin D from sunlight at latitudes above 37 degrees north or below 37 degrees south.

11.4.1 POTENTIAL CAUSAL MECHANISMS

Basic and preclinical animal studies provide clues as to how vitamin D may lower risk for psychosis, and how vitamin D deficiency may raise risk for psychosis and depression. These mechanisms include 25-OH vitamin D and calciferol, the renal metabolite of 25-OH D (1,25-OH D): 1) altering neurotrophic factors and monoamine levels [17,18], resulting in vitamin D-related behavioral phenotypes similar to those for depression and psychosis [19], 2) facilitating oxidative stress responses [20], 3) changing multiple neuroendocrine transmitters [21,23], and 4) regulating hormonal and serotonin pathway effects within the CNS [24,25].

TABLE 2: Unadjusted associations between subject characteristics and psychosis

Variable	Odds Ratio*	95% CI	P-Value
Age §	0.91	(0.69, 1.20)	0.51
25_OH_D §	0.95	(0.90, 0.99)	0.04
Vitamin D Deficient vs. Not Deficient	3.52	(1.38,8.95)	0.008
BMI §	0.99	(0.94, 1.06)	0.88
CHOL §	0.99	(0.96, 1.01)	0.23
Calcium §	1.70	(0.53, 5.46)	0.38
DBP §	1.01	(0.96, 1.06)	0.73
GLU §	1.02	(0.99, 1.05)	0.07
HDL §	0.98	(0.93, 1.03)	0.40
LDL §	0.99	(0.97, 1.02)	0.71
Pulse §	1.00	(0.97, 1.03)	0.88
SBP §	0.99	(0.96, 1.03)	0.81
Trigl §	0.99	(0.97, 1.01)	0.23
Gender Female vs. Male	0.60	(0.23, 1.58)	0.30
Extended Family Psychosis	2.32	(0.60, 8.99)	0.22
Immediate Family Psychosis	5.92	(1.52, 23.11)	0.01
Onset at Adolescence vs. Prepuberty	1.78	(0.68, 4.68)	0.24
Living in Urban vs. Rural/Suburban setting	1.40	(0.33, 5.89)	0.64
Inpatient vs. Outpatient Status	1.22	(0.77, 3.12)	0.69
Private Insurance vs. Medicaid	0.45	(0.18, 1.13)	0.09
Race			0.16
Black vs. White	0.95	(0.24, 3.79)	0.95
Other vs. White **	3.81	(1.08,13.42)	0.04
Smoking (Yes vs. No)	2.92	(0.94, 9.07)	0.06
Current Medication †			
Antidepressants	0.19	(0.006, 0.41)	0.004
Antipsychotics	1.44	(0.57, 3.70)	0.44
Anticonvulsants	0.88	(0.26, 2.98)	0.84
Benzodiazepines	0.62	(0.03, 4.08)	0.67
Other Medications	0.89	(0.33, 2.41)	0.82
Past Medication			
Antidepressants	1.22	(0.49,,3.02)	0.67
Antipsychotics	1.81	(0.63, 5.14)	0.27
Anticonvulsants	1.07	(0.35, 3.30)	0.91

TABLE 2: *Cont.*

Variable	Odds Ratio*	95% CI	P-Value
Benzodiazepines	6.78	(0.59, 78.15)	0.13
Other Medications	0.89	(0.17,,4.61)	0.89
Stimulants	0.58	(0.15, 2.20)	0.43

*Bolded text denotes significance at p < 0.05. *Odds ratios greater than one indicates increased odds of psychosis. § Odds ratio is expressed for a unit increase in the independent variable. ** Other includes Asian and Biracial. † Current Stimulants evidenced 0 cell count which resulted in questionable model fit.*

TABLE 3: Multiple regression model (adjusted) for association of subject characteristics and psychosis

Variable	Odds Ratio	95% CI	P-Value
Vitamin D Levels			
Deficient vs Not Deficient	3.26	(1.15 9.19)	0.03
Race			0.33
Black vs. White	0.59	(0.14, 2.6)	0.49
Other vs. White **	1.68	(0.52, 7.67)	0.27
Other vs. Black	3.65	(0.64, 20.83)	0.14

**Odds ratios greater than one indicates increased odds of psychosis. ** White includes Hispanic; Other includes Asian and Biracial.*

11.4.2 RACE, ETHNICITY, DIETARY INTAKE AND SUNLIGHT EXPOSURE

Dietary intake and sunlight exposure as sources of vitamin D are influenced by race. The NHANES found poor dietary intake of vitamin D and lower exercise in older African American and female Hispanic adolescents. Although not fully comparable due to different methodologies, our mentally ill non-Caucasian population also demonstrates more vitamin D deficiency, and for Asians and biracial subjects a greater rate of psychosis, but not after adjusting for vitamin D level. Small clinical studies to date suggest potential for a causal link between low vitamin D and mood disorders [8-11,16,26], necessitating that randomized controlled trials in carefully defined populations of interest be performed to better characterize the relationship between vitamin D deficiency and risk for depression and psychosis.

11.4.3 ALTERNATE HYPOTHESES

In addition to the possibility that vitamin D deficiency contributes to vulnerability to psychosis, other nutritional factors may play a role: adolescents eating a diet low in dairy products may also consume less of other nutrient-rich foods, including those with essential fatty acids. Adverse omega-3:omega-6 fatty acid ratios and/or other dietary micronutrient deficiencies that are commonly associated with vitamin D deficiency such as vitamin B12 may also contribute to emergence of psychotic symptoms.

11.4.4 IMPLICATIONS FOR FUTURE RESEARCH IN PSYCHIATRY

11.4.4.1 EFFECTS ON MENTAL ILLNESS

If a prospective association between psychotic features and vitamin D deficiency is confirmed, outstanding issues include: 1) how vitamin D affects monoamine function and the HPA axis and immune responses to stress and symptom production, 2) whether supplementation can be protective against incident depression or psychosis and their recurrence, and 3) whether supplementation improves symptoms in those with clinically diagnosed depression or psychosis, especially in populations with darker skin [26]. An open-label Swedish case-series suggests that depression is improved by vitamin D supplementation in adolescents [27]. Prevention studies in high-risk offspring would be highly novel. Thus, future studies could target both prevention of mental and comorbid physical illness, focusing on disparity and somatic treatment augmentation.

11.4.4.2 IMPORTANCE TO OVERALL HEALTH IN PSYCHIATRIC POPULATIONS

Normalizing vitamin D levels warrants study in those with severe mental illness to determine whether, and at what dose, vitamin D helps protect against metabolic side effects from psychopharmacologic treatment or reduces the development of comorbid physical illnesses such as diabetes, cardiovascular disease, and osteoporosis. Low vitamin D is associated with greater BMI, insulin resistance, and systolic blood pressure, lower HDL-C in obese adolescents and adults, and lower final height in young adult women [3,28-31]. Vitamin D status may be especially important in those with serious mental illness as they develop poorer metabolic health at earlier ages. Optimal vitamin D levels also may protect against several different cancers (breast, colon, pancreas, and prostate), and autoimmune disorders (lupus, multiple sclerosis, and Type I diabetes) [32]. Molecular mechanisms of vitamin D that are protective against cancer include reducing cellular oxidative stress [33]. Vitamin D supplementation may thus represent a low-cost population-based intervention capable of reducing utilization of more intensive physical and mental health treatments; multiple trials are underway assessing impact on a variety of physical health conditions including osteoporosis, insulin resistance, and cardiovascular risk. A large scale epidemiologic RCT (the Vitamin D and omega¬3 Trial; VITAL) is examining whether supplementation prevents chronic diseases (http://www.vitalstudy.org).

11.4.4.3 SUPPLEMENTATION ISSUES IN ADOLESCENTS

How should low vitamin D levels be corrected? Supplementation with over-the-counter or prescription vitamin D for those with low vitamin D is important, as natural dietary sources are few and include chiefly oily fish, irradiated mushrooms, egg yolks, and fortified milk, juices, cereal, and margarine   (http://dietary¬supplements.info.nih.gov/factsheets/vitamind. asp). Most adolescents, especially those who skip breakfast or are lactose intolerant, do not consume adequate amounts of these foods to maintain optimal vitamin D levels, and cannot meet their requirements through diet alone. Risk for developing vitamin D toxicity with supplements has been largely unsupported [34]; studies giving as much as 14,000 IU per week of D3 to adolescents over one year's time have shown no evidence of toxicity [35]. A serum level of more than 200 ng/ml 25-OHD may be necessary for symptoms of toxicity to occur. The Institute of Medicine in 2010 raised its daily intake recommendations based on evidence for skeletal growth and maintenance; the current recommended dietary allowance (RDA) is 600 IU per day for 1–70 years of age with an upper level intake of 4,000 IU per day [36]. The American Academy of Pediatrics had previously raised its recommended supplementation from 200 IU in 2003 to 400 IU per day in 2008 to prevent rickets in children and adolescents who do not obtain this goal through fortified foods [37]. Additional initial supplementation to return deficient individuals to normal may be indicated as dietary reference intake amounts recommended by the IOM may still be insufficient for bone health maintenance in many individuals [38]. The amount necessary to prevent breast and colon cancer, Type I diabetes, and multiple sclerosis has been speculated to be closer to 4,000-8,000 IU per day [32]. The amount appropriate for maintenance of best mental and physical health is therefore controversial, and is unknown in the chronically mentally ill, who may metabolize vitamin D more quickly due to added oxidative stress burden.

11.4.5 LIMITATIONS

This work is limited by a small sample size, cross-sectional method, in-patient sampling bias, and lack of formal research measures for diagnosis and severity of illness, family psychiatric history, sun exposure, and intake of Vitamin D and other dietary nutrients. No adolescents, however, were taking vitamin D supplementation. A winter sampling bias is present, potentially contributing to low rates of D-deficiency, however, this does not rule out that seasonal effects in illness severity and admission rates related to greater vitamin D deficiency may occur. Analysis of ultraviolet radiation for latitudes 0 to 80 degrees N found that for March through October, sites from 18 degrees to 44 degrees N (the majority of the continental United States) had equal amounts of vitamin D producing ultraviolet light; November through February only demonstrated decreases in vitamin D producing ultraviolet light [39]. Additional limitations include that adolescents were not screened for osteomalacia; serum parathyroid hormone values were not routinely checked in those who were D-deficient; however, several performed clinically were within normal ranges. Many confidence intervals are wide; confirmation of these results awaits a large sample study and more rigorous design. Probing smaller enriched clinical samples may be useful in providing biologic signals of relevance in populations with depression, for example, using neurocognitive tasks. Descriptive differences in a clinical population compared with population norms may also provide direction for further investigation related to both interactive effects of mental illness and ancestry.

11.5 CONCLUSION

Vitamin D deficiency is highly prevalent in this descriptive sample of acutely mentally ill adolescents, especially in African-American and Asian teens, and appears related to psychotic symptoms. This work is the first to report an association between psychosis and vitamin D deficiency in psychiatrically hospitalized adolescents [40] and confirms this association found previously in an adult population [13]. Our study also expands on similar deficiency findings from a Parisian inpatient adolescent cohort [15], providing clinical diagnoses of mood disorders in the great majority of inpatient teens with vitamin D deficiency, and further, finding lower risk for psychosis in the presence of antidepressant treatment. Both support the possibility that heightened vulnerability to psychotic features occurs in the substantial proportion of teens with mood disorders who are vitamin D deficient. Prospective trials of vitamin D supplementation are needed to address targeted mental health symptom domains as well as metabolic health variables in D-deficient severely mentally ill adolescents and adults, focusing on dose-finding and tolerability. Calls have been made for clinical monitoring in patients with psychiatric illness as well as randomized trials of vitamin D for depression [41,42]. Clinical screening for vitamin D deficiency in severely mentally ill adolescents is justified by their high risk for both chronic mental illness and early onset of cardiometabolic comorbidities, especially as vitamin D deficiency at mid-life appears a strong independent predictor of all-cause mortality (odds ratios 2.64, 95% CI 1.901 to 3.662. p<0.0001) [43]. A key clinical question raised by our work and supported by known safety data is whether psychiatrically hospitalized dark-complected adolescents, including African-Americans, Asians, and Muslim females in traditional covered dress, should be routinely supplemented with vitamin D until proven otherwise.

REFERENCES

1. Holick MF, Chen TC: Vitamin D deficiency: a worldwide problem with health consequences. Am J Clin Nutr 2008, 87:1080S-1086S. suppl
2. Gordon CM, DePeter KC, Feldman HA, Grace E, Emans SJ: Prevalence of vitamin D deficiency among healthy adolescents. Arch Pediatr Adolesc Med 2004, 158:531-537.
3. Kumar J, Muntner P, Kaskel FJ, Hailpern SM, Melamed ML: Prevalence and associations of 25-hydroxyvitamin D deficiency in US children: NHANES 2001–2004. Pediatrics 2009, 124:e362-e370.
4. Holick MF: Sunlight and vitamin D for bone health and prevention of autoimmune diseases, cancers, and cardiovascular disease. Am J Clin Nutr 2004, 80(6 Suppl):1678S-1688S.
5. McCann J, Ames B: Is there convincing biological or behavioral evidence linking vitamin D deficiency to brain dysfunction? FASEB J 2008, 22:982-1001.
6. McGrath J, Saari K, Hakko H, Jokelainen J, Jones P, Järvelin MR, Chant D, Isohanni M: Vitamin D supplementation during the first year of life and risk of schizophrenia: a Finnish birth cohort study. Schizophr Res 2004, 67(2–3):237-245.
7. Eskandari F, Martinez PE, Torvik S, Phillips TM, Sternberg EM, Mistry S, Ronsaville D, Wesley R, Toomey C, Sebring NG, Reynolds JC, Blackman MR, Calis KA, Gold PW, Cizza G: Low bone mass in premenopausal women with depression. Arch Intern Med 2007, 167:2329-2336.
8. Thys-Jacobs S, Silberton M, Alvir J, Paddison P, Rico M, Coldsmith R: Reduced bone mass in women with premenstrual syndrome. J Wom Health 1995, 4:161-168.
9. Wilkins C, Sheline Y, Roe C, Birge S, Morris J: Vitamin D deficiency is associated with low mood and worse cognitive performance in older adults. Am J Geriatr Psychiatr 2006, 14:1032-1040.
10. Gloth FM, Alam W, Hillis B: Vitamin D vs broad spectrum phototherapy in the treatment of seasonal affective disorder. J Nutr Health Aging 1999, 3(1):5-7.
11. Jorde R, Sneve M, Figenschau Y, Svartberg J, Waterloo K: Effects of vitamin D supplementation on symptoms of depression in overweight and obese subjects: randomized double blind trial. J Intern Med 2008, 264(6):599-609.

12. Norman AW, Bouillon R, Whiting SJ, Vieth R, Lips P: 13th workshop consensus for vitamin D nutritional guidelines. J Steroid Biochem Mol Biol 2007, 103(3–5):204-205.

13. Berg AO, Melle I, Torjesen PA, Lien L, Hauff E, Andreassen OA: A cross-sectional study of vitamin D deficiency among immigrants and Norwegians with psychosis compared to the general population. J Clin Psychiatr 2010, 71(12):1598-1604. Epub 2010 Apr 6

14. Zhang M, Cheng K, Fetmalani A, Rope R, Martin E: Do children with psychiatric disorders have a higher prevalence of hypovitaminosis D? In New Research Poster 01–67; Annual American Psychiatric Association Annual Meeting. , Honolulu, Hawaii; 2011.

15. Bonnot O, Inaoui R, Raffin-Viard M, Bodeau N, Coussieu C, Cohen D: Children and adolescents with severe mental illness need Vitamin D supplementation regardless of disease or treatment. J Child Adolesc Psychopharmacol 2011, 21(2):157-161.

16. Berk M, Jacka FN, Williams LF, Ng F, Dodd S, Pasco JA: Is this D vitamin to worry about? Vitamin D insufficiency in an inpatient sample. Aust New Zeal J Psychiatr 2008, 42:874-878.

17. Cass WA, Smith MP, Peters LE: Calcitriol protects against the dopamine- and serotonin-depleting effects of neurotoxic doses of methamphetamine. Ann NY Acad Sci 2006, 1074:261-271.

18. Baksi SN, Hughes MJ: Chronic vitamin D deficiency in the weanling rat alters catecholamine metabolism in the cortex. Brain Res 1982, 242:387-390.

19. Harms LR, Eyles DW, McGrath JJ, Mackay-Smith A, Burne THJ: Developmental vitamin D deficiency alters adult behavior in 129/SvJ and C57BL/6 J mice. Behav Brain Res 2008, 187:343-350.

20. Berk M, Ng F, Dean O, Dodd S, Bush AI: Glutathione: a novel treatment target in psychiatry. Trends Pharmacol Sci 2008, 29:346-351.

21. Stumpf WE, O'Brien LP: 1,25 (OH)2 vitamin D3 sites of action in the brain. An autoradiographic study. Histochemistry 1987, 87:393-406.

22. Stumpf WE: Vitamin D sites and mechanisms of action: a histochemical perspective. Reflections on the utility of autoradiography and cytopharmacology for drug targeting. Histochem Cell Biol 1995, 104:417-427.

23. Wion D, MacGrogan D, Neveu I, Jehan F, Houlgatte R, Brachet P: 1,25-Dihydroxyvitamin D3 is a potent inducer of nerve growth factor synthesis. J Neurosci Res 1991, 28:110-114.

24. Watson LC, Marx CE: New onset of neuropsychiatric symptoms in the elderly: possible primary hyperparathyroidism. Psychosomatics 2002, 43:413-417.

25. Partonen T: Vitamin D and serotonin in winter. Med Hypotheses 1998, 51:267-268.

26. Bertone-Johnson ER: Vitamin D and the occurrence of depression: causal association or circumstantial evidence? Nutr Rev 2009, 67(8):481-492.

27. Högberg G, Gustafsson S, Hällström T, Gustafsson T, Klawitter B, Petersson M: Depressed adolescents in a case-series were low in vitamin D and depression was ameliorated by vitamin D supplementation. Accepted article. Acta Paediatr

28. Smotkin-Tangorra M, Purushothaman R, Gupta A, Negati G, Anhalt H, Ten S: Prevalence of vitamin D insufficiency in obese children and adolescents. J Pediatr Endocrinol Metab 2007, 20(7):817-23.

29. McGill A, Stewart JM, Lithander FE, Strik CM, Poppitt SD: Relationships of low serum vitamin D3 with anthropometry and markers of the metabolic syndrome and diabetes in overweight and obesity. Nutr J 2008, 7:4.

30. Reis JP, von Muhlen D, Miller ER, Michos ED, Appel LJ: Vitamin D status and cardiometabolic risk factors in the United States adolescent population. Pediatrics 2009, 124(3):e371-379.

31. Kremer R, Campbell PP, Reinhardt Gilsanz V: Vitamin D status and its relationship to body fat, final height, and peak bone mass in young women. J Clin Endocrinol Metab 2009, 94:67-73.

32. Garland C, Garland F, Gorham E, Lipkin M, Newmark H, Mohr S: The role of vitamin D in cancer prevention. Am J Public Health 2006, 96:252-61.

33. Bao BY, Ting HJ, Hsu JW, Lee YF: Protective role of 1α, 25-dihydroxyvitamin D3 against oxidative stress in nonmalignant human prostate epithelial cells. Int J Cancer 2008, 122:26992706.

34. Vieth R, Chan P, MacFarlane GD: Efficacy and safety of vitamin D3 intake exceeding the lowest observed adverse effect level. Am J Clin Nutr 2001, 73:288-294.

35. Maalouf J, Nabulsi M, Vieth R, Kimball S, El-Rassi R, Mahfoud Z, Fuleihan GEH: Short- and Long-Term Safety of Weekly High-Dose Vitamin D3 Supplementation in School Children. J Clin Endocrinol Metab 2008, 93:2693-2701.

36. Ross AC, Taylor CL, Yaktine AL, Valle HB (Eds): Committee to Review Dietary Reference Intakes for Vitamin D and Calcium; Institute of Medicine. The National Academies Press, Washington, DC; 2011. Also: Institute of Medicine. Dietary Reference Intakes for Calcium and Vitamin D. November 30, 2010 http://www.iom.edu/Reports/2010/Dietary-Reference-Intakes-for-Calcium-and-Vitamin-D.aspx

37. Wagner CL, Greer FR: and the Section on Breastfeeding and Committee on Nutrition: Prevention of rickets and vitamin D deficiency in infants, children, and adolescents. Pediatrics 2008, 122:1142-1152. http://www.aap.org/new/VitaminDreport.pdf

38. Heaney RP, Holick MF: Why the IOM recommendations for Vitamin D are deficient. J Bone Miner Res 2011, 26:455-457.

39. Kimlin MG, Olds WJ, Moore MR: Location and vitamin D synthesis: Is the hypothesis validated by geophysical data? J Photochem Photobiol B Biol 2007, 86:234-239.

40. Gracious BL, Finucane TL, Campbell-Friedman M, Parkhurst MN, Messing S: 25-OH Vitamin D Deficiency Associated with Psychotic Features in Acutely Mentally Ill Adolescents. In New Research Poster 3.3, 57th Annual Meeting, American Academy of Child and Adolescent Psychiatry. , New York, NY; 2010.

41. Berk M, Sanders KM, Pasco JA, Jacka FN, Williams LJ, Hayles AL, Dodd S: Vitamin D deficiency may play a role in depression. Med Hypotheses 2007, 69:1316-1319.

42. Young SN: Has the time come for randomized controlled trials of vitamin D for depression? J Psychiatr Neurosci 2009, 34(1):3.

43. Vacek JL, Vanga SR, Good M, Lai SM, Lakkireddy D, Howard PA: Vitamin D deficiency and supplementation and relation to cardiovascular health. Am J Cardiol 2012, 109(3):359-63.Epub 2011 Nov 8

PART III

NUTRITIONAL INTERVENTIONS FOR IMPROVED COGNITIVE FUNCTION

CHAPTER 12

THE EFFECTS OF BREAKFAST ON BEHAVIOR AND ACADEMIC PERFORMANCE IN CHILDREN AND ADOLESCENTS

KATIE ADOLPHUS, CLARE L. LAWTON, AND LOUISE DYE

12.1 INTRODUCTION

Breakfast is widely acknowledged to be the most important meal of the day. Children who habitually consume breakfast are more likely to have favorable nutrient intakes including higher intake of dietary fiber, total carbohydrate and lower total fat and cholesterol (Deshmukh-Taskar et al., 2010). Breakfast also makes a large contribution to daily micronutrient intake (Balvin Frantzen et al., 2013). Iron, B vitamins (folate, thiamine, riboflavin, niacin, vitamin B6, and vitamin B12) and Vitamin D are approximately 20–60% higher in children who regularly eat breakfast compared with breakfast skippers (Gibson, 2003). Consuming breakfast can also contribute to maintaining a body mass index (BMI) within the normal range. Two systematic reviews report that children and adolescents who habitually consume breakfast [including ready-to-eat-cereal (RTEC)]

The Effects of Breakfast on Behavior and Academic Performance in Children and Adolescents. © *Adolphus K, Lawton CL, and Dye L.* Frontiers in Human Neuroscience *7,425 (2013); doi: 10.3389/ fnhum.2013.00425. Licensed under Creative Commons Attribution 3.0 Unported License, http://creativecommons.org/licenses/by/3.0/.*

have reduced likelihood of being overweight (Szajewska and Ruszczyn-ski, 2010; de la Hunty et al., 2013). Breakfast consumption is also associated with other healthy lifestyle factors. Children who do not consume breakfast are more likely to be less physically active and have a lower cardio respiratory fitness level (Sandercock et al., 2010). Moreover, there is evidence that breakfast positively affects learning in children in terms of behavior, cognitive, and school performance (Hoyland et al., 2009).

The assumptions about the benefit of breakfast for children's learning are largely based on evidence which demonstrates acute effects of breakfast on children's cognitive performance from laboratory based experimental studies. Although the evidence is quite mixed, studies generally demonstrate that eating breakfast has a positive effect on children's cognitive performance, particularly in the domains of memory and attention (Wesnes et al., 2003, 2012; Widenhorn-Muller et al., 2008; Cooper et al., 2011; Pivik et al., 2012). Additionally, the positive effects of breakfast are more demonstrable in children who are considered undernourished, typically defined as one standard deviation below normal height or weight for age using the US National Center for Health Statistics (NCHS) reference (Pollitt et al., 1996; Cueto et al., 1998). More recent evidence compares breakfast meals that differ in Glycaemic Load (GL), Glycaemic Index (GI) or both. This evidence generally suggests that a lower postprandial glycaemic response is beneficial to children's cognitive performance (Benton and Jarvis, 2007; Ingwersen et al., 2007; Micha et al., 2011; Cooper et al., 2012) however the evidence is equivocal (Brindal et al., 2012). Moreover, it remains unclear whether this effect is specifically due to GI or GL, or both, or to other effects unrelated to glycaemic response.

Studies rarely investigate the acute effects of breakfast on behavior in the classroom and there remains a lack of research in this area. This may be, in part, attributed to the complicated nature of the measures used to assess behavior in class and the need to develop standardized, validated, and comparable coding systems to measure behavior. Similarly, few studies examine the effects of breakfast on tangible academic outcomes such as school grades or standardized achievement tests relative to cognitive outcomes. Whilst crude measures of academic performance may not provide the most sensitive indicator of the effects of breakfast, direct measures of academic performance are ecologically valid, have most relevance to pupils, parents, teachers, and educational policy makers and as a result may produce most impact.

Cognitive, behavioral, and academic outcomes are not independent. Changes in cognitive performance are likely to be reflected by changes in behavior. An increase in attention following breakfast, compared with no breakfast, may be reflected by an increase in on-task behavior during lessons. Similarly, changes in cognitive performance may also impact school performance and academic outcomes in a cumulative manner. The beneficial effects of eating breakfast on cognitive performance are expected to be short term and specific to the morning on which breakfast is eaten and to selective cognitive functions. These immediate or acute effects might translate to benefits in academic performance with habitual or regular breakfast consumption, but this has not been evaluated in most studies. Short term changes in cognitive function during lessons (e.g., memory and attention) may therefore translate, with habitual breakfast consumption, to meaningful changes in school performance by an increased ability to attend to and remember information during lessons. In class behavior also has important implications for school performance. This is because a prerequisite for academic learning is the ability to stay on task and sustain attention in class. Greater attention in class and engagement in learning activities (referred to as on-task behavior) are likely to be associated with a more productive learning environment which may impact academic outcomes in the long term.

Children may be particularly vulnerable to the nutritional effects of breakfast on brain activity and associated cognitive, behavioral, and academic outcomes. Children have a higher brain glucose metabolism compared with adults. Positron Emission Tomography studies indicate that cerebral metabolic rate of glucose utilization is approximately twice as high in children aged 4–10 years compared with adults. This higher rate of glucose utilization gradually declines from age 10 and usually reaches adult levels by the age of 16–18 years (Chugani, 1998). Average cerebral blood flow and cerebral oxygen utilization is 1.8 and 1.3 times higher in children aged 3–11 years compared with adults, respectively (Kennedy and Sokoloff, 1957; Chiron et al., 1992). Moreover, the longer overnight fasting period, due to higher sleep demands during childhood and adolescence compared with adults, can deplete glycogen stores overnight (Thorleifsdottir et al., 2002). To maintain this higher metabolic rate, a continuous supply of energy derived from glucose is needed, hence breakfast consumption may be vital in providing adequate energy for the morning. Nevertheless, breakfast is the most frequently skipped meal. Between 20–30% of children and adolescents skip breakfast in the developed world (Deshmukh-Taskar et al., 2010; Corder et al., 2011).

Despite intense public and scientific interest and a widely promoted consensus that breakfast improves concentration and alertness, Hoyland et al. (2009) were only able to identify 45 studies on the effects of breakfast on objectively measured cognitive performance in the period of 1950–2008 in their systematic review. They concluded that breakfast consumption is more beneficial than skipping breakfast to cognitive outcomes, effects which were more apparent in children who are considered undernourished. They did not consider ecologically valid outcomes of behavior (in-class or at school) and academic performance. This article complements the Hoyland et al. (2009) review by considering the evidence on the effect of breakfast on behavior (in-class or at school) and academic performance in children and considers the methodological challenges in isolating the effects of breakfast from other factors. Findings will be discussed dependent on outcome measure and study design with effects evaluated based on breakfast manipulation where possible. The effects of breakfast in different populations will be considered, including children, adolescents who are undernourished or well-nourished and from differing socio-economic status (SES) backgrounds. The habitual and acute effects of breakfast will be considered along with the effects of school breakfast programs (SBPs).

12.2 METHODS

The literature was searched for original articles and reviews published between 1950–2013 on databases: Ovid MEDLINE, Pubmed, Web of Science, the Cochrane Library, EMBASE databases and PsychINFO. The search was conducted using the key words "breakfast" or "school breakfast" combined with "children" or "adolescents" combined with "behavio$," "on-task," "off-task," "concentration," "attention," "school performance," "academic performance," "scholastic performance," "academic achievement," "school grades," "school achievement," and "educational achievement" using the Boolean operator "and." The $ symbol was used for truncation to ensure the search included all keywords associated with behavior ("behavior," "behaviour," "behavioural," "behavioral"). Studies are limited to these outcomes in children and adolescents (<18 years). The reference lists of existing reviews and identified articles were examined individually to supplement the electronic search. The presentation of the results are organized by two main outcomes: In-class behavior/behavior at school and academic performance with corresponding summary tables which detail design, sample, breakfast intervention/dietary assessment, assessment of outcomes and reported results for each article. A total of 36 studies are included. Fourteen studies included behavior measures, seventeen studies included academic performance measures, and five studies examined both behavior and academic performance.

12.3 RESULTS

12.3.1 IN-CLASS BEHAVIOR AND BEHAVIOR AT SCHOOL

Nineteen studies employed behavioral measures to examine the effects of breakfast on behavior at school, either by use of classroom observations or rating scales usually completed by teachers (Table (Table1).1). Four studies included both classroom observations and rating scales (Kaplan et al., 1986; Milich and Pelham, 1986; Rosen et al., 1988; Richter et al., 1997).

12.3.2 OBSERVATIONS OF BEHAVIOR IN THE CLASSROOM

Direct measures of classroom behavior were utilized in 11 studies. Although there are inconsistent findings, the evidence indicated a mainly positive effect of breakfast on on-task behavior in the classroom in children. Seven of the eleven studies demonstrated a positive effect of breakfast on on-task behavior. This was apparent in children who were either well-nourished, undernourished and/or from low SES or deprived backgrounds. Two studies carried out in undernourished samples (Chang et al., 1996; Richter et al., 1997) and three studies in children from low SES backgrounds (Bro et al., 1994, 1996; Benton et al., 2007) demonstrated positive effects on on-task behavior following breakfast. One study reported a negative effect of a SBP on behavior in undernourished children (Cueto and Chinen, 2008) and three studies in children with behavioral problems demonstrated no effect of breakfast composition on behavior (Kaplan et al., 1986; Milich and Pelham, 1986; Wender and Solanto, 1991). Most studies included small samples of the order of 10–30 children which, although limited in terms of power and generalizability to the larger population, are more feasible and appropriate given the nature of the data and extensive coding methods required.

Intervention studies. Four intervention studies demonstrated a positive effect of SBPs on on-task behavior in undernourished and low SES children. Richter et al. (1997) reported a significant positive change in behavior from pre to post intervention in undernourished children aged 8 years. Following a 6-week SBP providing approximately 267 Kcal per day at breakfast, children in the intervention group displayed significantly less off-task and out of seat behavior and significantly more class participation (Richter et al., 1997). Concomitant teacher ratings of hyperactivity also declined significantly in the intervention group, however teachers reported no change in attention. This effect has also been demonstrated in adolescents. Two studies in small samples of adolescents aged 14–19 years showed an increase in on-task behavior in the classroom following an unstandardized teacher led SBP in vocational schools in USA (Bro et al., 1994, 1996). More recent evidence failed to show the same benefit in undernourished children (≤ -2 SD height-for-age of the NCHS reference) aged 11 years. Cueto and Chinen (2008) observed a reduction in on-task behavior following a 3-year SBP measured using time per day spent in the classroom as an indirect proxy measure. The design of the intervention required teachers to dedicate time to providing the breakfast mid-morning. This unexpected negative impact on on-task behavior is unlikely to occur when breakfast is delivered before school by non-teaching staff and when direct measures of classroom behavior are employed.

Acute experimental studies. Seven studies employed a within-subjects acute experimental design to examine the effects of breakfast on classroom behavior across the morning. The findings were inconsistent, with three of the seven studies showing an advantage of breakfast on on-task behavior (Chang et al., 1996; Benton and Jarvis, 2007; Benton et al., 2007).

Benton et al. (2007) observed classroom behavior and reaction to frustration following three isocaloric breakfast meals of high, medium or low GL in a sample of young children (mean age: 6 years 10 months) from a school in an economically disadvantaged area. Children spent significantly more time on-task following a low GL breakfast meal compared with medium and high GL breakfast meals. This effect was specific to the first 10 min of the observation. Children also displayed fewer signs of frustration during a video game observation, but again, effects were short lived and specific to the initial observation period. No significant effects were found for distracted behavior. Although meals aimed to be isocaloric, actual intake across conditions was variable and the macronutrient content differed between conditions. Consequently, the difference in classroom behavior may be due to differences in macronutrient content rather than GL. Four studies failed to find a similar advantage for on-task behavior in children with Attention Deficit Disorder with hyperactivity (ADD-H) or behavioral problems (Kaplan et al., 1986; Milich and Pelham, 1986; Wender and Solanto, 1991) or in primary school children without behavioral problems (Rosen et al., 1988) following breakfast meals that differed in sugar content.

Mixed results were reported when comparing the effects of breakfast vs. no breakfast in undernourished children. Chang et al. (1996) examined the effects of breakfast on classroom behavior in 57 undernourished (< −1 SD weight-for-age of the NCHS reference) and 56 adequately nourished children in Jamaican rural schools. A significant increase in on-task behavior was observed following a 520 Kcal breakfast, which was seen only in the well-equipped school. In the three less well-equipped schools, behavior deteriorated following breakfast with an observed increase in off-task behavior (talking, movement). The well-equipped school had separate classrooms for each class and each child had their own desk, an environment probably more conducive to positive in-class behavior. The deterioration of behavior following breakfast in the less well-equipped schools could reflect greater difficulties in accurately observing whether children are on-task or off-task when they do not have their own desk or are in overcrowded classrooms. In developed high income countries where school infrastructure is more standardized and where classrooms are not overcrowded, this possibly spurious effect is less likely to occur (Murphy et al., 2011; Ni Mhurchu et al., 2013). However, negative effects on behavior have also been reported in UK primary and secondary school children within deprived areas following a SBP (Shemilt et al., 2004). Therefore, other factors, including the breakfast club environment, delivery, and staff engagement with the SBP may have also influenced the impact of breakfast on behavior, as well as school structure. For example, activities during the breakfast club and general atmosphere may promote negative and excitable behavior. Nutritional status did not influence the results of Chang et al's study, however, the degree of undernourishment was mild. It is possible that positive effects may be more demonstrable in children who are more severely undernourished. In addition, an appropriate environment in terms of classroom structure and equipment is needed to accurately observe the effects of breakfast.

One study examined the effects of breakfast size with or without a mid-morning snack (Benton and Jarvis, 2007). The results indicated that children who consumed a small breakfast (<150 Kcal) spent significantly more time on-task when a mid-morning snack was also eaten. This effect was not evident in children who consumed more energy at breakfast (151–230 Kcal and >230 Kcal). Correspondingly, children who consumed <150 Kcal at breakfast spent significantly more time off-task when no snack was eaten compared with children who consumed more energy at breakfast. This suggests a mid-morning snack is only beneficial for children who have skipped or eaten very little for breakfast and corrects the energy deficiency.

12.3.3 RATING SCALES AND QUESTIONNAIRES

Twelve studies utilized teacher completed rating scales to assess children's behavior at school following breakfast. These studies usually employed global scales to assess a range of behavioral domains including: attention, disruptive behavior, hyperactivity, pro-social behavior, and aggression. The majority used standardized, established measures of behavior comparable across studies. Measures included the Strength and Difficulties Questionnaire (SDQ), Social Skills Rating System (SSRS), Child Behavior Checklist (CBCL) Conners Teacher Rating Scale (CTRS), and The Attention Deficit Disorder—Hyperactivity Comprehensive Teacher's Rating Scale (ACTeRS). Of the 12 studies that utilized rating scales and questionnaires, only two studies used unstandardized questionnaires and interviews with teachers to measure behavior (Wahlstrom and Begalle, 1999; Overby and Hoigaard, 2012). Six of the twelve studies demonstrated a positive effect of breakfast on behavior at school, which was mainly hyperactivity and disruptive behavior.

Intervention studies. Six intervention studies reported mixed evidence for the effects of SBPs on behavior at school. Two studies in low SES and undernourished children aged 8–10 years reported beneficial effects on hyperactivity (Richter et al., 1997; Murphy et al., 1998). In a longitudinal analysis of a 4-month SBP, Murphy et al. (1998) found significantly greater decreases in CTRS hyperactivity scores in children who increased participation in the SBP compared with children whose participation was unchanged. Similarly, results from a 6-week SBP in undernourished children indicated a significant decline in ACTeRS hyperactivity scores following the SBP, but no change in attention, social skills and oppositional behavior during lessons (Richter et al., 1997). Wahlstrom and Begalle (1999) reported an increase in social behavior and readiness to learn from interviews with teachers following a 3-year SBP. Their results also indicated a decrease in overall discipline referrals following the SBP. Whilst this evidence indicates an apparent benefit of SBPs on school behavior, methodological shortcomings, including a lack of randomization and the inclusion of an appropriate control group, cannot preclude the effects of confounding factors.

Three recent robust randomized control trials (RCT) that address the above inadequacies failed to find a similar benefit for school behavior measured by the SDQ following a 1 year intervention. Both Ni Mhurchu et al. (2013) and Murphy et al. (2011) reported no significant effects of a 1 year SBP on hyperactivity, inattention, emotional symptoms, conduct and peer relationship problems, and pro-social behavior in children. However, in both trials, SBP attendance was low and variable, limiting the potential impact on behavior. The barriers to participation in SBPs include a lack of parental support, a lack of teaching support, social stigma, busy morning schedules, transport issues preventing children from getting to school early and breakfast clubs causing children to arrive late to the first lesson (Reddan et al., 2002; McDonnell et al., 2004; Greves et al., 2007; Lambert et al., 2007). Furthermore, the proportion of children eating breakfast everyday remained unchanged whilst the proportion of children eating breakfast at home decreased, suggestive of a shift in consumption from at-home to at-school, rather than a change/increase in consumption. This may account for the lack of observed effects on behavior. Shemilt et al. (2004) indicated a negative impact of a SBP on behavior in both primary and secondary school children within deprived areas. Although this study aimed to employ a RCT design, contamination between treatment arms necessitated a longitudinal observational analysis of behavioral outcomes and SBP attendance, rather than the planned intention to treat analysis. Results at 1 year follow up indicated that children who attended the breakfast club had a higher incidence of borderline or abnormal conduct, prosocial, and total difficulties compared to children who did not attend the breakfast club (Shemilt et al., 2004). Teachers also indicated that children were more energetic, less well-behaved and were difficult to control in the classroom as a result of attending the breakfast club. Parallel qualitative data from teachers, breakfast club staff and researchers who observed the breakfast club suggested that children's behavior deteriorated during the breakfast club as a result of inadequate supervision and training, and a lack of teaching staff who seemed to be regarded with more authority by children. Observations of the breakfast club indicated behavior was often boisterous or disruptive and there was a general lively atmosphere. This suggests that factors associated with the delivery of the SBP had more impact on behavioral outcomes than the subtle nutritional effects of breakfast in this study. In addition, this study epitomizes the difficulties in isolating the independent effects of breakfast.

Acute experimental studies. Three acute experimental studies examined the effects of breakfast meals that differed in sugar content on CTRS hyperactivity, inattention/over-activity and aggression subscales. Both Milich and Pelham (1986) and Kaplan et al. (1986) showed no effect of the sugar content of breakfast and behavior in children with ADD-H or behavioral problems. However, Rosen et al. (1988) observed a small significant increase in hyperactivity scores following a breakfast with high sugar content compared with low sugar in children without behavior problems (Rosen et al., 1988).

Cross-sectional studies. Two cross-sectional studies in well-nourished adolescent populations reported a significant association between habitual breakfast consumption and behavior. Overby and Hoigaard (2012) found that frequency of breakfast was significantly associated with less self-reported disruptive behavior during lessons in adolescents (mean age 14.6 years). Adolescents who habitually consumed breakfast (>5 days/per week) had significantly reduced likelihood of disruptive behavior [Odds Ratio (OR): 0.29, 95% CI: 0.15–0.55] compared with those who ate breakfast less frequently (≤5 times per week). A similar association was also evident between breakfast quality based on the number of food groups within the breakfast meal and CBCL scores (higher score indicates poor behavior) in adolescents (O'Sullivan et al., 2009). Higher breakfast quality scores were most strongly associated with lower CBLC externalizing behavior scores (which indicates aggression and delinquency). The results indicated a stepwise decrease in total scores on the CBCL with increasing breakfast quality, indicative of a possible dose-response relationship.

Prospective cohort studies. Although there is some associative evidence of a relationship between habitual breakfast consumption and behavior in adolescents, the same relationship was not apparent in a well-controlled prospective cohort study. Miller et al. (2012) reported no association between frequency of breakfast and negative behavior (e.g., arguing, fighting, angry, and disruptive) in 21,400 school children aged 5–15 years following a 10 years follow up and adjustment for extensive confounders.

12.3.4 ACADEMIC PERFORMANCE

Twenty-two studies employed academic performance measures to investigate the effects of breakfast on academic outcomes (Table (Table2).2). The academic performance outcomes employed by studies included either school grades or standardized achievement tests. Twenty-one studies demonstrated that habitual breakfast (frequency and quality) and SBPs have a positive effect on children and adolescents' academic performance.

12.3.5 AVERAGE SCHOOL GRADES

Ten studies examined the effects of breakfast on average school grades. The majority produced a composite score from school reported grades across a range of subjects, usually considered "core" subjects. Two studies relied on self-reported school grades (Lien, 2007) or self-reported subjective ratings of school performance (So, 2013). Seven of the ten studies were in 12–18 year olds, reflecting the schooling system in which grading is more common in older pupils. Only three studies were carried out in primary school children aged 7–11 years (Murphy et al., 1998; Kleinman et al., 2002; Rahmani et al., 2011). One study included children of low SES (Murphy et al., 1998) and two studies included undernourished children (Kleinman et al., 2002; Gajre et al., 2008). All 10 studies identified demonstrated that habitual breakfast (frequency and quality) and SBPs have a positive effect on children and adolescents' school performance, with three studies observing clearest effects on mathematics grades (Murphy et al., 1998; Kleinman et al., 2002; Morales et al., 2008).

Intervention studies. Three intervention studies demonstrated positive effects of SBPs on school grades, particularly mathematics grades in both well-nourished, undernourished and low SES children aged 7–10 years. Effects were demonstrable after an intervention period of 3–6 months. A significant increase in school grades was apparent following an intervention providing 250 ml 2.5% fat milk at breakfast, which was apparent in girls only (Rahmani et al., 2011). Although it was not clear if the sample included undernourished children, the effect coincided with a significant increase in weight of the girls following the intervention in schools which received the intervention compared to control schools. Supportive evidence from Kleinman et al. (2002) found that following a 6-month SBP, children who had improved their nutritional status from at risk (energy and/or >2 nutrients <50% RDA) to adequate significantly increased their mathematics grades. Murphy et al. (1998) reported that following a 4-month SBP, children who increased participation were significantly more likely to increase their mathematics grades compared to those who had decreased or maintained participation.

Cross-sectional studies. Seven cross-sectional studies demonstrated a consistent positive association between habitual breakfast and school grades in adolescents.

Frequency of breakfast consumption was associated with school performance in five studies. Breakfast skipping (eating breakfast <5 days/week) was associated with lower average annual school grades in a sample of 605 Dutch adolescents aged 11–18 years who were in higher educational streams (Boschloo et al., 2012). This association was evident in both sexes and independent of age. Additionally, breakfast skipping was associated with more self-reported attention problems, which partially mediated this relationship. A larger cohort of nearly 6500 Korean adolescents of similar age range (10–17 years) demonstrated a similar association across all ages. However, the association was stronger in younger children (10–11 and 13–14 years) than older children (16–17 years) (Kim et al., 2003). Effects were seen in both genders, except for in 10–11 year olds, where the significant association between regular breakfast intake and school performance was only apparent in boys.

This association is also evident in undernourished adolescents (Gajre et al., 2008). Gajre et al. (2008) demonstrated that eating breakfast >4 days/week significantly predicted total average grades in a sample of children aged 11–13 years, a third of whom were undernourished. Analysis of individual subject domains indicated that regular breakfast eaters had significantly higher grades for science and English, but not mathematics compared to children who never ate breakfast (Gajre et al., 2008).

Lien (2007) demonstrated, in a large sample of adolescents aged 15–16 years, that those who never ate breakfast were twice as likely to have lower self-reported school grades compared with those who consumed breakfast every day (7 days/week). This finding was consistent in boys and girls. Moreover, the odds of having lower self-reported school grades decreased with successive quintiles of breakfast eating frequency suggestive of a dose-response relationship. Recent evidence from an internet based study demonstrated a similar relationship between habitual breakfast and self-rated academic performance in over 75,500 adolescents aged 12–18 years (So, 2013). Regular breakfast eaters (7 days/week) had increased likelihood of rating their school performance as higher compared with breakfast skippers (0 day/week).

Two studies demonstrated a consistent association between breakfast composition derived from energy and food groups provided and school grades in adolescents aged 12–17 years. Morales et al. (2008) found that adolescents who habitually ate breakfast that provided >25% of total estimated energy needs and included four or more foods groups from dairy, cereals, fruit, and fat were more likely to achieve higher grades than those consuming no breakfast or breakfast lacking the specified food groups. Analysis of individual subject domains indicated that mathematics, chemistry and social science grades were highest in full (>25% of total energy needs and ≥4 food groups) and good (<25% energy and three food groups) quality breakfast groups compared with no breakfast. Physical education, biology and languages grades were highest in the no breakfast group compared with full and good quality breakfast groups. Supportive findings from Herrero Lozano and Fillat Ballesteros (2006) indicated that higher average grades were obtained in adolescents who habitually consumed a breakfast containing three food groups from dairy, cereals and fruit compared with those consuming no breakfast or breakfast providing one of the specified food groups. The contribution of a mid-morning snack to breakfast quality was also considered in the analysis, which indicated a positive association between a mid-morning snack and school grades specific to children who had consumed no breakfast.

12.3.6 STANDARDIZED ACHIEVEMENT TESTS

Age specific standardized achievement tests are routinely administered by schools in developed countries for monitoring and provide an overall indication of intellectual level. Various sub-tests are included, usually literacy/reading, numeracy/arithmetic and reasoning. Standardized achievement tests employed by studies include the Wide Range Achievement test (WRAT), the National Assessment Program—Literacy and Numeracy (NAPLAN), Measure of Academic Progress (MAP), Scholastic Aptitude Test (SAT), and Assessment Tool for Teaching and Learning (asTTle). Twelve studies used standardized achievement tests to measure school performance. Two studies conducted in developing countries used unstandardized achievement tests developed for the purpose of the research to account for variability in curriculum and school environment (Cueto and Chinen, 2008; Acham et al., 2012). Studies were generally conducted in children aged 6–13 years with 10 of the 12 studies in children younger than 13 years. Evidence indicated a positive effect of SBPs on test scores, with clearest effects on arithmetic scores in both well-nourished and undernourished samples. Evidence also indicated a positive association between habitual breakfast frequency and quality, and test scores.

Intervention studies. Six of the seven intervention studies demonstrated positive effects of SBPs on standardized achievement tests in children aged 4–14 years, with clearest effects on arithmetic scores in undernourished children. Four of the seven studies demonstrated a benefit of breakfast on arithmetic scores (Powell et al., 1998; Simeon, 1998; Wahlstrom and Begalle, 1999; Cueto and Chinen, 2008). Four of the studies were carried out in samples which included undernourished children (Jacoby et al., 1996; Powell et al., 1998; Simeon, 1998; Cueto and Chinen, 2008) and two studies included low SES samples (Meyers et al., 1989; Ni Mhurchu et al., 2013). Effects were demonstrable after an intervention period of at least 1 month and up to 3 years.

Two studies found positive effects on arithmetic test scores from the WRAT following a relatively large breakfast meal (>500 Kcal) compared with a low energy control in undernourished and well-nourished children (Powell et al., 1998; Simeon, 1998). Cueto and Chinen (2008) examined the effects of a mid-morning SBP providing 600 Kcal and 60% of the daily requirements for several vitamins and minerals and 100% of the daily requirement for iron in a large sample of children, two thirds of whom were undernourished (≤ -2 SD height-for-age of the NCHS reference). Higher arithmetic and reading scores were demonstrated following the SBP in intervention schools compared to control schools, particularly in schools which tended to have higher levels of poverty, undernourished children and lower achievement. Comparable results were reported by Jacoby et al. (1996) following the same breakfast intervention for 1 month in children where the majority were below height-for-age but relatively overweight (due to increased body water and weight-for-height classification). Children in intervention schools of higher weight (and therefore likely to be undernourished) increased vocabulary scores post intervention. No effects were observed in normal weight children who were therefore likely to be well nourished.

In children aged 8–12 years from low SES backgrounds, Meyers et al. (1989) reported greater increases in language and total test scores in SBP attendees compared with non-attendees. Wahlstrom and Begalle (1999) also demonstrated an increase in scores for reading and mathematics from pre to post intervention. However, both studies were not well-controlled. A recent large RCT in pupils from low SES schools in New Zealand failed to show any benefit of a 1 year SBP on school achievement tests for literacy and numeracy and self-reported reading ability (Ni Mhurchu et al., 2013).

Cross-sectional studies. Four cross-sectional studies demonstrated a consistent positive association between habitual breakfast consumption and achievement test scores in children, including undernourished children.

Frequency of breakfast consumption was associated with achievement scores in two studies. Acham et al. (2012) demonstrated in well-nourished and undernourished 9–15 year olds predominantly considered low ability, that those who had consumed breakfast and a mid-day meal were almost twice as likely to score highly on achievement tests compared to those who only had one meal. This association was specific to boys, and consuming breakfast alone was not associated with school performance (Acham et al., 2012). This gender difference is not consistent across studies with evidence demonstrating increased odds of having lower self-reported school grades when skipping breakfast compared with habitually consuming breakfast in both genders (Lien, 2007). Edwards et al. (2011) indicated that higher mean mathematics MAP scores were associated with habitually eating breakfast (≥5 days/week) compared with less frequent consumption (<5 days/week). No association was found between breakfast frequency and reading MAP scores.

Two studies demonstrated an association between breakfast composition (energy, food group, and micronutrient content) and achievement scores in children aged 8–13 years. Habitually consuming a breakfast providing ≤20% of total energy needs was associated with poorer total SAT performance, particularly logical reasoning in 9–11 year olds (Lopez-Sobaler et al., 2003). However, SES was not controlled. O'Dea and Mugridge (2012) demonstrated a significant association between habitual breakfast quality according to food groups (carbohydrate and protein) and micronutrients (vitamin C and calcium) and NAPLAN literacy scores in children aged 8–13 years. No significant association was found between breakfast quality and numeracy scores.

Prospective cohort studies. Miller et al. (2012) demonstrated, in a large cohort of 21,400 school children aged 5–15 years, a non-significant association between breakfast eating frequency and scores on standardized achievement tests for reading, mathematics and science following adjustment for an extensive set of confounders. This was specific to breakfast that was eaten with the family rather than total breakfast intake.

12.4 DISCUSSION

12.4.1 THE EFFECTS OF BREAKFAST ON BEHAVIOR

12.4.1.1 OVERVIEW OF FINDINGS

This review identified 19 studies that examined the effects of breakfast on behavior in children and adolescents of which 11 studies demonstrated a positive effect of breakfast on behavior. The evidence suggests a mainly positive effect of breakfast on on-task behavior in the classroom. This effect was apparent in children irrespective of whether they were well-nourished and undernourished or from low SES or deprived backgrounds. However, most of the research on the impact of breakfast on behavior has taken the form of SBP evaluations, which lack scientific rigor. Three RCTs have not found similar benefits for behavior using standardized measures following a 1 year SBP, although, participation in the SBP was consistently low in some trials, which is likely to account for the lack of effects. In order for SBPs to impact on behavioral outcomes, the barriers to participation need to be addressed. Studies in children with pre-existing behavior problems (e.g., ADD-H) demonstrated no benefit of breakfast of differing sugar content. Findings for other behavioral outcomes including off-task behavior, distractibility, hyperactivity, and disruptive behavior are inconsistent. The frequent null findings reported suggest the effects of breakfast may be specific to selective behavioral domains.

The increase in on-task behavior following breakfast may indicate that children who eat breakfast are more able to concentrate, pay attention and are more alert at school. This is supported by evidence that demonstrates positive effects of breakfast on cognitive performance including attention and memory (Hoyland et al., 2009). Similarly, more on-task behavior in the classroom may be associated with improvements in academic performance supported by the positive association between habitual breakfast intake and academic performance (Boschloo et al., 2012; So, 2013). Moreover, an improvement in classroom behavior has the potential to reduce disruption and produce a more productive learning environment.

12.4.1.2 METHODOLOGICAL ISSUES

Behavioral measures. Classroom behavior was typically measured by coding observed behavior into predefined domains. Most of the studies focus primarily on on-task and off-task behavior within the classroom. Other behavioral domains measured less frequently include: being distracted, disruptive behavior, positively, or negatively interacting with peers, interacting with teacher, and reaction to frustration. One study did not directly observe classroom behavior and measured overall time spent in the classroom as a proxy measure for on-task behavior, which is an inadequate assessment of behavior (Cueto and Chinen, 2008). The measures used to code classroom behavior are often non-validated, unstandardized coding methods developed for the purpose of the research, and often inter-rater reliability is unspecified or merely recorded as acceptable. Overall, the general theme is the subjective nature of these studies and reliance on interpretation of behavior. There is a lack of studies that use systematic, validated, and reliable coding systems to measure classroom behavior. Two recent studies have demonstrated effects on on-task behavior following school lunch manipulations using a validated observation protocol (Golley et al., 2010; Storey et al., 2011). Future studies investigating the effects of breakfast on behavior should adopt validated and reliable, focused coding schemes to measure classroom behavior. Given the subjective nature of the methods to assess behavior, observers should also be blind to treatment condition.

Observational methods: Real-time vs. Recorded observations. Several issues concern the observational methods used to assess behavior. Real-time classroom observations carried out by teachers or researchers were common. Only four studies utilized video recorded classroom observations likely to produce more accurate and ecologically valid behavioral measures and offer the possibility of post hoc verification by independent observers (Milich and Pelham, 1986; Wender and Solanto, 1991; Richter et al., 1997; Benton et al., 2007). Video recorded classroom observations are therefore a more accurate and reliable behavioral measure. During real-time classroom observations, the researcher is required to observe multiple pupils within the lesson. The dual processing of watching and recording in the classroom is a complex task. The use of a video recorded classroom observation may have the advantage of increased accuracy via the ability to replay, review, and control observer fatigue (Haidet et al., 2009). Secondly, due to the reactive nature of the observation process, the Hawthorne effect may be present, such that children and teachers change their behavior because they are under observation (Roethlisberger and Lombard, 1977). Not having observers present during the observation or utilizing video recorded observation methods may limit this anticipated behavior change. Finally, the habituation period, where cameras/observers are introduced, is often not reported. This habituation period may allow children to become familiar to the presence of observers/cameras in order to reduce reactive behavior change. Future studies should consider, when possible, a video recorded observation to yield a more accurate, reliable observation whilst maintaining ethical safeguards.

Design. Various breakfast manipulations are employed. There are few direct comparisons of breakfasts varying in composition precluding conclusions about the effects of breakfast composition on behavior. Additionally, many studies lack randomization and the inclusion of an appropriate comparable control group. Most studies are based on small samples and limited to children aged <13 years, with fewer studies in adolescents. Metabolic and behavioral effects of breakfast may be different in older children aged >13 years. Classroom behavior is dynamic and can be different across year groups and ages. Previous research has found differences in behavior between older and younger children in the classroom following school lunch manipulations, where younger children tend to be more distracted when working alone with the reverse true for older children and adolescents (Golley et al., 2010; Storey et al., 2011). The influence of gender on behavior is also not considered by most studies. For example, Chang et al. (1996) demonstrated that girls talked and displayed more movement compared with boys in a set task classroom situation. Further research in this field should include larger samples providing sufficient power and also include older children >13 years and consider the effects of gender on behavior.

12.4.2 THE EFFECT OF BREAKFAST ON ACADEMIC PERFORMANCE

12.4.2.1 OVERVIEW OF FINDINGS

This review identified 21 studies that demonstrated suggestive evidence that habitual breakfast (frequency and quality) and SBPs are associated with children and adolescents' academic performance. This effect was apparent in both well-nourished or undernourished samples and/or children from low SES backgrounds. Increased frequency of habitual breakfast was consistently positively associated with improved school performance. Some evidence suggested that increased quality of habitual breakfast in terms of providing a greater variety of food groups (3–4) and adequate energy (>20–25% of total estimated energy needs) is positively related to school performance.

Evidence suggested a positive effect of SBPs on arithmetic test scores and mathematic grades. Three studies demonstrated clearest effects on mathematic grades (Murphy et al., 1998; Kleinman et al., 2002; Morales et al., 2008) and four studies demonstrated a benefit of breakfast on arithmetic scores (Powell et al., 1998; Simeon, 1998; Wahlstrom and Begalle, 1999; Cueto and Chinen, 2008; Edwards et al., 2011). However, some of the evidence was inconsistent (Gajre et al., 2008; O'Dea and Mugridge, 2012). Gajre et al. (2008) found that regular breakfast eaters (>4 days per week) had significantly higher marks for science and English compared to those who never eat breakfast, but there was no difference in mathematics marks. However, total marks, which included mathematics, were significantly higher in the regular breakfast group compared with the no breakfast group. Similarly, the majority of studies employing composite measures of school grades across subject domains show a positive association which, may be related to increased power afforded by composite measures.

Some evidence suggested that effects may be more apparent in undernourished children who improved their nutritional status from at risk to adequate following a SBP (Kleinman et al., 2002). Cueto and Chinen (2008) reported that positive effects on achievement test scores following a SBP, particularly in schools which tended to have more undernourished children and lower achievement. In support, studies that were carried out in samples including undernourished children demonstrated consistent positive effects of breakfast on school performance (Jacoby et al., 1996; Powell et al., 1998; Simeon, 1998; Cueto and Chinen, 2008). This is suggestive of a possible mechanism by which breakfast may improve school performance. The observed increase in school performance may be facilitated by correction of nutritional deficiencies due to the fortification of many breakfast products, particularly with iron and iodine which have largely been implicated in improving cognitive function which may influence school performance (Tiwari et al., 1996; Grantham-McGregor and Ani, 2001; Falkingham et al., 2010). Whilst nutritional influences may have contributed toward the improved school performance, school attendance also increased in many studies following which may account for most of the improvement in school grades (Hoyland et al., 2009; Defeyter et al., 2010).

12.4.2.2 METHODOLOGICAL ISSUES

Influence of confounders. Research on breakfast and educational outcomes is a particularly difficult area given the potential for confounding. The majority of studies that employ academic outcomes are cross-sectional, so adjustment of potential confounders is critical. Adequate control for confounders varied within the studies identified. An important potential confound is SES. It is likely that children and adolescents who eat breakfast differ from those who do not eat breakfast in ways that also influence educational outcomes. There is a consistent evidence that SES is associated with breakfast eating, with children from higher SES backgrounds more likely to regularly eat breakfast than children from lower SES backgrounds, an effect which is consistent across gender and age (Delva et al., 2006; Moore et al., 2007; Doku et al., 2011; Hallström et al., 2011, 2012; Overby et al., 2011). Similarly, there is well established consistent evidence that SES is a central determinant of academic performance and cognitive ability (Brooks-Gunn and Duncan, 1997; McLoyd, 1998; McCulloch and Joshi, 2001; Machin and Vignoles, 2004). However, some studies failed to adequately adjust for SES in their analysis or used various proxy measures of SES which may be inadequate. If SES is not accounted for in the analysis, it is likely associations observed are because children select into both high breakfast consumption frequency and higher school grades as a result of SES. Further work investigating the effects of breakfast on school performance should carefully consider the role of confounding, and apply adequate controls in the analysis, particularly for SES.

Academic performance measures. Studies employed a wide range of outcomes as academic performance indicators, either by use of average school grades or standardized achievement tests. Two studies relied on self-reported school grades (Lien, 2007) or self-reported subjective ratings of school performance (So, 2013) which are open to socially desirable and inaccurate reporting. Moreover, direct measures of academic performance, although ecologically valid are however, crude measures that may be insensitive to the effects of breakfast. Although many confounders are controlled for in the studies reviewed, it may be inappropriate to use broad measures of scholastic achievement such as end of year grades since many other factors interplay to determine grades. There are multiple, modifiable, and unmodifiable, determinants of academic performance that may act over and above the subtle nutritional effects of breakfast.

Design. The evidence is based on studies investigating the effects of either habitual breakfast consumption or SBPs on academic performance. The majority of studies on habitual breakfast intake are cross-sectional. The dominance of cross-sectional evidence, although offering a unique opportunity to establish the effects of habitual breakfast on academic performance, provides no indication of causality or temporality. Only one well controlled prospective cohort study has been published to date (Miller et al., 2012). This study focused on breakfast that was eaten with the family rather than total breakfast intake, however this may still be reflective of habitual breakfast consumption particularly in younger children who are more likely to have family meals (Fulkerson et al., 2006) and since most regular breakfast eaters have breakfast at home (Hoyland et al., 2012).

SBP intervention studies also present difficulties in attributing the direct effects of the breakfast meal or the regime of providing a free school breakfast in a breakfast club environment to academic outcomes (Defeyter et al., 2010). Many studies lack details of the composition and amount of food provided and consumed, precluding conclusions regarding breakfast type. SBPs are often associated with increased attendance (Jacoby et al., 1996; Simeon, 1998; Kleinman et al., 2002) punctuality (Murphy et al., 1998), readiness to learn (Wahlstrom and Begalle, 1999), decreased dropout rates (Cueto and Chinen, 2008) better behavior in the classroom (Bro et al., 1994; Richter et al., 1997) and increased pro-social behavior (Shemilt et al., 2004), all of which are likely to impact school performance concurrently. The positive effects of SBPs on other outcomes that will also influence academic performance make it difficult to attribute the effects either to the breakfast meal or as an artifact of increased attendance and punctuality. Furthermore, the intervention duration is particularly important in relation to academic performance because it is likely that a stable period of operation is needed to impact both breakfast eating behavior and academic outcomes. Two studies following a 1 year SBP reported no increase in the total number of children eating breakfast (Murphy et al., 2011; Ni Mhurchu et al., 2013). Clearly, the increase in school performance reported in studies that do not impact breakfast eating behavior is likely to be an artifact of other outcomes.

Dietary assessment. Studies that examine the effects of habitual breakfast consumption on scholastic outcomes also have limitations in terms of how breakfast is measured and defined. Varying definitions of breakfast and classifications of habitual consumption are used. Often dichotomous classifications using different cut-offs (e.g., ≥5 days/week, <5 days/week) to define habitual breakfast consumption are employed precluding comparisons between these categories. This crude indication of habitual consumption is unlikely to reflect true intake of breakfast.

Measurements of habitual breakfast intake are normally brief dietary assessments, given their use in situations for to measure specific aspects of diet. One item questionnaires (e.g., breakfast yes/no) are often used which may yield an inadequate assessment of habitual intake. Additionally there is a lack of validation studies examining the accuracy of brief dietary assessment or measures of specific meals compared with other methods which tend to examine total diet. Different measurement periods are used to define habitual breakfast and studies do not differentiate between weekday and weekend breakfast consumption, despite the importance for school performance where weekday (school-days) breakfast meals may be more important. Measures focus on either frequency or composition and it is rare both to be considered. Self-report measures also have limitations because breakfast is often subjectively defined and interpreted by the respondent, allowing for bias, inaccurate recall, and misreporting. Furthermore, all food and drink consumed as part of breakfast may not be considered. For example, food consumed on the way to school or food that is not traditionally consumed for breakfast may be excluded.

The majority of studies on habitual breakfast intake are based on adolescent samples aged 12–18 years. Accurate nutritional assessment in adolescents is problematic and challenging compared with younger children, who are more likely to eat breakfast at home (Hoyland et al., 2012). There is an overall trend of increased inaccuracy and underreporting of food intake with age (Livingstone et al., 2004). Validation studies show dietary records provide unbiased and accurate estimates of diet in normal weight children up until the age of 9 years whereas adolescents and older children are more likely to underreport dietary energy intake by approximately 20% (Livingstone et al., 1992; Bandini et al., 1997). Adolescence is a period of rapid growth, increasing body image concerns, changing eating habits, increased independence over diet, greater peer influence and decreased cooperation with authority, all of which may decrease compliance and reporting accuracy in this population (Livingstone et al., 2004).

Further work should consider, both frequency and composition of breakfast as well as differentiating between weekday and weekend breakfast when measuring habitual breakfast intake. A longer measurement period to define habitual breakfast (e.g., at least 7 days) is needed to adequately measure breakfast intake and a dichotomous classification system to define habitual breakfast is insufficient.

12.4.3 SUMMARY OF THE EFFECT OF BREAKFAST ON BEHAVIOR AND ACADEMIC PERFORMANCE

Overall, the evidence suggests beneficial effects of breakfast for on-task behavior in the classroom, mainly in younger children <13 years. This effect was apparent in children who were well-nourished, undernourished and/or from deprived or low SES backgrounds. For school performance outcomes, evidence suggests a positive association between habitual breakfast frequency and quality on school grades or achievement test scores. Similarly, evidence from SBPs suggest a positive effect on school performance, particularly mathematics grades and arithmetic scores and in undernourished children and/or children from deprived or low SES backgrounds. The positive effects of breakfast on academic performance appear clearer than those on behavior, probably due to the difficulties surrounding accurate measures of behavior which are inherently subjective in nature. These outcomes are ecologically valid, have more relevance to pupils, parents, teachers, and educational policy makers and as a result may produce most impact.

REFERENCES

1. Acham H., Kikafunda J., Malde M., Oldewage-Theron W., Egal A. (2012). Breakfast, midday meals and academic achievement in rural primary schools in Uganda: implications for education and school health policy. Food Nutr. Res. 56 10.3402/fnr. v3456i3400.11217
2. Balvin Frantzen L., Treviño R. P., Echon R. M., Garcia-Dominic O., Dimarco N. (2013). Association between frequency of ready-to-eat cereal consumption, nutrient intakes, and body mass index in fourth- to sixth-grade low-income minority children. J. Acad. Nutr. Diet. 113, 511–519 10.1016/j.jand.2013.01.006
3. Bandini L. G., Cyr H., Must A., Dietz W. H. (1997). Validity of reported energy intake in preadolescent girls. Am. J. Clin. Nutr. 65, 1138S–1141S
4. Benton D., Jarvis M. (2007). The role of breakfast and a mid-morning snack on the ability of children to concentrate at school. Physiol. Behav. 90, 382–385 10.1016/j. physbeh.2006.09.029

5. Benton D., Maconie A., Williams C. (2007). The influence of the glycaemic load of breakfast on the behaviour of children in school. Physiol. Behav. 92, 717–724 10.1016/j.physbeh.2007.05.065

6. Boschloo A., Ouwehand C., Dekker S., Lee N., De Groot R., Krabbendam L., et al. (2012). The relation between breakfast skipping and school performance in adolescents. Mind Brain Educ. 6, 81–88 10.1111/j.1751-228X.2012.01138.x

7. Brindal E., Baird D., Danthiir V., Wilson C., Bowen J., Slater A., et al. (2012). Ingesting breakfast meals of different glycaemic load does not alter cognition and satiety in children. Eur. J. Clin. Nutr. 66, 1166–1171 10.1038/ejcn.2012.99

8. Bro R. T., Shank L., Williams R., McLaughlin T. F. (1994). The effects on an in class breakfast program on attendance and on task behaviour of high school students. Child Fam. Behav. Ther. 16, 1–8 10.1300/J019v16n03_01

9. Bro R. T., Shank L. L., McLaughlin T. F., Williams R. L. (1996). Effects of a breakfast program on on-task behaviors of vocational high school students. J. Educ. Res. 90, 111–115 10.1080/00220671.1996.9944452

10. Brooks-Gunn J., Duncan G. J. (1997). The effects of poverty on children. Future Child. 7, 55–71 10.2307/1602387

11. Chang S. M., Walker S. P., Himes J., Grantham-McGregor S. M. (1996). Effects of breakfast on classroom behaviour in rural Jamaican schoolchildren. Food Nutr. Bull. 17, 248–257

12. Chiron C., Raynaud C., Maziere B., Zilbovicius M., Laflamme L., Masure M. C., et al. (1992). Changes in regional cerebral blood flow during brain maturation in children and adolescents. J. Nucl. Med. 33, 696–703

13. Chugani H. T. (1998). A critical period of brain development: studies of cerebral glucose utilization with PET. Prev. Med. 27, 184–188 10.1006/pmed.1998.0274

14. Cooper S. B., Bandelow S., Nevill M. E. (2011). Breakfast consumption and cognitive function in adolescent schoolchildren. Physiol. Behav. 103, 431–439 10.1016/j.physbeh.2011.03.018

15. Cooper S. B., Bandelow S., Nute M. L., Morris J. G., Nevill M. E. (2012). Breakfast glycaemic index and cognitive function in adolescent school children. Br. J. Nutr. 107, 1823–1832 10.1017/S0007114511005022

16. Corder K., van Sluijs E. M. F., Steele R. M., Stephen A. M., Dunn V., Bamber D., et al. (2011). Breakfast consumption and physical activity in British adolescents. Br. J. Nutr. 105, 316–321 10.1017/S0007114510003272

17. Cueto S., Chinen M. (2008). Educational impact of a school breakfast programme in rural Peru. Int. J. Educ. Dev. 28, 132–148 10.1016/j.ijedudev.2007.02.007

18. Cueto S., Jacoby E., Pollitt E. (1998). Breakfast prevents delays of attention and memory functions among nutritionally at-risk boys. J. Appl. Dev. Psychol. 19, 219–233 10.1016/S0193-3973(99)80037-9

19. Defeyter M. A., Graham P. L., Walton J., Apicella T. (2010). NEWS AND VIEWS: breakfast clubs: availability for British schoolchildren and the nutritional, social and academic benefits. Nutr. Bull. 35, 245–253 10.1111/j.1467-3010.2010.01843.x

20. de la Hunty A., Gibson S., Ashwell M. (2013). Does regular breakfast cereal consumption help children and adolescents stay slimmer? A systematic review and meta-analysis. Obes. Facts 6, 70–85 10.1159/000348878

21. Delva J., O'Malley P. M., Johnston L. D. (2006). Racial/ethnic and socioeconomic status differences in overweight and health-related behaviors among American students: national trends 1986-2003. J. Adolesc. Health 39, 536–545 10.1016/j.jadohealth.2006.02.013

22. Deshmukh-Taskar P. R., Nicklas T. A., O'Neil C. E., Keast D. R., Radcliffe J. D., Cho S. (2010). The relationship of breakfast skipping and type of breakfast consumption with nutrient intake and weight status in children and adolescents: the National Health and Nutrition Examination Survey 1999-2006. J. Am. Diet. Assoc. 110, 869–878 10.1016/j.jada.2010.03.023

23. Doku D., Koivusilta L., Raisamo S., Rimpela A. (2011). Socio-economic differences in adolescents' breakfast eating, fruit and vegetable consumption and physical activity in Ghana. Public Health Nutr. 27, 1–9

24. Edwards J. U., Mauch L., Winkelman M. R. (2011). Relationship of nutrition and physical activity behaviors and fitness measures to academic performance for sixth graders in a Midwest City school District. J. Sch. Health 81, 65–73 10.1111/j.1746-1561.2010.00562.x

25. Falkingham M., Abdelhamid A., Curtis P., Fairweather-Tait S., Dye L., Hooper L. (2010). The effects of oral iron supplementation on cognition in older children and adults: a systematic review and meta-analysis. Nutr. J. 9, 1475–2891

26. Fulkerson J. A., Story M., Mellin A., Leffert N., Neumark-Sztainer D., French S. A. (2006). Family dinner meal frequency and adolescent development: relationships with developmental assets and high-risk behaviors. J. Adolesc. Health 39, 337–345 10.1016/j.jadohealth.2005.12.026

27. Gajre N. S., Fernandez S., Balakrishna N., Vazir S. (2008). Breakfast eating habit and its influence on attention-concentration, immediate memory and school achievement. Indian Pediatr. 45, 824–828

28. Grantham-McGregor S., Ani C. (2001). A review of studies on the effect of iron deficiency on cognitive development in children. J. Nutr. 131, 649S–668S

29. Gibson S. (2003). Micronutrient intakes, micronutrient status and lipid profiles among young people consuming different amounts of breakfast cereals: further analysis of data from the National Diet and Nutrition Survey of Young People aged 4 to 18 years. Public Health Nutr. 6, 815–820 10.1079/PHN2003493

30. Golley R., Baines E., Bassett P., Wood L., Pearce J., Nelson M. (2010). School lunch and learning behaviour in primary schools: an intervention study. Eur. J. Clin. Nutr. 64, 1280–1288 10.1038/ejcn.2010.150

31. Greves H., Lozano P., Liu L., Busby K., Cole J., Johnston B. (2007). Immigrant families' perceptions on walking to school and school breakfast: a focus group study. Int. J. Behav. Nutr. Phys. Act. 4:64 10.1186/1479-5868-4-64

32. Haidet K. K., Tate J., Divirgilio-Thomas D., Kolanowski A., Happ M. B. (2009). Methods to improve reliability of video-recorded behavioral aata. Res. Nurs. Health 32, 465–474 10.1002/nur.20334

33. Hallström L., Vereecken C. A., Labayen I., Ruiz J. R., Le Donne C., Garcia M. C., et al. (2012). Breakfast habits among European adolescents and their association with sociodemographic factors: the HELENA (Healthy Lifestyle in Europe by Nutrition in Adolescence) study. Public Health Nutr. 15, 1879–1889 10.1017/S1368980012000341

34. Hallström L., Vereecken C. A., Ruiz J. R., Patterson E., Gilbert C. C., Catasta G., et al. (2011). Breakfast habits and factors influencing food choices at breakfast in relation to socio-demographic and family factors among European adolescents. The HELENA Study. Appetite 56, 649–657 10.1016/j.appet.2011.02.019

35. Herrero Lozano R., Fillat Ballesteros J. C. (2006). A study on breakfast and school performance in a group of adolescents. Nutr. Hosp. 21, 346–352

36. Hoyland A., Dye L., Lawton C. L. (2009). A systematic review of the effect of breakfast on the cognitive performance of children and adolescents. Nutr. Res. Rev. 22, 220–243 10.1017/S0954422409990175

37. Hoyland A., McWilliams K. A., Duff R. J., Walton J. L. (2012). Breakfast consumption in UK schoolchildren and provision of school breakfast clubs. Nutr. Bull. 37, 232–240 10.1111/j.1467-3010.2012.01973.x

38. Ingwersen J., Defeyter M. A., Kennedy D. O., Wesnes K. A., Scholey A. B. (2007). A low glycaemic index breakfast cereal preferentially prevents children's cognitive performance from declining throughout the morning. Appetite 49, 240–244 10.1016/j.appet.2006.06.009

39. Jacoby E., Cueto S., Pollitt E. (1996). Benefits of a school breakfast programme among Andean children in Huaraz, Peru. Food Nutr. Bull. 17, 54–64

40. Kaplan H. K., Wamboldt F. S., Barnhart M. (1986). Behavioural effects of dietary sucrose in disturbed children. Am. J. Psychiatry 143, 944–945

41. Kennedy C., Sokoloff L. (1957). An adaptation of the nitrous oxide method to the study of the cerebral circulation in children - normal values for cerebral blood flow and cerebral metabolic rate in childhood. J. Clin. Invest. 36, 1130–1137 10.1172/JCI103509

42. Kim H. Y. P., Frongillo E. A., Han S. S., Oh S. Y., Kim W. K., Jang Y. A., et al. (2003). Academic performance of Korean children is associated with dietary behaviours and physical status. Asia Pac. J. Clin. Nutr. 12, 186–192

43. Kleinman R. E., Hall S., Green H., Korzec-Ramirez D., Patton K., Pagano M. E., et al. (2002). Diet, breakfast, and academic performance in children. Ann. Nutr. Metab. 46, 24–30 10.1159/000066399

44. Lambert L. G., Raidl M., Carr D. H., Safaii S., Tidwell D. K. (2007). School nutrition directors' and teachers' perceptions of the advantages, disadvantages, and barriers to participation in the school breakfast program. J. Child Nutr. Manag. 31 Available online at: http://docs.schoolnutrition.org/newsroom/jcnm/07fall/lambert/

45. Lien L. (2007). Is breakfast consumption related to mental distress and academic performance in adolescents? Public Health Nutr. 10, 422–428

46. Livingstone M. B., Prentice A. M., Coward W. A., Strain J. J., Black A. E., Davies P. S., et al. (1992). Validation of estimates of energy intake by weighed dietary record and diet history in children and adolescents. Am. J. Clin. Nutr. 56, 29–35

47. Livingstone M. B., Robson P. J., Wallace J. M. W. (2004). Issues in dietary intake assessment of children and adolescents. Br. J. Nutr. 92, S213–S222 10.1079/BJN20041169

48. Lopez-Sobaler A. M., Ortega R. M., Quintas M. E., Navia B., Requejo A. M. (2003). Relationship between habitual breakfast and intellectual performance (logical reasoning) in well-nourished schoolchildren of Madrid (Spain). Eur. J. Clin. Nutr. 57, S49–S53

49. Machin S., Vignoles A. (2004). Educational inequality: the widening socio-economic gap. Fisc. Stud. 25, 107–128 10.1111/j.1475-5890.2004.tb00099.x

50. McCulloch A., Joshi H. E. (2001). Neighbourhood and family influences on the cognitive ability of children in the British National Child Development Study. Soc. Sci. Med. 53, 579–591 10.1016/S0277-9536(00)00362-2

51. McDonnell E., Probart C., Weirich J. E., Hartman T., Birkenshaw P. (2004). School breakfast programs: perceptions and barriers. J. Child Nutr. Manag. 28 Available online at: http://docs.schoolnutrition.org/newsroom/jcnm/04fall/mcdonnell/

52. McLoyd V. C. (1998). Socioeconomic disadvantage and child development. Am. Psychol. 53, 185–204 10.1037/0003-066X.53.2.185

53. Meyers A. F., Sampson A. E., Weitzman M., Rogers B. L., Kayne H. (1989). School breakfast program and school performance. Am. J. Dis. Child. 143, 1234–1239

54. Micha R., Rogers P. J., Nelson M. (2011). Glycaemic index and glycaemic load of breakfast predict cognitive function and mood in school children: a randomised controlled trial. Br. J. Nutr. 106, 1552–1561 10.1017/S0007114511002303

55. Milich R., Pelham W. E. (1986). Effects of sugar ingestion on the classroom and playgroup behaviour of attention deficit disordered boys. J. Consult. Clin. Psychol. 54, 714–718 10.1037/0022-006X.54.5.714

56. Miller D. P., Waldfogel J., Han W.-J. (2012). Family meals and child academic and behavioral outcomes. Child Dev. 83, 2104–2120 10.1111/j.1467-8624.2012.01825.x

57. Moore G. F., Tapper K., Murphy S., Lynch R., Raisanen L., Pimm C., et al. (2007). Associations between deprivation, attitudes towards eating breakfast and breakfast eating behaviours in 9-11-year-olds. Public Health Nutr. 10, 582–589 10.1017/S1368980007699558

58. Morales I. F., Vilas M. V. A., Vega C. J. M., Para M. C. M. (2008). Relation between the breakfast quality and the academic performance in adolescents of Guadalajara (Castilla-La Mancha). Nutr. Hosp. 23, 383–387

59. Murphy S., Moore G. F., Tapper K., Lynch R., Clarke R., Raisanen L., et al. (2011). Free healthy breakfasts in primary schools: a cluster randomised controlled trial of a policy intervention in Wales, UK. Public Health Nutr. 14, 219–226 10.1017/S1368980010001886

60. Murphy J. M., Pagano M. E., Nachmani J., Sperling P., Kane S., Kleinman R. E. (1998). The relationship of school breakfast to psychosocial and academic functioning: cross-sectional and longitudinal observations in an inner-city school sample. Arch. Pediatr. Adolesc. Med. 152, 899–907 10.1001/archpedi.152.9.899

61. Ni Mhurchu C., Gorton D., Turley M., Jiang Y., Michie J., Maddison R., et al. (2013). Effects of a free school breakfast programme on children's attendance, academic achievement and short-term hunger: results from a stepped-wedge, cluster randomised controlled trial. J. Epidemiol. Community Health 67, 257–264 10.1136/jech-2012-201540

62. O'Dea J. A., Mugridge A. C. (2012). Nutritional quality of breakfast and physical activity independently predict the literacy and numeracy scores of children after adjusting for socioeconomic status. Health Educ. Res. 27, 975–985 10.1093/her/cys069

63. O'Sullivan T. A., Robinson M., Kendall G. E., Miller M., Jacoby P., Silburn S. R., et al. (2009). A good-quality breakfast is associated with better mental health in adolescence. Public Health Nutr. 12, 249–258 10.1017/S1368980008003935

64. Overby N., Hoigaard R. (2012). Diet and behavioral problems at school in Norwegian adolescents. Food Nutr. Res. 56, 28 10.3402/fnr.v56i0.17231

65. Overby N., Stea T. H., Vik F. N., Klepp K. I., Bere E. (2011). Changes in meal pattern among Norwegian children from 2001 to 2008. Public Health Nutr. 14, 1549–1554 10.1017/S1368980010003599

66. Pivik R. T., Tennal K. B., Chapman S. D., Gu Y. (2012). Eating breakfast enhances the efficiency of neural networks engaged during mental arithmetic in school-aged children. Physiol. Behav. 106, 548–555 10.1016/j.physbeh.2012.03.034

67. Pollitt E., Jacoby E., Cueto S. (1996). School breakfast and cognition among nutritionally at-risk children in the Peruvian Andes. Nutr. Rev. 54, S22–S26

68. Powell C. A., Walker S. P., Chang S. M., Grantham-McGregor S. M. (1998). Nutrition and education: a randomized trial of the effects of breakfast in rural primary school children. Am. J. Clin. Nutr. 68, 873–879

69. Rahmani K., Djazayery A., Habibi M. I., Heidari H., Dorosti-Motlagh A. R., Pourshahriari M., et al. (2011). Effects of daily milk supplementation on improving the physical and mental function as well as school performance among children: results from a school feeding program. J. Res. Med. Sci. 16, 469–476

70. Reddan J., Wahlstrom K., Reicks M. (2002). Children's perceived benefits and barriers in relation to eating breakfast in schools with or without universal school breakfast. J. Nutr. Educ. Behav. 34, 47–52 10.1016/S1499-4046(06)60226-1

71. Richter L. M., Rose C., Griesel R. D. (1997). Cognitive and behavioural effects of a school breakfast. S. Afr. Med. J. 87, 93–100

72. Roethlisberger F. J., Lombard G. F. F. (1977). The Elusive Phenomena: an Autobiographical Account of My Work in the Field of Organizational Behavior at the Harvard Business School. Boston; Cambridge, MA: Division of Research, Graduate School of Business Administration, Harvard University; ditributed by Harvard University Press

73. Rosen L. A., Bender M. E., Sorrell S., Booth S. R., McGrath M. L., Drabman R. S. (1988). Effects of sugar (sucrose) on childrens behaviour. J. Consult. Clin. Psychol. 56, 583–589 10.1037/0022-006X.56.4.583

74. Sandercock G. R. H., Voss C., Dye L. (2010). Associations between habitual schoolday breakfast consumption, body mass index, physical activity and cardiorespiratory fitness in English schoolchildren. Eur. J. Clin. Nutr. 64, 1086–1092 10.1038/ejcn.2010.145

75. Shemilt I., Harvey I., Shepstone L., Swift L., Reading R., Mugford M., et al. (2004). A national evaluation of school breakfast clubs: evidence from a cluster randomized controlled trial and an observational analysis. Child Care Health Dev. 30, 413–427 10.1111/j.1365-2214.2004.00453.x

76. Simeon D. T. (1998). School feeding in Jamaica: a review of its evaluation. Am. J. Clin. Nutr. 67, 790S–794S

77. So W.-Y. (2013). Association between frequency of breakfast consumption and academic performance in healthy Korean adolescents. Iran. J. Public Health 42, 25–32

78. Storey H. C., Pearce J., Ashfield-Watt P. A. L., Wood L., Baines E., Nelson M. (2011). A randomized controlled trial of the effect of school food and dining room modifications on classroom behaviour in secondary school children. Eur. J. Clin. Nutr. 65, 32–38 10.1038/ejcn.2010.227

79. Szajewska H., Ruszczynski M. (2010). Systematic review demonstrating that break-fast consumption influences body weight outcomes in children and adolescents in Europe. Crit. Rev. Food Sci. Nutr. 50, 113–119 10.1080/10408390903467514

80. Thorleifsdottir B., Björnsson J. K., Benediktsdottir B., Gislason T., Kristbjarnarson H. (2002). Sleep and sleep habits from childhood to young adulthood over a 10-year period. J. Psychosom. Res. 53, 529–537 10.1016/S0022-3999(02)00444-0

81. Tiwari B. D., Godbole M. M., Chattopadhyay N., Mandal A., Mithal A. (1996). Learning disabilities and poor motivation to achieve due to prolonged iodine defi-ciency. Am. J. Clin. Nutr. 63, 782–786

82. Wahlstrom K. L., Begalle M. S. (1999). More than test scores: results of the univer-sal school breakfast pilot in Minnesota. Top. Clin. Nutr. 15, 17–29

83. Wender E. H., Solanto M. V. (1991). Effects of sugar on aggressive and inattentive behavior in children with attention deficit disorder with hyperactivity and normal children. Pediatrics 88, 960–966

84. Wesnes K. A., Pincock C., Richardson D., Helm G., Hails S. (2003). Breakfast re-duces declines in attention and memory over the morning in schoolchildren. Appe-tite 41, 329–331 10.1016/j.appet.2003.08.009

85. Wesnes K. A., Pincock C., Scholey A. (2012). Breakfast is associated with enhanced cognitive function in schoolchildren. An internet based study. Appetite 59, 646–649

86. Widenhorn-Muller K., Hille K., Klenk J., Weiland U. (2008). Influence of having breakfast on cognitive performance and mood in 13- to 20-year-old high school stu-dents: results of a crossover trial. Pediatrics 122, 279–284 10.1542/peds.2007-0944

There are two tables that are not available in this version of the article. To view them, please use the citation on the first page of this chapter.

CHAPTER 13

DIETARY LEVELS OF PURE FLAVONOIDS IMPROVE SPATIAL MEMORY PERFORMANCE AND INCREASE HIPPOCAMPAL BRAIN-DERIVED NEUROTROPHIC FACTOR

CATARINA RENDEIRO, DAVID VAUZOUR, MARCUS RATTRAY,
PIERRE WAFFO-TÉGUO, JEAN MICHEL MÉRILLON,
LAURIE T. BUTLER, CLAIRE M. WILLIAMS,
AND JEREMY P. E. SPENCER

13.1 INTRODUCTION

Phytochemical–rich foods, particularly those rich in flavonoids, have been shown to be effective in reversing age-related deficits in memory and learning [1]–[6]. In particular, studies using *Camellia sinensis* (tea) [7]–[12], *Gingko Biloba* [13]–[15], *Theobroma cacao* (cocoa) [16]–[18] and *Vaccinium spp* (blueberry) [19]–[23] have demonstrated beneficial effects on memory and learning in both humans and animal models. Whilst these studies clearly demonstrate the efficacy of flavonoid-rich foods in

Dietary Levels of Pure Flavonoids Improve Spatial Memory Performance and Increase Hippocampal Brain-Derived Neurotrophic Factor. © *Rendeiro C, Vauzour D, Rattray M, Waffo-Téguo P, Méril-lon JM, Butler LT, Williams CM, and Spencer JPE. PLoS ONE* **8**,*5 (2013); doi:10.1371/journal. pone.0063535. Licensed under Creative Commons Attribution 3.0 Unported License, http://creative-commons.org/licenses/by/3.0/.*

promoting cognitive performance, they fall short of providing evidence that flavonoids themselves are the causal agents in driving beneficial effects on memory, learning and neuro-cognitive performance. Because each of these foods contains large array of macro- and micro-nutrients and a diverse phytochemical profile (flavonoids, hydroxycinnamates, phenolic acids), to date it has been difficult to assign specific biological functions to a single flavonoids or even specific flavonoid groups.

Several studies have indicated that absorbed flavonoids and their metabolites are able to transverse the blood-brain-barrier [24]–[26] and may exert neuropharmacological actions at the molecular level, influencing signalling pathways, gene expression and protein function [27]–[30]. For instance, the beneficial effects of green tea, blueberry and *Gingko Biloba* on spatial memory have been shown to involve increases in hippocampal brain-derived neurotrophic factor (BDNF) [23], [31]–[33]. The conversion of short-term memory (STM) into long-term memory (LTM) is regulated at the molecular level in neurons [34]–[36] and involves the synthesis of new proteins that control neuronal morphology and connectivity [37]. A growing body of evidence indicates that BDNF plays a key role in the regulation of both short-term synaptic function and long-term activity-dependent synaptic plasticity during memory formation [38]–[40]. Furthermore, declines in hippocampal BDNF levels occur during aging [41]–[43] and appear to negatively impact on memory performance [44], whilst both exercise and diet have been shown to influence BDNF expression in the hippocampus [45], [46].

We have previously shown that blueberry intervention induces both spatial memory improvements and BDNF signalling in young and old animals [23], [47]. However, despite evidence for the functional and molecular actions of blueberry and other flavonoid-rich foods, limited data exist with regards to the actions of pure flavonoids on memory [48]–[51]. For example, Maher et al (2006) [51] reported that administration of pure fisetin improves recognition memory in rodents, although the underpinning mechanisms were investigated ex-vivo in hippocampal slices. In addition, the administration of pure (−)-epicatechin has been shown to improve the retention of spatial memory in the Morris Water Maze (MWM) [50], albeit at doses above those considered to be dietary. In the present study, we have extended these studies by examining the impact of dietary quantities of pure anthocyanins and the flavanols (similar to those present in blueberry) on spatial working memory and BDNF modulation in the hippocampus of aged rats (18-month old).

13.2 MATERIALS AND METHODS

13.2.1 MATERIALS

Antibodies used were anti-GAPDH (New England Biolabs, Hitchin, UK); anti-BDNF (Santa Cruz Biotechnology, Santa Cruz, CA); anti-pro-BDNF, (Millipore, Warford, UK). Horseradish peroxidase-conjugated goat anti-rabbit secondary antibody (Sigma, UK), ECL reagent and Hyperfilm-ECL were purchased from Amersham Biosciences (Amersham, UK). Pure standards of (−)-epicatechin and (+) catechin were purchased from Sigma (Poole, UK) and standards of anthocyanins and anthocyanidins were obtained from Extrasynthese (Genay, France). HPLC-grade hexane, acetone, glacial acetic, acetonitrile, methanol, water, and hydrochloric acid were purchased from Fischer Scientific (Loughborough, UK). Standard AIN-76A purified diet for rodents was purchased from Research Diets (New Jersey, USA). All other reagents were obtained from Sigma or Merck (Poole, UK).

13.2.2 INTERVENTION DIETS

Diets were prepared by Research Diets Inc. (USA) by incorporating either a) blueberry powder, b) pure anthocyanins or c) pure flavanols into the standard AIN-76A purified diet for rodents (Research Diets, USA) and made into dry pellets for animal consumption. The blueberry powder was prepared as follows: whole fresh Highbush blueberries (A.G. Axon and Sons, UK) were blended, freeze dried, powdered using a miller (APEX Construction, UK), sieve size 0.027 inches, and then incorporated into the standard rodent feed (AIN-76A) at the level of 2% (w/w), similar to that previously used [22], [23]. The pure anthocyanin extract was prepared by extracting anthocyanins directly from the blueberries giving rise to a pre-purified extract, containing 62.4% anthocyanins expressed as malvidin-3-O-β-glucopyranoside equivalents (as analyzed by HPLC). Both anthocyanin and flavanol diets were prepared by incorporating either the anthocyanin extract or pure flavanols, (+)-catechin and (−)-epicatechin (Sigma, UK), into the standard rodent feed at a level equivalent to that found in the blueberry diet (2% w/w). The blueberry powder and the anthocyanin extract were analysed for their flavonoid content prior to incorporation into the diets as described previously [52]–[54].

The blueberry-supplemented feed contained approximately 253.1 µg flavonoids/g feed (179.0 µg anthocyanins; 74.1 µg flavanols). The pure anthocyanin diet contained approximately 179.0 µg of anthocyanins (69.9 µg of delphinidin-3-O-β-glucopyranoside; 12.2 µg of cyanidin-3-O-β-glucopyranoside; 34.7 µg of petunidin-3-O-β-glucopyranoside; 2.60 µg of peonidin 3-O-β-glucopyranoside; 62.6 µg of malvidin-3-O-β-glucopyranoside). The flavanol diet contained 14.8 µg of pure (−)-epicatechin and 59.3 µg of (+)-catechin. The control diet was prepared by matching the AIN-76A purified diet for the levels sugars (glucose, fructose and sucrose) and vitamin C present in the blueberry diet. No flavonoids were detected in the control diet. All diets were prepared by Research Diets Inc., USA and were iso-caloric and matched as far as possible for macro- and micro-nutrients (such as sugars and vitamins).

13.2.3 ANIMALS AND SUPPLEMENTATION

All procedures were conducted according to the specifications of the United Kingdom Animals (Scientific Procedures) Act, 1986. The programme of work, of which the experiments described here were a part, was reviewed by the University of Reading Local Ethical Review Panel and was given a favorable ethical opinion for conduct. Utmost effort was utilized to prevent suffering and minimize the numbers of rats required for this experiment. Four groups of adult, male Wistar (n = 8 per group, Harlan, UK) were housed in groups of 2 and maintained on a 12 h light-dark cycle (lights on at 10 a.m.). All rats were 18 months old at the start of the experiment. After the habituation and shaping sessions period (described below) animals were administered one of 4 diets for 6 weeks: A) Control diet;

B) 2% (w/w) Blueberry diet; C) Anthocyanin Extract and D) Flavanols (−)-epicatechin and (+)-catechin. All diets were kept in a dry and dark place and administered fresh each day to the animals. Food intake was monitored daily (around 10 am) by weighting the amount of food administered to each cage and the amount remaining in the cage in the following day. Animal weight was monitored daily. During the supplementation period, all animals were tested once a week on a standard X-maze alternation task (described below).

13.2.4 SPATIAL MEMORY TESTING

13.2.4.1 HABITUATION AND SHAPING SESSIONS.

Rats were tested in a cross-maze apparatus as described previously [55]. Extramaze cues (laboratory furniture, lights and several prominent visual features on the walls) were held constant throughout the experiment. Rats were first habituated to the maze apparatus for 4 consecutive days. During the habituation period the rats were starved overnight in order to motivate them to collect pellets of food from the maze, after which starvation overnight was ceased. Following habituation, rats received 6 weeks of shaping sessions to assure that the animals could reliably collect rewards from the end of the maze arms before testing and supplementation begun. As such, each rat received two shaping sessions per week. Each shaping session consisted of six trials. During each shaping trial, rats were trained to enter an open goal arm and collect a reward pellet from the food well of that goal arm (entry to the alternate goal arm was restricted). This process was repeated until the rat had completed 6 trials. Across each shaping session, the 'open' goal arm was varied between trials according to a pseudorandom schedule.

13.2.4.2 ALTERNATION TASK.

Immediately after completion of the 6-week shapping period, test sessions were started. Each test session (8 trials) contained a pseudo-random sequence of correct choices between the two arms, as well as a pseudo-random sequence for the start arm during the choice phase. All rats were un-fasted during the procedure as the reward pellets provided sufficient motivation to ensure a high level of responding in the animals. Testing sessions were performed as described previously [23] with each animal receiving 8 trials per test session, with 5 minutes interval between trials. Here, each trial consisted of a sample phase and a choice phase. During the sample phase, a rat was placed in the start arm and allowed access to only one goal arm, entry to the goal arm was rewarded with a pellet in the food well. Access to the alternate goal arm was restricted during this phase. Once the reward pellet had been collected and eaten, the sample phase was over and the animal was placed back on the start arm for 10 seconds. During the choice phase, both goal arms could be accessed and the animal was allowed to make a free choice between these 2 arms. However, the rat was only rewarded for entering the arm that it had not visited during the sample phase. An animal was deemed to have selected an arm when it had placed a hind foot down that arm; retracing before the hind foot crossed the line was measured as a failure on the task. If the animal chose the correct arm, it was rewarded with a pellet in the food well. The animal was then returned to its cage for 5 minutes, before the next trial. The maze was cleaned with 50% ethanol solution between trials to remove any olfactory clues. For each trial, choice accuracy was measured. The number of correct choices (max 8 out of 8 trials) was recorded for each testing session. Rats were given 6 test sessions in total on the cross-maze, one test session per week with the first session being administered immediately before supplementation was started (baseline). The weight of all animals was measured over course of the experiment, as well as the daily amount of food consumed. During the experiment a total of three animals died of natural causes, one from the control-diet group (leaving the control group with a total of 7 subjects) and two from the blueberry-supplemented group (leaving the blueberry group with a total of 6 subjects).

13.2.5 TISSUE COLLECTION

Following the final test session animals were sacrificed by decapitation and their brains were immediately extracted and halved. Half the brain was frozen in dry ice at −80°C until it was sectioned for in situ hybridization (see below), the remaining half brain had the hippocampus dissected out and this was frozen at −80°C until used for Western immunoblotting analysis.

13.2.6 WESTERN IMMUNOBLOTTING

Proteins were extracted using the Trizol method [56], as described previously [47] and optimized for the extraction of BDNF. Protein concentration was determined by a Lowry based protein assay [57] (Bio-Rad RC DC Protein Assay) (Bio-Rad, UK). For analysis of proteins by Western Immunoblotting, samples were incubated for 2 min at 95°C in boiling buffer (final concentration: 62.5 mM Tris, pH 6.8; 2% SDS; 5% 2-mercaptoethanol; 10% glycerol and 0.0025% bromophenol blue). Samples were stored at −80°C until analysis. Six animals per group were used for the Western Blotting Analysis, representing the total number of blueberry-fed animals and six animals (out of 7/8) randomly chosen from control, anthocyanins and flavanols diet groups. Protein samples from these animals (40–80 μg/lane) were run on 9–12% SDS-polyacrylamide gels and then transferred to nitrocellulose membranes (Hybond-ECL®; Amersham) by semi-dry electroblotting ($1.5mA/cm^2$), as described previously [23], [47]. Blots were then incubated with either anti-BDNF pAb (1:1000), anti-pro-BDNF pAb (1:1000) or anti-GAPDH pAb (1:5000).Bands were analyzed using the band analysis software UVISoft Band. Molecular weights of the bands were calculated from comparison with pre-stained molecular weight markers (MW 27,000–180,000 and MW 6,500–45,000, BioRad) that were run in parallel with the samples. GAPDH levels were used to normalize pro-BDNF and BDNF protein levels, as such relative band intensities were calculated as a ratio of BDNF or pro-BDNF and GAPDH levels.

13.2.7 PREPARATION OF BRAIN SECTIONS

Coronal sections (10 μm) containing the dorsal hippocampus were cut using a cryostat, Bright Cryostat model OTF (Huntingdon, UK), and mounted onto poly-L-lysine coated microscope slides (VWR, UK). Sections were fixed for 15 min in 4% paraformaldehyde in DEPC-PBS (phosphate buffered saline, pH 7.4, which had been treated overnight with 0.1% diethylpyrocarbonate and autoclaved before use), followed by two 10 min incubations in DEPC–PBS (pH 7.4). Sections were then acetylated (0.1 M triethanolamine, 0.25%acetic anhydride in DEPC-treated 0.9% NaCl), dehydrated through a graded series of ethanols (70%, 95%, 100%), delipidated for 5 min in chloroform and placed in 95% ethanol for 5 min. Sections were then air dried and stored frozen at −80°C.

13.2.8 IN SITU HYBRIDIZATION RIBOPROBES

The methodology used was adapted from that described previously in [58]. Plasmid containing a fragment of rat BDNF cDNA (460bp cloned between the EcoRI and Sph1 site of pGEM4Z) [59] was cut with EcoRI. The cDNA template was purified using a GFX column (GE Healthcare, UK), quantified in a NanoDrop Spectrophotometer (Thermoscientific, UK) and purity confirmed by ratio $A_{260}/A_{280} \geq 1.8$. The riboprobes (Antisense and Sense) were transcribed from cDNA template using T7 RNA polymerase and simultaneously labeled with fluoroscein-12-UTP (Boehringer Mannheim, UK). The probe was kept at −80°C. Just before being used the probe was diluted (1/500) in hybridization buffer (0.02% bovine serum albumin, 0.02% polyvinyl pyrrolidone, 0.02% ficoll, 10% dextran sulfate, 50% formamide, 50 mM polyadenylitic acid, 100 mg/ml herring sperm DNA, 600 mM NaCl, 60 mM sodium citrate, pH 7.4), incubated at 65°C for 15 min and placed on ice.

13.2.9 IN SITU HYBRIDIZATION

In situ hybridization was conducted as described previously [47]. The relative mRNA levels in hippocampus and cortex were assessed by optical density measurements. Images were captured using a CCD camera AxioCam MR3 (Zeiss, UK) connected to Microscope Zeiss – Imager A1 Axio (Zeiss, UK). All the microscope parameters were kept constant for all the sections (Scaling 10X; Exposure 2.6 ms). The densiometric analysis was carried out using Image J. The optical density of the several hippocampal subfields (Dentate Gyrus- DG; Polymorphic cell layer- PCL; Cornu Ammonis 1- CA1; Cornu Ammonis3 – CA3) and cortex was measured from two sections per animal and 6 animals per group. The mean optical density from each region in each section was corrected by subtracting the mean optical density of the background. The data is presented as mean ($\pm$ S.E.M) of the corrected optical density measurement within each group.

13.2.10 STATISTICS

For the behavioral data, "choice accuracy", defined as the number of correct choices in the X-maze, was subjected to two-way analysis of variance (ANOVA) for repeated measures with diet group (Control, Blueberry, Anthocyanins, Flavanols) and time (0,1, 2, 3, 4, 5, 6 weeks) as main factors. This was followed by post-hoc Tukey tests where appropriate. The BDNF in situ hybridization data was subjected to a one-way ANOVA for each brain region (DG, PCL, CA1, CA3, Cortex) with diet group (Control, Blueberry, Anthocyanins, Flavanols) as the main factor. Post-hoc Tukey tests were subsequently used to examine differences between individual treatments. For Immunoblot data, statistical comparisons were carried out using to a one-way ANOVA with diet group as the main factor. Post-hoc comparisons were made using Tukey's test. Correlation coefficients were calculated using the Pearson product-moment correlation coefficient. All the data is expressed as mean $\pm$ S.E.M and was analyzed using SPSS.

13.3 RESULTS

13.3.1 WEIGHT AND FOOD INTAKE

There was no significant increase in weight among the animals over the time course of the experiment ($F_{12, 312} = 1.347$, NS), and no difference in weight between diet groups was observed ($F_{1, 26} = 1.162$, NS). On average, animals weighed 486.8 (± 8.3) g throughout the experiment. In addition, there were no significant changes in food intake for any of the 4 diet groups (P>0.05), with the control group consuming on average 29.1 g of food per day, the blueberry group 31.2 g of food/day, the anthocyanin group 31.3 g of food/day and the flavanol group 31.2 g of food/day. On average, the blueberry-supplemented group consumed 7.89 mg/day/rat of flavonoids (5.58 mg of anthocyanins; 2.31 mg of total flavanols), the anthocyanin group consumed on average 5.60 mg/day/rat anthocyanins, and the flavanols group consumed on average 2.31 mg/day/rat flavanols (0.46 mg of (−)-epicatechin and 1.85 mg of (+)-catechin).

13.3.2 SPATIAL WORKING MEMORY

At baseline, the choice accuracy for all four diet groups was similar, showing approximately 59% accuracy (Fig. 1). There was a highly significant difference in performance between the 4 dietary groups (F 1, 25 = 7.915, P<0.001), and a highly significant effect of time (F 6, 150 = 5.354, P<0.001) but no significant interaction was seen between diet and time (F 18, 150 = 0.789, NS) (Fig. 1 A). Subsequent post hoc Tukey tests examining specific differences in performance between the individual diet groups indicated that there was a significant increase in choice accuracy between the control group and each diet (control vs. blueberry: P<0.005; control vs. anthocyanin: P<0.01; control vs. flavanol: P<0.005). Although we observed an apparent decline in performance in the control group in the first two weeks of intervention in comparison to baseline performance, this was not statistically significance (F 6, 48 = 1.239, NS). As such, the control group maintained an average score of 60% correct choices throughout the experiment, whilst the blueberry-, anthocyanin- and flavanol-diets induced an improvement in choice accuracy over the course of the intervention period, with all groups achieving between 75–80% choice accuracy by the end of the intervention period (Fig. 1B). Post-hoc analysis indicated that the significant improvements in choice accuracy observed achieved significance (in relation to baseline) by the 4th week of supplementation (P<0.05), and were maintained throughout the remainder of the intervention (week 5 and 6, P<0.05) (Fig. 1B).

A

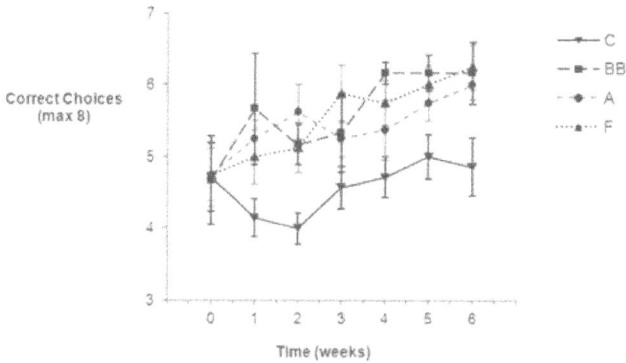

B

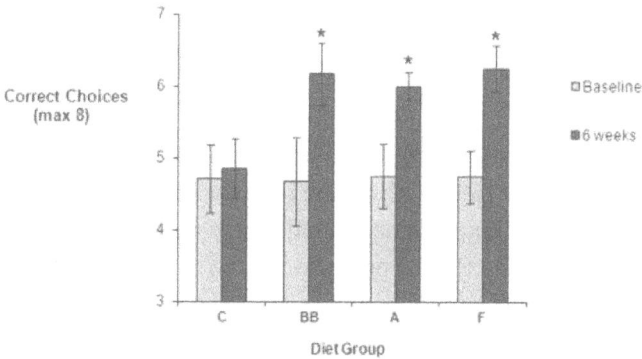

FIGURE 1: Effect of 6 weeks blueberry (BB), Anthocyanins Extract (A) and Flavanols (F) on spatial working memory in aged rats (18 months old). A) Effect of flavonoid-rich diets (BB, A or F) on correct choices (± standard error of the mean) in a X-maze Alternation Task: a significant increase in choice accuracy was observed between the control group and the blueberry group (P<0.005); the control and the anthocyanins groups (P<0.01) and the control and the flavanols groups (P<0.005). Maximum score is 8 correct choices (Control group: Triangle 'down'; Blueberry group: Square; Anthocyanins group: Circle; Flavanols group: Triangle 'up'). B) Comparison between animals performance at baseline and following 6 week supplementation with either a Control, Blueberry, Anthocyanins or Flavanol diet. * Indicates a significant increase in number of correct choices in comparison to baseline performance, P<0.05.

13.3.3 MODULATION OF BDNF AND PRO-BDNF PROTEIN LEVELS IN THE HIPPOCAMPUS

Levels of hippocampal pro- and mature BDNF were assessed by Western immunoblotting and normalized against GAPDH protein levels (Fig. 2A). A one way-ANOVA revealed significant differences in BDNF levels between the diet groups (F 3, 23 = 5.751, P<0.005), although no significant changes were observed for pro-BDNF (F 3,23 = 1.40, NS). Further post-hoc comparisons (Tukey test) between diet groups revealed significant increases in BDNF levels in the hippocampus of the blueberry (P<0.05), anthocyanin (P<0.05), and flavanol (P<0.01) fed groups compared to the control group. In addition, there was a significant positive correlation between hippocampal BDNF levels in individual animals from all dietary groups and their performance on the spatial memory task (R = 0.46, P<0.01) (Fig. 2B).

13.3.4 CHANGES IN HIPPOCAMPAL BDNF MRNA LEVELS

The hybridization pattern obtained for the BDNF probe was similar to that detected previously [60], with all the principal hippocampal layers exhibiting BDNF mRNA expression, including the dentate granule cell layer in the dentate gyrus. On RNase pre-treated sections, the hybridization signal was very low or absent, with RNase treated sections significantly lower in signal than the non-treated sections for all regions in the hippocampus and in cortex (P<0.001) (Fig. 3). An initial one-way ANOVA revealed that there was a significant difference in BDNF mRNA levels between the 4 diets in the dentate gyrus (F 3,24 = 3.293, P<0.05) (Fig. 3A), PCL (F 3, 24 = 3.925, P<0.05) (Fig. 3A), CA1 (F 3, 25 = 3.460, P<0.05) (Fig. 3C) and CA3 region (F 3,24 = 3.868, P<0.05) (Fig. 3D). In contrast, no significant changes in BDNF mRNA expression were detected in the cortex (F 3, 25 = 1.218, NS) following intervention with any of the 4 diets (Fig. 3B). Post-hoc analysis revealed that only the pure anthocyanin intervention led to a significant elevation of BDNF mRNA expression relative to the control group, and that this increase was observed in the DG, PCL, CA1 and CA3 hippocampal regions (P<0.05) (Fig. 3). The greatest anthocyanin-induced increase was observed in the in CA1 region, which exhibited an approximate 81% increase in BDNF mRNA expression compared to the control group (Fig. 3C).

Whilst the blueberry and the pure flavanol diet failed to significantly increase hippocampal levels of BDNF mRNA in the DG, PCL and CA3 regions, both were observed to increase BDNF expression relative to control in the CA1 region, by about 52% and 38% respectively, albeit non-significantly (Fig. 3C). Despite the fact that BDNF mRNA changes in response to blueberry and flavanols were non-significant, we observed significant correlations between hippocampal BDNF protein levels and BDNF mRNA levels in all of the hippocampal regions: DG (R = 0.59, P<0.01), CA1 (R = 0.55, P<0.01) and CA3 (R = 0.46, P<0.05).

13.4 DISCUSSION

Flavonoid-rich foods such as blueberry, green tea and *Gingko biloba* have been shown to be highly effective at reversing age-related deficits in spatial memory and in the enhancement of different aspects of synaptic plasticity, [19], [32], [61]–[63], a process severely affected by ageing [64], [65]. For example, we have previously shown that intervention with a 2% (w/w) blueberry diet resulted in significant improvements in spatial working memory that were mediated through the activation of the ERK-CREB-BDNF pathway, a pivotal pathway for the control of synaptic plasticity [23]. In the present study, we have shown that dietary levels of pure flavanol monomers (−)-epicatechin and (+)-catechin and a pure anthocyanin mixture (reflective of those found in blueberries) are also capable of mediating improvements in spatial working memory in aged animals. Indeed, the changes in spatial memory induced by the pure flavonoids mimicked those induced by whole blueberry, suggesting that the flavonoids are likely to be responsible for the efficacy induced by the whole fruit in vivo.

A

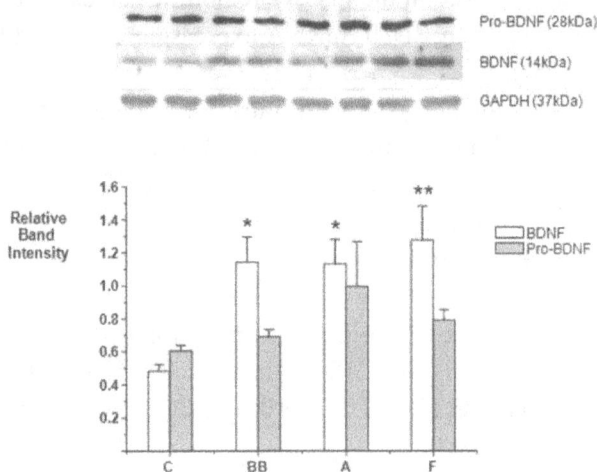

B

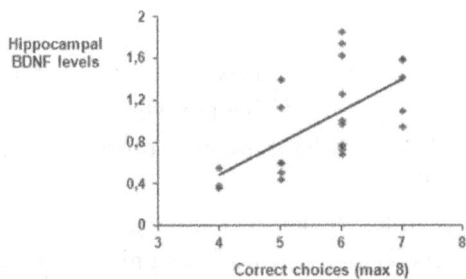

FIGURE 2: Levels of brain-derived neurotrophic factor (BDNF) in the hippocampus. A) Dissected hippocampal tissue lysates were probed for levels of pro-BDNF and BDNF using antibodies that detect the pro-domain of the BDNF protein and the mature protein. Representative immunoblots showing protein levels in 2 animals on the control diet (C), 2 animals supplemented with 2% BB diet (BB), 2 animals supplemented with Anthocyanins Extract (A) and 2 animals supplemented with Flavanols ((−) Epicatechin and (+) Catechin) (F) are presented. Pro-BDNF (grey bars) and mature BDNF (white bars). * Indicates a significant increase in BDNF levels in Blueberry and Anthocyanins groups relative to the control group, P<0.05; n = 6. ** Indicates a significant increase in BDNF levels in Flavanols group relative to control, P<0.01, n = 6. Pro-BDNF and mature BDNF were normalized against GAPDH. B) Correlation between choice accuracy (number of correct choices) in spatial memory task after 6 weeks of dietary interventions (C, BB, A and F) and levels of hippocampal BDNF protein levels, n = 24.

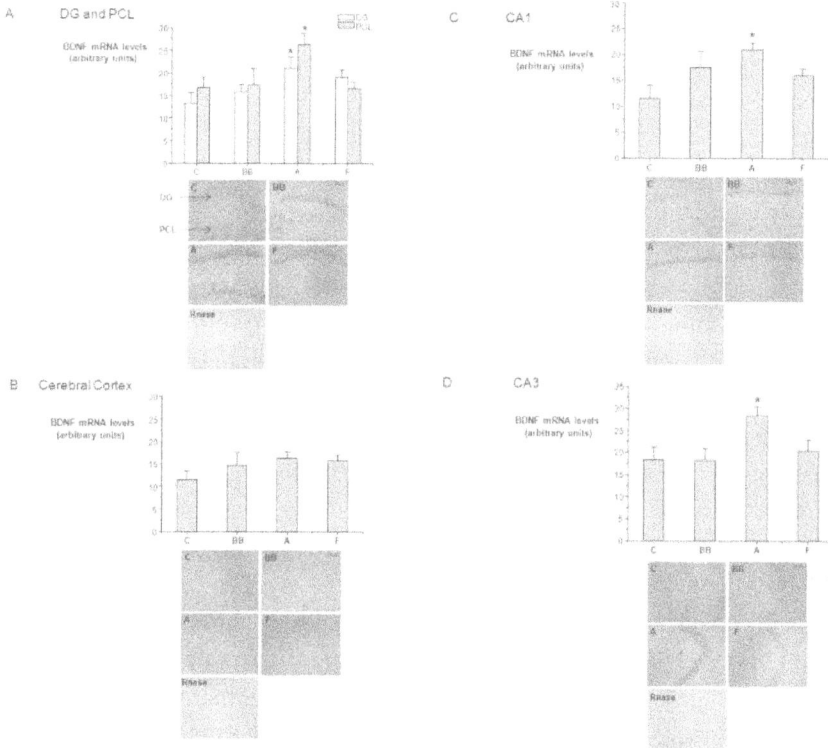

FIGURE 3: Effects of blueberry supplementation in BDNF mRNA levels in the hippocampus and cortex. A) Dentate Gyrus (DG) (white bars) and Polymorphic Cell Layer (PCL) (grey bars) of the hippocampus, B) Cortex, C) CA1 D) CA3. Representative pictures of hippocampal and cortical sections showing BDNF mRNA expression from 1 animal from the control (C) group, one from the BB group (BB), one from the Anthocyanins group (A) and one from the Flavanols group (F) are presented. * Indicates a significant increase in BDNF mRNA levels in the anthocyanins group in comparison to control in DG, PCL, CA1 and CA3, P<0.05. No significant differences between the four diet groups were observed in the cerebral cortex. Optical density levels are shown as mean ± SEM derived from at least 6 animals per group. Representative Rnase treated sections are presented for each hippocampal region. The scale presented represents 100 μm.

These findings were supported by observations that enhancements in spatial memory induced by the flavonoid-rich diets also significantly correlated with increases in hippocampal BDNF protein levels, suggesting that the effect of flavonoids on this neurotrophin may underpin performance on memory tasks. Our data agree with previous findings indicating that (−)-epicatechin dosed at 125 mg/kg of body weight (BW) per day for 6 weeks, is capable of enhancing synaptic plasticity; a crucial process during spatial learning [50]. However, our data indicates that such changes in spatial memory are also induced by significantly lower doses of flavonoids, more reflective of normal dietary intake [Human equivalent dose (mg/kg): flavanols = 4.75 mg/kg ×(6/37) = 0.77 mg/kg or 54 mg for a 70 Kg adult; anthocyanins = 130 mg for a 70 Kg adult] [66].

There is solid evidence indicating that hippocampal BDNF expression, in response to spatial memory training, is associated with memory performance [44], [67], [68]. BDNF has been shown to play a crucial role in synaptic plasticity, where it controls the stability of the hippocampal circuitry through its action in promoting changes in neuronal spine density and morphology [69]–[71]. Such morphological changes, stimulated by BDNF, dictate the efficiency of the synaptic connections and consequently affect spatial learning outputs [72]. Additionally, increases in neurotrophin expression may be also be important in determining neurogenesis [50], with some data suggestive that BDNF plays an important role in modelling the neurovascular niche, particularly in the formation and maintenance of the vascular tube, which affects new neuronal proliferation and differentiation [73], [74].

The elevation of hippocampal protein levels of BDNF by blueberry and pure flavonoids is particularly relevant as BDNF expression in the hippocampus is known to decrease with age in several mammalian species, including humans [42], [43], [75], with these decreases associated with a decline in spatial memory [41], [44], [76]. Furthermore, these age-related alterations in BDNF expression appear to be region-and circuit specific [77], [78]. We observed the greatest regulation of BDNF mRNA expression by pure anthocyanins in the CA1 region of the hippocampus, although levels were significantly increased in all hippocampal regions assessed. In contrast, blueberry and flavanol interventions did not appear to affect mRNA BDNF expression, despite the increases in protein levels detected in the hippocampus. Despite this, we observed a significant correlation between hippocampal protein levels of BDNF and levels of BDNF mRNA in the DG, CA1 and CA3 regions following intervention with all three of the flavonoid-containing diets, suggesting that the changes in BDNF protein are at least partly dependent on flavonoid-induced BDNF mRNA expression.

Alternatively, flavanols present in the blueberry diet may act to increase hippocampal BDNF levels via alternative mechanisms, such as through BDNF stabilization rather than its de novo synthesis. BDNF protein levels in the neurons originate from the cleavage of pro-BDNF into mature BDNF by the tPA/plasmin enzyme system, which is expressed at the hippocampal synapses [79]. Spatial learning is known to strongly increase the conversion of pro-BDNF into BDNF in both young and aged animals, with this process being typically down-regulated by ageing. As such, changes in BDNF protein levels in neurons do not always directly reflect changes in BDNF mRNA levels [80]. The increased expression of hippocampal protein BDNF levels seen after intervention with pure flavanols may be mediated by increases pro-BDNF metabolism during learning rather than via increases in pro-BDNF mRNA expression. In support of this, we observed lower levels of pro-BDNF in the flavanol group in comparison to the anthocyanin group (albeit not significantly), suggesting increased pro-BDNF metabolism during learning for the flavanol group.

Previously, we have observed an increase of mRNA BDNF in different regions of the hippocampus in young healthy animals, followed by an increase in both pro-BDNF and BDNF protein levels, suggesting that the flavonoids present in blueberry have the potential to stimulate both BDNF expression as well as BDNF stabilization [47]. Since in an aged rat both these processes are typically down regulated [81], the data emanating for this study suggest that flavanols given in a pure form are more efficient in regulating BDNF metabolism/stabilization during learning whilst pure anthocyanins may play an important role at stimulating de novo BDNF expression. However, a direct comparison between the effects of flavonoids in these two experiments is not trivial as the rats species used were different and age-dependent changes in BDNF are known to differ among rat species [81]. Thus, such an analysis would be valuable in future work to better understand how age differences impact on the potential effects of flavonoids on brain health.

Although, the mechanisms by which flavonoids act in the brain are not clear, there is evidence to suggest that blueberry flavonoids can cross the blood-brain barrier (BBB) and reach the central nervous system, where they have the potential to directly regulate gene and protein expression in neurons [23], [24], [82]. However, at present it is unclear as to whether flavonoid-induced memory improvements are mediated exclusively centrally or whether other mechanisms such as stimulations in endothelial function and peripheral blood flow [83] also contribute. Such vascular effects are significant since it has been reported that increased cerebrovascular blood flow facilitates proliferation of neuronal cells in the hippocampus and this may influence memory [84].

Our study presents evidence that dietary quantities of pure flavanols, (−)-epicatechin and (+)-catechin and pure anthocyanins are capable of inducing beneficial effects on memory in aged rats. As such, our data add weight to the evidence suggesting that flavonoids are the causal agents in determining the cognitive benefits of flavonoid-rich foods such as blueberry. Our data further support the view that such effects of flavonoids are determined at the molecular level in the hippocampus, where they are able to increase the expression of BDNF in specific regions of the hippocampus. Most notably, our data suggest that dietary amounts of flavanols and anthocyanins are capable of inducing both molecular and behavioral changes linked to memory in rats. As such, these compounds represent potential therapeutics that can counteract age-associated cognitive decline through dietary intervention or most importantly can play a crucial role in preventing age-related cognitive impairment.

REFERENCES

1.   Letenneur L, Proust-Lima C, Le Gouge A, Dartigues JF, Barberger-Gateau P (2007) Flavonoid intake and cognitive decline over a 10-year period. Am J Epidemiol 165: 1364–1371. doi: 10.1093/aje/kwm036
2.   Patel AK, Rogers JT, Huang X (2008) Flavanols, mild cognitive impairment, and Alzheimer's dementia. Int J Clin Exp Med 1: 181–191.

3. Beking K, Vieira A (2010) Flavonoid intake and disability-adjusted life years due to Alzheimer's and related dementias: a population-based study involving twenty-three developed countries. Public Health Nutr 13: 1403–1409. doi: 10.1017/s1368980009992990

4. Lamport DJ, Dye L, Wightman JD, Lawton CL (2012) The effects of flavonoid and other polyphenol consumption on cognitive performance: A systematic research review of human experimental and epidemiological studies. Nutrition and Aging 1: 5–25.

5. Saunders C, Spencer JPE (2012) Metabolic and immune risk factors for dementia and their modification by flavonoids: New targets for the prevention of cognitive impairment? Nutrition and Aging 1: 69–88.

6. Carey AN, Poulose SM, Shukitt-Hale B (2012) The beneficial effects of tree nuts on the aging brain. Nutrition and Aging 1: 55–67.

7. Chan YC, Hosoda K, Tsai CJ, Yamamoto S, Wang MF (2006) Favorable effects of tea on reducing the cognitive deficits and brain morphological changes in senescence-accelerated mice. J Nutr Sci Vitaminol (Tokyo) 52: 266–273. doi: 10.3177/jnsv.52.266

8. Haque AM, Hashimoto M, Katakura M, Tanabe Y, Hara Y, et al. (2006) Long-term administration of green tea catechins improves spatial cognition learning ability in rats. J Nutr 136: 1043–1047.

9. Kaur T, Pathak CM, Pandhi P, Khanduja KL (2008) Effects of green tea extract on learning, memory, behavior and acetylcholinesterase activity in young and old male rats. Brain Cogn 67: 25–30. doi: 10.1016/j.bandc.2007.10.003

10. Kuriyama S, Hozawa A, Ohmori K, Shimazu T, Matsui T, et al. (2006) Green tea consumption and cognitive function: a cross-sectional study from the Tsurugaya Project 1. Am J Clin Nutr 83: 355–361.

11. Lai HC, Chao WT, Chen YT, Yang VC (2004) Effect of EGCG, a major component of green tea, on the expression of Ets-1, c-Fos, and c-Jun during angiogenesis in vitro. Cancer Lett 213: 181–188. doi: 10.1016/j.canlet.2004.04.031

12. Unno K, Takabayashi F, Yoshida H, Choba D, Fukutomi R, et al. (2007) Daily consumption of green tea catechin delays memory regression in aged mice. Biogerontology 8: 89–95. doi: 10.1007/s10522-006-9036-8

13. Oliveira DR, Sanada PF, Saragossa Filho AC, Innocenti LR, Oler G, et al. (2009) Neuromodulatory property of standardized extract Ginkgo biloba L. (EGb 761) on memory: behavioral and molecular evidence. Brain Res 1269: 68–89. doi: 10.1016/j.brainres.2008.11.105

14. Shif O, Gillette K, Damkaoutis CM, Carrano C, Robbins SJ, et al. (2006) Effects of Ginkgo biloba administered after spatial learning on water maze and radial arm maze performance in young adult rats. Pharmacol Biochem Behav 84: 17–25. doi: 10.1016/j.pbb.2006.04.003

15. Williams B, Watanabe CM, Schultz PG, Rimbach G, Krucker T (2004) Age-related effects of Ginkgo biloba extract on synaptic plasticity and excitability. Neurobiol Aging 25: 955–962. doi: 10.1016/j.neurobiolaging.2003.10.008

16. Fisher ND, Sorond FA, Hollenberg NK (2006) Cocoa flavanols and brain perfusion. J Cardiovasc Pharmacol 47 Suppl 2S210–214. doi: 10.1097/00005344-200606001-00017

17. Francis ST, Head K, Morris PG, Macdonald IA (2006) The effect of flavanol-rich cocoa on the fMRI response to a cognitive task in healthy young people. J Cardiovasc Pharmacol 47 Suppl 2S215–220. doi: 10.1097/00005344-200606001-00018

18. Dinges DF (2006) Cocoa flavanols, cerebral blood flow, cognition, and health: going forward. J Cardiovasc Pharmacol 47 Suppl 2S221–223. doi: 10.1097/00005344-200606001-00019

19. Casadesus G, Shukitt-Hale B, Stellwagen HM, Zhu X, Lee HG, et al. (2004) Modulation of hippocampal plasticity and cognitive behavior by short-term blueberry supplementation in aged rats. Nutr Neurosci 7: 309–316. doi: 10.1080/10284150400020482

20. Shukitt-Hale B, Lau FC, Joseph JA (2008) Berry fruit supplementation and the aging brain. J Agric Food Chem 56: 636–641. doi: 10.1021/jf072505f

21. Krikorian R, Shidler MD, Nash TA, Kalt W, Vinqvist-Tymchuk MR, et al. (2010) Blueberry supplementation improves memory in older adults. J Agric Food Chem 58: 3996–4000. doi: 10.1021/jf9029332

22. Joseph JA, Shukitt-Hale B, Denisova NA, Bielinski D, Martin A, et al. (1999) Reversals of age-related declines in neuronal signal transduction, cognitive, and motor behavioral deficits with blueberry, spinach, or strawberry dietary supplementation. J Neurosci 19: 8114–8121.

23. Williams CM, El Mohsen MA, Vauzour D, Rendeiro C, Butler LT, et al. (2008) Blueberry-induced changes in spatial working memory correlate with changes in hippocampal CREB phosphorylation and brain-derived neurotrophic factor (BDNF) levels. Free Radic Biol Med 45: 295–305. doi: 10.1016/j.freeradbiomed.2008.04.008

24. Kalt W, Blumberg JB, McDonald JE, Vinqvist-Tymchuk MR, Fillmore SA, et al. (2008) Identification of anthocyanins in the liver, eye, and brain of blueberry-fed pigs. J Agric Food Chem 56: 705–712. doi: 10.1021/jf0719981

25. Milbury PE, Kalt W (2010) Xenobiotic metabolism and berry flavonoid transport across the blood-brain barrier. J Agric Food Chem 58: 3950–3956. doi: 10.1021/jf903529m

26. Andres-Lacueva C, Shukitt-Hale B, Galli RL, Jauregui O, Lamuela-Raventos RM, et al. (2005) Anthocyanins in aged blueberry-fed rats are found centrally and may enhance memory. Nutr Neurosci 8: 111–120. doi: 10.1080/10284150500078117

27. Williams RJ, Spencer JP, Rice-Evans C (2004) Flavonoids: antioxidants or signalling molecules? Free Radic Biol Med 36: 838–849. doi: 10.1016/j.freeradbiomed.2004.01.001

28. Schroeter H, Bahia P, Spencer JP, Sheppard O, Rattray M, et al. (2007) (-)Epicatechin stimulates ERK-dependent cyclic AMP response element activity and up-regulates GluR2 in cortical neurons. J Neurochem 101: 1596–1606. doi: 10.1111/j.1471-4159.2006.04434.x

29. Vauzour D, Vafeiadou K, Rice-Evans C, Williams RJ, Spencer JP (2007) Activation of pro-survival Akt and ERK1/2 signalling pathways underlie the anti-apoptotic effects of flavanones in cortical neurons. J Neurochem 103: 1355–1367. doi: 10.1111/j.1471-4159.2007.04841.x

30. Spencer JP (2008) Food for thought: the role of dietary flavonoids in enhancing human memory, learning and neuro-cognitive performance. Proc Nutr Soc 67: 238–252. doi: 10.1017/s0029665108007088

31. Li Q, Zhao HF, Zhang ZF, Liu ZG, Pei XR, et al. (2009) Long-term administration of green tea catechins prevents age-related spatial learning and memory decline in C57BL/6 J mice by regulating hippocampal cyclic amp-response element binding protein signaling cascade. Neuroscience 159: 1208–1215. doi: 10.1016/j.neuroscience.2009.02.008

32. Li Q, Zhao HF, Zhang ZF, Liu ZG, Pei XR, et al. (2009) Long-term green tea catechin administration prevents spatial learning and memory impairment in senescence-accelerated mouse prone-8 mice by decreasing Abeta1-42 oligomers and upregulating synaptic plasticity-related proteins in the hippocampus. Neuroscience 163: 741–749. doi: 10.1016/j.neuroscience.2009.07.014

33. Hou Y, Aboukhatwa MA, Lei DL, Manaye K, Khan I, et al. (2010) Anti-depressant natural flavonols modulate BDNF and beta amyloid in neurons and hippocampus of double TgAD mice. Neuropharmacology 58: 911–920. doi: 10.1016/j.neuropharm.2009.11.002

34. Igaz LM, Bekinschtein P, Vianna MM, Izquierdo I, Medina JH (2004) Gene expression during memory formation. Neurotox Res 6: 189–204. doi: 10.1007/bf03033221

35. Athos J, Impey S, Pineda VV, Chen X, Storm DR (2002) Hippocampal CRE-mediated gene expression is required for contextual memory formation. Nat Neurosci 5: 1119–1120. doi: 10.1038/nn951

36. Izquierdo I, Medina JH (1997) Memory formation: the sequence of biochemical events in the hippocampus and its connection to activity in other brain structures. Neurobiol Learn Mem 68: 285–316. doi: 10.1006/nlme.1997.3799

37. McGaugh JL (2000) Memory – a century of consolidation. Science 287: 248–251. doi: 10.1126/science.287.5451.248

38. Bekinschtein P, Cammarota M, Igaz LM, Bevilaqua LR, Izquierdo I, et al. (2007) Persistence of long-term memory storage requires a late protein synthesis- and BDNF- dependent phase in the hippocampus. Neuron 53: 261–277. doi: 10.1016/j.neuron.2006.11.025

39. Bekinschtein P, Cammarota M, Katche C, Slipczuk L, Rossato JI, et al. (2008) BDNF is essential to promote persistence of long-term memory storage. Proc Natl Acad Sci U S A 105: 2711–2716. doi: 10.1073/pnas.0711863105

40. Poo MM (2001) Neurotrophins as synaptic modulators. Nat Rev Neurosci 2: 24–32. doi: 10.1038/35049004

41. Hwang IK, Yoo KY, Jung BK, Cho JH, Kim DH, et al. (2006) Correlations between neuronal loss, decrease of memory, and decrease expression of brain-derived neurotrophic factor in the gerbil hippocampus during normal aging. Exp Neurol 201: 75–83. doi: 10.1016/j.expneurol.2006.02.129

42. Hayashi M, Mistunaga F, Ohira K, Shimizu K (2001) Changes in BDNF-immunoreactive structures in the hippocampal formation of the aged macaque monkey. Brain Res 918: 191–196. doi: 10.1016/s0006-8993(01)03002-5

43. Hattiangady B, Rao MS, Shetty GA, Shetty AK (2005) Brain-derived neurotrophic factor, phosphorylated cyclic AMP response element binding protein and neuropeptide Y decline as early as middle age in the dentate gyrus and CA1 and CA3 subfields of the hippocampus. Exp Neurol 195: 353–371. doi: 10.1016/j.expneurol.2005.05.014

44. Schaaf MJ, Workel JO, Lesscher HM, Vreugdenhil E, Oitzl MS, et al. (2001) Correlation between hippocampal BDNF mRNA expression and memory performance in senescent rats. Brain Res 915: 227–233. doi: 10.1016/s0006-8993(01)02855-4

45. Garza AA, Ha TG, Garcia C, Chen MJ, Russo-Neustadt AA (2004) Exercise, antidepressant treatment, and BDNF mRNA expression in the aging brain. Pharmacol Biochem Behav 77: 209–220. doi: 10.1016/j.pbb.2003.10.020

46. Berchtold NC, Castello N, Cotman CW (2010) Exercise and time-dependent benefits to learning and memory. Neuroscience 167: 588–597. doi: 10.1016/j.neuroscience.2010.02.050

47. Rendeiro C, Vauzour D, Kean RJ, Butler LT, Rattray M, et al. (2012) Blueberry supplementation induces spatial memory improvements and region-specific regulation of hippocampal BDNF mRNA expression in young rats. Psychopharmacology (Berl) 223: 319–330. doi: 10.1007/s00213-012-2719-8

48. Augustin S, Rimbach G, Augustin K, Cermak R, Wolffram S (2009) Gene Regulatory Effects of Ginkgo biloba Extract and Its Flavonol and Terpenelactone Fractions in Mouse Brain. J Clin Biochem Nutr 45: 315–321. doi: 10.3164/jcbn.08-248

49. Jin CH, Shin EJ, Park JB, Jang CG, Li Z, et al. (2009) Fustin flavonoid attenuates beta-amyloid (1-42)-induced learning impairment. J Neurosci Res 87: 3658–3670. doi: 10.1002/jnr.22159

50. van Praag H, Lucero MJ, Yeo GW, Stecker K, Heivand N, et al. (2007) Plant-derived flavanol (−)epicatechin enhances angiogenesis and retention of spatial memory in mice. J Neurosci 27: 5869–5878. doi: 10.1523/jneurosci.0914-07.2007

51. Maher P, Akaishi T, Abe K (2006) Flavonoid fisetin promotes ERK-dependent long-term potentiation and enhances memory. Proc Natl Acad Sci U S A 103: 16568–16573. doi: 10.1073/pnas.0607822103

52. Rodriguez-Mateos A, Cifuentes-Gomez T, Tabatabaee S, Lecras C, Spencer JP (2012) Procyanidin, Anthocyanin, and Chlorogenic Acid Contents of Highbush and Lowbush Blueberries. J Agric Food Chem.

53. Robbins RJ, Leonczak J, Johnson JC, Li J, Kwik-Uribe C, et al. (2009) Method performance and multi-laboratory assessment of a normal phase high pressure liquid chromatography-fluorescence detection method for the quantitation of flavanols and procyanidins in cocoa and chocolate containing samples. J Chromatogr A 1216: 4831–4840. doi: 10.1016/j.chroma.2009.04.006

54. Kelm MA, Johnson JC, Robbins RJ, Hammerstone JF, Schmitz HH (2006) High-performance liquid chromatography separation and purification of cacao (Theobroma cacao L.) procyanidins according to degree of polymerization using a diol stationary phase. J Agric Food Chem 54: 1571–1576. doi: 10.1021/jf0525941

55. Aggleton JP, Hunt PR, Nagle S, Neave N (1996) The effects of selective lesions within the anterior thalamic nuclei on spatial memory in the rat. Behav Brain Res 81: 189–198. doi: 10.1016/s0166-4328(96)89080-2

56. Banerjee S, Smallwood A, Chambers AE, Nicolaides K (2003) Quantitative recovery of immunoreactive proteins from clinical samples following RNA and DNA isolation. Biotechniques 35: 450–452, 454, 456.

57. Lowry OH, Rosebrough NJ, Farr AL, Randall RJ (1951) Protein measurement with the Folin phenol reagent. J Biol Chem 193: 265–275.

58. Rattray M, Michael GJ, Lee J, Wotherspoon G, Bendotti C, et al. (1999) Intraregional variation in expression of serotonin transporter messenger RNA by 5-hydroxytryptamine neurons. Neuroscience 88: 169–183. doi: 10.1016/s0306-4522(98)00231-0

59. Phillips HS, Hains JM, Laramee GR, Rosenthal A, Winslow JW (1990) Widespread expression of BDNF but not NT3 by target areas of basal forebrain cholinergic neurons. Science 250: 290–294. doi: 10.1126/science.1688328

60. Conner JM, Lauterborn JC, Yan Q, Gall CM, Varon S (1997) Distribution of brain-derived neurotrophic factor (BDNF) protein and mRNA in the normal adult rat CNS: evidence for anterograde axonal transport. J Neurosci 17: 2295–2313.

61. Cohen-Salmon C, Venault P, Martin B, Raffalli-Sebille MJ, Barkats M, et al. (1997) Effects of Ginkgo biloba extract (EGb 761) on learning and possible actions on aging. J Physiol Paris 91: 291–300. doi: 10.1016/s0928-4257(97)82409-6

62. Wang Y, Wang L, Wu J, Cai J (2006) The in vivo synaptic plasticity mechanism of EGb 761-induced enhancement of spatial learning and memory in aged rats. Br J Pharmacol 148: 147–153. doi: 10.1038/sj.bjp.0706720

63. Coultrap SJ, Bickford PC, Browning MD (2008) Blueberry-enriched diet ameliorates age-related declines in NMDA receptor-dependent LTP. Age (Dordr) 30: 263–272. doi: 10.1007/s11357-008-9067-y

64. Burke SN, Barnes CA (2006) Neural plasticity in the ageing brain. Nat Rev Neurosci 7: 30–40. doi: 10.1038/nrn1809

65. Rosenzweig ES, Barnes CA (2003) Impact of aging on hippocampal function: plasticity, network dynamics, and cognition. Prog Neurobiol 69: 143–179. doi: 10.1016/s0301-0082(02)00126-0

66. Reagan-Shaw S, Nihal M, Ahmad N (2008) Dose translation from animal to human studies revisited. FASEB J 22: 659–661. doi: 10.1096/fj.07-9574lsf

67. Hall J, Thomas KL, Everitt BJ (2000) Rapid and selective induction of BDNF expression in the hippocampus during contextual learning. Nat Neurosci 3: 533–535.

68. Falkenberg T, Mohammed AK, Henriksson B, Persson H, Winblad B, et al. (1992) Increased expression of brain-derived neurotrophic factor mRNA in rat hippocampus is associated with improved spatial memory and enriched environment. Neurosci Lett 138: 153–156. doi: 10.1016/0304-3940(92)90494-r

69. Alonso M, Medina JH, Pozzo-Miller L (2004) ERK1/2 activation is necessary for BDNF to increase dendritic spine density in hippocampal CA1 pyramidal neurons. Learn Mem 11: 172–178. doi: 10.1101/lm.67804

70. Tyler WJ, Alonso M, Bramham CR, Pozzo-Miller LD (2002) From acquisition to consolidation: on the role of brain-derived neurotrophic factor signaling in hippocampal-dependent learning. Learn Mem 9: 224–237. doi: 10.1101/lm.51202

71. Tolwani RJ, Buckmaster PS, Varma S, Cosgaya JM, Wu Y, et al. (2002) BDNF overexpression increases dendrite complexity in hippocampal dentate gyrus. Neuroscience 114: 795–805. doi: 10.1016/s0306-4522(02)00301-9

72. Leuner B, Falduto J, Shors TJ (2003) Associative memory formation increases the observation of dendritic spines in the hippocampus. J Neurosci 23: 659–665.

73. Li Q, Ford MC, Lavik EB, Madri JA (2006) Modeling the neurovascular niche: VEGF- and BDNF-mediated cross-talk between neural stem cells and endothelial cells: an in vitro study. J Neurosci Res 84: 1656–1668. doi: 10.1002/jnr.21087

74. Cheng A, Wang S, Cai J, Rao MS, Mattson MP (2003) Nitric oxide acts in a positive feedback loop with BDNF to regulate neural progenitor cell proliferation and differentiation in the mammalian brain. Dev Biol 258: 319–333. doi: 10.1016/s0012-1606(03)00120-9

75. Phillips HS, Hains JM, Armanini M, Laramee GR, Johnson SA, et al. (1991) BDNF mRNA is decreased in the hippocampus of individuals with Alzheimer's disease. Neuron 7: 695–702. doi: 10.1016/0896-6273(91)90273-3

76. Gooney M, Messaoudi E, Maher FO, Bramham CR, Lynch MA (2004) BDNF-induced LTP in dentate gyrus is impaired with age: analysis of changes in cell signaling events. Neurobiol Aging 25: 1323–1331. doi: 10.1016/j.neurobiolaging.2004.01.003

77. Gallagher M (2003) Aging and hippocampal/cortical circuits in rodents. Alzheimer Dis Assoc Disord 17 Suppl 2S45–47. doi: 10.1097/00002093-200304002-00004

78. Smith TD, Adams MM, Gallagher M, Morrison JH, Rapp PR (2000) Circuit-specific alterations in hippocampal synaptophysin immunoreactivity predict spatial learning impairment in aged rats. J Neurosci 20: 6587–6593.

79. Pang PT, Teng HK, Zaitsev E, Woo NT, Sakata K, et al. (2004) Cleavage of proBDNF by tPA/plasmin is essential for long-term hippocampal plasticity. Science 306: 487–491. doi: 10.1126/science.1100135

80. Silhol M, Arancibia S, Maurice T, Tapia-Arancibia L (2007) Spatial memory training modifies the expression of brain-derived neurotrophic factor tyrosine kinase receptors in young and aged rats. Neuroscience 146: 962–973. doi: 10.1016/j.neuroscience.2007.02.013

81. Tapia-Arancibia L, Aliaga E, Silhol M, Arancibia S (2008) New insights into brain BDNF function in normal aging and Alzheimer disease. Brain Research Reviews 59: 201–220. doi: 10.1016/j.brainresrev.2008.07.007

82. Abd El Mohsen MM, Kuhnle G, Rechner AR, Schroeter H, Rose S, et al. (2002) Uptake and metabolism of epicatechin and its access to the brain after oral ingestion. Free Radic Biol Med 33: 1693–1702. doi: 10.1016/s0891-5849(02)01137-1

83. Schroeter H, Heiss C, Balzer J, Kleinbongard P, Keen CL, et al. (2006) (−)-Epicatechin mediates beneficial effects of flavanol-rich cocoa on vascular function in humans. Proc Natl Acad Sci U S A 103: 1024–1029. doi: 10.1073/pnas.0510168103

84. Palmer TD, Willhoite AR, Gage FH (2000) Vascular niche for adult hippocampal neurogenesis. J Comp Neurol 425: 479–494. doi: 10.1002/1096-9861(20001002)425:4<479::aid-cne2>3.0.co;2-3

CHAPTER 14

CAMEL MILK AS A POTENTIAL THERAPY AS AN ANTIOXIDANT IN AUTISM SPECTRUM DISORDER (ASD)

LAILA Y. AL-AYADHI AND NADRA ELYASS ELAMIN

14.1 INTRODUCTION

Autism spectrum disorder (ASD) is a severe neurodevelopment disorder with onset prior to 3 years of age [1, 2]. It is characterized by impairments in social orientation, communication, and repetitive behaviors [3, 4]. In addition to behavioural impairment, ASD is associated with high prevalence of autoimmune disease [5, 6], gastrointestinal disease and dysbiosis [7], and mental retardation [8].

The prevalence of autism has increased over the last several decades. The incidence of ASD in United States increased in 2008 to 1 in 88 children [9]. Prevalence of autism spectrum disorders in Saudi Arabia is estimated to be 6 : 1000 [10]. Increased prevalence has great effects on public health implications and has stimulated intense research into potential etiologic factors.

Camel Milk as a Potential Therapy as an Antioxidant in Autism Spectrum Disorder (ASD). © AL-Ayadhi LY and Elamin NE. Evidence-Based Complementary and Alternative Medicine **2013** *(2013); http://dx.doi.org/10.1155/2013/602834. Licensed under Creative Commons Attribution 3.0 Unported License, http://creativecommons.org/licenses/by/3.0/.*

Although the aetiology and pathology is poorly understood, different factors have been suggested to affect autism, for example, immune factors, environmental, neurochemical, and genetic factors [3, 10, 11], oxidative stress [10–13].

Extensive studies have demonstrated that oxidative stress plays a vital role in the pathology of several neurological diseases such as Alzheimer's disease [14], Down syndrome [15], Parkinson's disease [16], schizophrenia [17], bipolar disorder [18], and autism [10, 14].

Oxidative stress occurs when reactive oxygen species (ROS) levels exceed the antioxidant capacity of a cell. It acts as a mediator in brain injury, strokes, and neurodegenerative diseases [19–21]; thus, the control of ROS production is necessary for physiologic cell function. The ROS within the cells are neutralized by antioxidant defence mechanisms, including superoxide dismutase (SOD), catalase, and glutathione peroxidise (GSH-Px) enzymes. The increased production of ROS both centrally (in the brain) and peripherally (in the plasma) may result in the reduction of brain cell number leading to autism pathology and apoptosis [14, 22].

Several studies have suggested the contribution of oxidative stress to the development of autism. These studies demonstrated the alteration of antioxidant enzymes like GSH-Px, MPO, and SOD, lipid peroxidation, antioxidant proteins as ceruloplasmin and transferrin, and detoxifying metabolites like GSH, as well as antioxidant nutrient vitamins and minerals [10, 11, 13, 23–26].

Camel milk has emerged to have potential therapeutic effects in many diseases such as food allergy, diabetes mellitus [27, 28], hepatitis B [29], autism [30], and other autoimmune diseases [31]. It has a unique composition that differs from other ruminants' milk. It contains lower fat, cholesterol, and lactose than cow milk, higher minerals (calcium, iron, magnesium, copper, zinc, and potassium) and vitamins A, B2, E, and C compared to cow milk [32, 33], and it contains no beta lactoglobulin and beta casein which are the main causative of allergy in cow's milk [34]. Furthermore, camel milk contains various protective proteins, mainly enzymes which exert antibacterial, antiviral, and immunological properties [35, 36]; these include immunoglobulins, lysozymes, lactoferrin, lactoperoxidase, N-acetyl-§-glucosaminidase (NAGase), and peptidoglycan recognition protein (PGRP) [34], which are crucial in preventing food allergy and rehabilitating the immune system [31]. Camel milk proved its potential effect in the treatment of food allergies, due to its inflammation-inhibiting proteins, and hypoallergenic properties, in addition to its smaller size nanobodies, which are different than those found in human. Camel milk nanobodies, as a single domain, show many promising and therapeutic potencies in infection and immunity [37].

The aim of the current study was to evaluate the effect of camel milk consumption on oxidative stress biomarkers in autistic children, by measuring the plasma levels of glutathione, superoxide dismutase, and myeloperoxidase.

14.2 MATERIALS AND METHODS

14.2.1 SUBJECTS

The present study included 60 subjects with ASD, especially those with known allergies or food intolerances, aged 2–12 years. Clinical diagnosis was based on the criteria for autistic disorder as defined in the Diagnostic and Statistical Manual of Mental Disorders, Fourth Edition, Text Revision (DSM-IV) [2]. Subjects were recruited from the Autism Research and Treatment Center, Faculty of Medicine, King Saud University.

The study protocol received the ethical approval from the Institutional Review Board of Faculty of Medicine, King Saud University. A written informed consent was obtained from all parents/guardians before being enrolled in the study.

14.2.2 STUDY DESIGN

The study was a double-blinded, randomized clinical trial (RCT). The participants were randomly divided into three groups: Group I (n = 24) received raw camel milk; Group II (n = 25) received boiled camel milk; and Group III (n = 11) received cow milk as a placebo. All groups received the same instructions, volume of milk, and containers to preserve the blinding of the study.

Parents were instructed to include the average of 500 mL of camel milk in their children's regular daily diet for a period of 2 weeks. Parents were asked to continue with the children's daily routines. They were not allowed to add or remove any interventions such as diet plans, supplements, or pharmacotherapies throughout the study period. Group I was also instructed to drink cold milk, beginning with small quantities that increase gradually, until 500 mL per day was consumed to avoid any risk of diarrhoea.

14.2.3 CHILDHOOD AUTISM RATING SCALE (CARS)

The Childhood Autism Rating Scale (CARS) was administered as a measure of symptom severity [11]. The Wing Subgroups Questionnaire (WSQ) [12] is a questionnaire with 13 behavioral domains (e.g., communication, social approach, play, imitation, motor behavior, and resistance to change) on which parents rate their child's behavior. A summary score is calculated for each subtype (i.e., aloof, passive, and active but odd), and the highest summary score is considered to indicate the subtype.

14.2.4 BLOOD SAMPLING

After overnight fast, ten mL blood samples were collected in EDTA tubes from autistic children before and 2 weeks after camel milk consumption. Centrifugation was done; plasma and red blood cells were obtained and deep frozen (at −80°C) until further analysis.

14.2.5 METHODS

14.2.5.1 MEASUREMENT OF GLUTATHIONE

This was done by using commercially available ELISA kit (Wuhan Eiaab Science Inc., China) specific for measurement of plasma glutathione levels according to the manufacturer's instructions. Briefly, the microtiter plate has been precoated with an antibody specific to GSH. Standards and samples were pipetted into the wells with a biotin-conjugated polyclonal antibody specific for GSH. Next, avidin conjugated to horseradish peroxidase (HRP) was added and incubated. A substrate solution was added and colour developed in proportion to the amount of GSH. The colour development was stopped, and the intensity of the colour was measured.

14.2.5.2 MEASUREMENT OF SUPEROXIDE DISMUTASE

This assay employs the quantitative sandwich enzyme immunoassay technique for the assessment of human superoxide dismutase in plasma (Wuhan Eiaab Science Inc., China). A monoclonal antibody specific for SOD has been precoated onto a microplate. Standards and samples were pipetted into the wells, followed by addition of a second antibody specific for SOD. Then, a substrate solution was added to the wells and colour developed in proportion to the amount of SOD bound in the initial step. The colour development was stopped, and the intensity of the color was measured.

14.2.5.3 MEASUREMENT OF MYELOPEROXIDASE

Plasma myeloperoxidase level was measured using double antibody sandwich ELISA (GenWay biotech, USA) according to the manufacturer's instructions. This method is based upon formation of enzyme-labeled antibodies complex followed by addition of chromogenic substrate to develop a color that is proportionate to the myeloperoxidase concentration.

14.2.6 STATISTICAL ANALYSIS

The data were analyzed and presented as mean ± SEM (standard error of the mean). Statistical differences in each measurement before and 2 weeks after milk therapy were determined with P values, and $P < 0.5$ was considered significant. The receiver operating characteristics (ROC) curve as a fundamental tool for biomarkers evaluation was performed using the same computer program. In a ROC curve, the true positive rate (sensitivity) is plotted in function of the false positive rate (100-specificity) for different cut-off points of a parameter. Each point on the ROC curve represents a sensitivity/specificity pair corresponding to a particular decision threshold. The area under the ROC curve is a measure of how well a parameter can distinguish between camel-milk-treated and untreated autistic subjects.

14.3 RESULTS

The present study was performed to study the effect of camel milk consumption on oxidative stress on ASD subjects by measuring the plasma levels of glutathione, superoxide dismutase, and myeloperoxidase.

Table 1 and Figure 1 show plasma levels of GSH, SOD, and MPO together with CARS of autistic children, before and 2 weeks after camel milk consumption. All measured parameters showed significant changes after camel milk consumption.

TABLE 1: Glutathione, superoxide dismutase, and myeloperoxidase in plasma of autistic children together with CARS before and 2 weeks after camel milk consumption.

	Raw milk (N = 24)		Boiled milk (N = 25)		Placebo (N = 11)	
	Mean ± SEM	P value	Mean ± SEM	P value	Mean ± SEM	P value
Glutathione						
Before	0.37 ± 0.03	0.05	0.34 ± 0.03	0.02	0.36 ± 0.02	0.5
After	0.41 ± 0.01		0.45 ± 0.02		0.35 ± 0.04	
SOD						
Before	0.54 ± 0.03	0.2	0.49 ± 0.02	0.007	0.52 ± 0.03	0.5
After	0.59 ± 0.02		0.57 ± 0.02		0.54 ± 0.03	
MPO						
Before	2.65 ± 0.17	0.05	2.44 ± 0.13	0.02	2.11 ± 0.37	0.2
After	3.22 ± 0.24		3.08 ± 0.19		2.62 ± 0.16	
CARS						
Before	37.63 ± 6.31	0.004	36.82 ± 3.27	0.001	34.18 ± 3.25	0.772
After	34.54 ± 5.19		33.80 ± 4.91		34.41 ± 3.25	

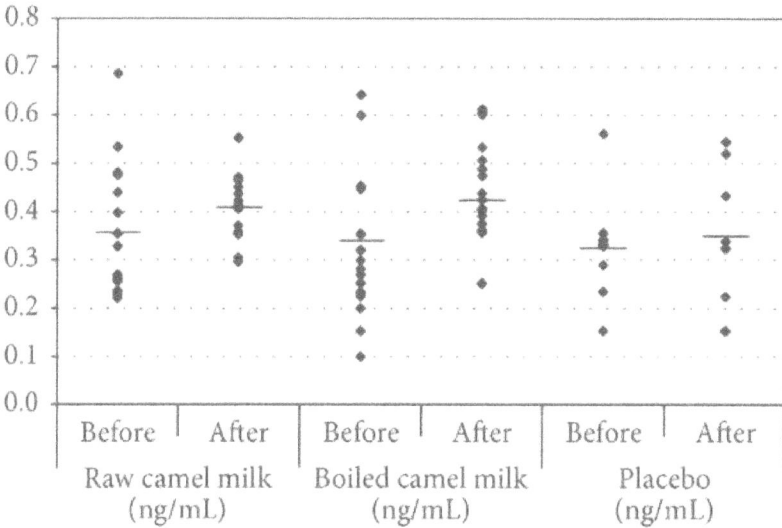

FIGURE 1: Levels of (a) GSH, (b) SOD, (c) MPO, and (d) CARS in autistic patients before and after treating with the camel milk. The mean value for each group is designated by a line.

Plasma GSH levels were significantly increased in group I and group II (P = 0.05, P = 0.02, resp.), but not in group III, following 2 weeks of camel milk consumption. In addition, plasma levels of SOD demonstrated no significant differences in group I (P = 0.2) and group III (P = 0.5). On the other hand, group II demonstrated a highly statistically significant change following 2 weeks of boiled camel milk consumption (P = 0.007). Furthermore, there was a significant elevation of MPO in both group I, the raw camel milk (P = 0.02), and group II, the boiled camel milk (P = 0.05), but not in group III, the placebo group (P = 0.2).

Table 2 and Figures 2(a)–2(d) demonstrate ROC analysis of the 4 measured variants. It could be easily noticed that GSH, SOD, MPO, and CARS show higher area under the curve (AUC), % specificity, and sensitivity in groups I and II than in group III.

TABLE 2: ROC curve of GSH, SOD, MPO, and CARS of autistic patients before and after treatment with camel milk.

Parameters		Raw camel milk	Boiled Camel milk	Placebo
GSH	Area under the curve	0.677	0.723	0.504
	Best cut-off value	0.357	0.356	0.326
	Sensitivity%	83.3	88.0	45.5
	Specificity%	62.5	72.0	72.7
SOD	Area under the curve	0.642	0.706	0.591
	Best cut-off value	0.453	0.562	0.585
	Sensitivity%	95.8%	56.0%	54.5
	Specificity%	41.7%	88.0%	72.7
MPO	Area under the curve	0.584	0.703	0.702
	Best cut-off value	3.17	2.385	2.180
	Sensitivity%	45.8%	76.0%	90.9%
	Specificity%	79.2%	64.0%	54.4%
CARS	Area under the curve	0.729	0.682	0.512
	Best cut-off value	35.5	33.75	37.25
	Sensitivity%	70.8	44.0	81.8
	Specificity%	70.8	96.0	36.4

14.4 DISCUSSION

The present study aimed at evaluating the effect of camel milk on oxidative stress among subjects with autism spectrum disorders by measuring the levels of antioxidant enzymes: SOD, MPO, and GSH.

Several studies have suggested an increased vulnerability of subjects with ASD to oxidative stress. Oxidative stress and the consequent damage occur when antioxidant defence mechanisms fail to effectively counter endogenous or exogenous sources of reactive oxygen species [38]. Increased oxidative stress might contribute to behavioural aberrations, sleep disorder, and gastrointestinal disturbances in autistic children [39, 40].

Low plasma antioxidant enzymes, GSH-Px [25] and SOD [23], were reported. Low level of antioxidant enzymes indicated increased vulnerability to oxidative stress due to impaired antioxidant defence mechanisms, which lead to harmful effects of free radicals that could have an important role in the aetiology of autism. Moreover, increased oxidative stress in autistic subjects leads to a decrease in the levels of nonenzymatic antioxidants like GSH, vitamin E and C [13], which in turn leads to impairment of metabolic pathways and may contribute to the developmental delays which occur in autism; this could be corrected by micronutrient supplementation [41]. In addition, lower plasma levels of glutathione and cysteine in subjects with ASD were documented [42, 43].

Camel milk has been reported to improve clinical outcomes of ASD [31]. The effect of camel milk consumption on autistic behaviour was documented through significant changes in the Childhood Autism Rating Scale (CARS) scoring results [44], as casein- and gluten-free diet has been reported to improve autistic behavior [31], possibly by reducing excess central opioid effects [45].

Glutathione is one of the most important intracellular antioxidants, responsible for maintaining the reducing intracellular microenvironment that is essential for normal cellular function and viability. It also exerts neuroprotective properties and reduces neuropathy and hence decreases oxidative stress.

Subjects with ASD were shown to exhibit abnormal plasma levels of metabolites in the pathway of glutathione redox metabolism, due to inefficient detoxification system [12]. The concentration of reduced glutathione (GSH) was found to be significantly decreased compared to control [10, 25], which reflects increased oxidative stress due to the impaired defense mechanisms against ROS.

The results of the present study show a significant increase in GSH level after camel milk consumption; this could be attributed to the antioxidant nutrients constituents of camel milk. Magnesium is known to reduce oxidative stress and enhance vitamin E and C absorption [44], whereas zinc increases total glutathione, GSHPx, and SOD levels. Moreover, vitamin E has been suggested to enhance glutathione levels [46]. Taken together, high levels of Mg and Zn and vitamin E in camel milk might help to increase glutathione production and enzymes production and hence to decrease the oxidative stress in autistic subjects.

Superoxide dismutase is an antioxidant enzyme that inhibits lipid peroxidation by catalyzing the conversion of superoxide into hydrogen peroxide (H_2O_2) and oxygen (O_2) [13] and acts as a primary defence, as it prevents further generation of free radicals. Insufficient capacity of SOD to metabolize the resulting H_2O_2 may lead to toxicity [10].

It was shown that the SOD activity was significantly higher in autistic children compared to control, in response to oxidative stress. The increased activity may be an adaptive response to eliminate superoxide that was excessively produced [10]. In contrast, other studies reported significant decrease of SOD levels in autistic children compared to controls [24, 43], due to the impairment of the defence mechanism against oxidative stress. Low SOD may also contribute to the nutritional status as some of the antioxidant nutrient levels affect the status of the antioxidant enzymes. For example, adequate amounts of superoxide dismutase are produced when the body receives an adequate and balanced intake of copper and zinc. Copper deficiency was reported to reduce the level of superoxide dismutase [23, 46], whereas zinc deficient diet decreases superoxide dismutase, glutathione peroxidase, total glutathione, and vitamin E [47]. Other studies suggested that the low zinc levels have been associated with autism and related to lower SOD levels, due to the lower zinc to copper ratio in autistic children compared to controls [23, 48].

In the present study, SOD level was significantly increased after camel milk consumption; this could be attributed to the high contents of zinc, copper, magnesium, and vitamin E in camel milk.

Myeloperoxidase is a biomarker of oxidative stress that is responsible for microbicidal activity against a wide range of organisms and one of the indicators of inflammation [49]. Elevated superoxide generated from dysfunctional mitochondria promotes the formation of excessive H_2O_2, the substrate for MPO-mediated hypochlorous acid synthesis, which is then converted to the inflammatory biomarker, 3-chlorotyrosine (3-CT), in activated immune cells during an inflammatory response [38].

Elevated expression of MPO has previously been demonstrated in chronic neurological disease states, such as Alzheimer's disease [50], Parkinson's disease [51], multiple sclerosis [52], and autism spectrum disorder [53].

It has been demonstrated that autistic children with severe GI disease have low serum levels of MPO, which is directly linked with GI pathology seen in this group [54]. The present study demonstrated a significant increase in the plasma myeloperoxidase level following camel milk consumption, which could be a consequence of increased level of SOD. MPO and SOD work synergistically to protect the cell contents against oxidizing activity by destroying anions and hydrogen peroxide [50]; superoxide dismutase catalyzes the conversion of superoxide radicals to H_2O_2, with catalase neutralizing H_2O_2 and then myeloperoxidase converting H_2O_2 to highly reactive hypochlorous acid [23]. Another possibility might be the improvement of GI problems due to the deprivation of camel milk from beta lactoglobulin and beta casein, the major cause for food allergy and GI disease in autistic subjects [7, 54, 55].

Various studies demonstrated a remarkable improvement of some symptoms in ASD subjects following a gluten- and casein- free diet [34], glutathione supplementation [22], antioxidant supplementation such as vitamin E, C, and selinum [22–24], or magnesium and zinc supplementation [43]. These molecules are essential for glutathione synthesis, antioxidant enzymes activities, antioxidant vitamins absorption, and effective antioxidant defence mechanism and hence they play an important role in decreasing oxidative stress as confirmed in various studies.

In light of this information, the role of camel milk in decreasing oxidative stress and treatment of ASD could be explained on the basis that it contains high level of antioxidant vitamins C, A, and E and is very rich in antioxidant minerals magnesium and zinc. Antioxidant vitamins are useful in reducing the oxidative stress. Vitamin E and magnesium have been suggested to enhance glutathione biosynthesis. Magnesium deficiency has been associated with the production of reactive oxygen species [46]. On the other hand, zinc is essential for the activity of many enzymes in living organisms such as SOD and GPx. It has been reported that zinc can prevent cell damage through activation of the antioxidant system [47, 56]. Taken together, these nutrients enhance the production of detoxifying molecules, absorption of antioxidant vitamins, and activation of antioxidant enzymes which in turn activate the detoxification system and reduce the exerted oxidative stress. Another possibility is that camel milk can help to combat and treat gastrointestinal problems, which are frequently associated with ASD, due to its inflammation-inhibiting constituents and hypoallergenic properties, in addition to its smaller size antibodies which are similar to human antibodies [7, 37], and thus improve some autistic behaviours.

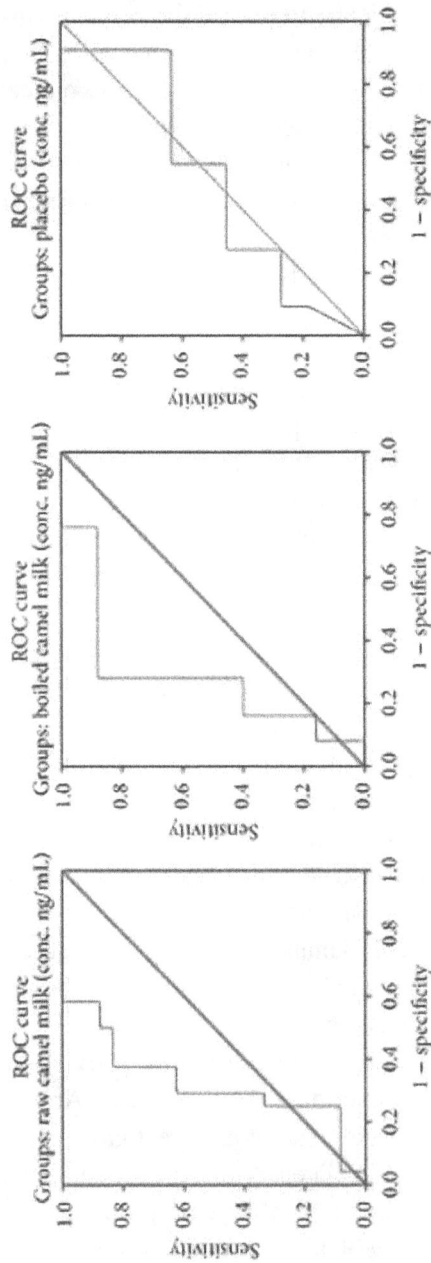

FIGURE 2: ((a)–(d)): ROC curves showing specificity, sensitivity, and area under the curves for (a) GSH, (b) SOD, (c) MPO, and (d) CARS.

The role of the measured parameters in the etiology of autistic features could be also ascertained in this study. The amelioration induced by raw and camel milk on GSH, SOD, and MPO was accompanied by a significant improvement in the behaviour of the autistic children after two weeks of camel milk consumption. CARS was significantly lower after camel milk consumption than before.

Table 2 and Figures 2(a)–2(d) demonstrate that although the four measured parameters did not show very high specificity and sensitivity, GSH and CARS show satisfactory values of both measures. This could help to suggest GSH as a predictive biomarker to follow the potency of camel milk treatment in parallel with the measurement of CARS as a behavioural and cognitional measure.

In conclusion, our findings suggest that camel milk could play an important role in decreasing oxidative stress by alteration of antioxidant enzymes and nonenzymatic antioxidant molecules levels and improvement of autistic behaviour. A larger scale study considering the period and dosage of camel milk is needed to determine the effect of camel milk on oxidative stress biomarkers and hence the treatment of ASD. In addition, other parameters representing different signalling pathways related to the pathology of autism are recommended. Screening for a predictive marker which might record higher specificity and sensitivity than those of the present study is critically needed.

REFERENCES

1. C. Lord, E. H. Cook, B. L. Leventhal, and D. G. Amaral, "Autism spectrum disorders," Neuron, vol. 28, no. 2, pp. 355–363, 2000.
2. American Psychiatric Association, "Diagnostic and statistical manual of mental disorders," Tech. Rep. DSM-IV-TR, American Psychiatric Association, Washington, DC, USA, 2000.
3. N. Momeni, J. Bergquist, L. Brudin et al., "A novel blood-based biomarker for detection of autism spectrum disorders," Translational Psychiatry, vol. 2, article e91, 2012.
4. J. Veenstra-VanderWeele and E. H. Cook Jr., "Molecular genetics of autism spectrum disorder," Molecular Psychiatry, vol. 9, no. 9, pp. 819–832, 2004.
5. P. Ashwood, P. Krakowiak, I. Hertz-Picciotto, R. Hansen, I. Pessah, and J. Van de Water, "Elevated plasma cytokines in autism spectrum disorders provide evidence of

immune dysfunction and are associated with impaired behavioral outcome," Brain, Behavior, and Immunity, vol. 25, no. 1, pp. 40–45, 2011.

6.   L. Y. AL-Ayadhi and G. A. Mostafa, "A lack of association between elevated serum levels of S100B protein and autoimmunity in autistic children," Journal of Neuroinflammation, vol. 9, article 54, 2012.

7.   J. F. White, "Intestinal pathophysiology in autism," Experimental Biology and Medicine, vol. 228, no. 6, pp. 639–649, 2003.

8.   S. Bölte and F. Poustka, "The relation between general cognitive level and adaptive behavior domains in individuals with autism with and without co-morbid mental retardation," Child Psychiatry and Human Development, vol. 33, no. 2, pp. 165–172, 2002.

9.   J. Baio, "Prevalence of Autism spectrum disorders—autism and developmental disabilities monitoring network, 14 Sites, United States, 2008," Morbidity and Mortality Weekly Report, vol. 61, no. 3, pp. 1–19, 2012.

10. Y. Al-Gadani, A. El-Ansary, O. Attas, and L. Al-Ayadhi, "Metabolic biomarkers related to oxidative stress and antioxidant status in Saudi autistic children," Clinical Biochemistry, vol. 42, no. 10-11, pp. 1032–1040, 2009.

11. E. Schopler, R. J. Reichler, and B. R. Renner, "The childhood autism rating scale," Western Psychology Services, Los Angeles, Calif, USA.

12. P. Castelloe and G. Dawson, "Subclassification of children with autism and pervasive developmental disorder: a questionnaire based on Wing's subgrouping scheme," Journal of Autism and Developmental Disorders, vol. 23, no. 2, pp. 229–242, 1993.

13. A. Chauhan, V. Chauhan, W. T. Brown, and I. Cohen, "Oxidative stress in autism: increased lipid peroxidation and reduced serum levels of ceruloplasmin and transferrin—the antioxidant proteins," Life Sciences, vol. 75, no. 21, pp. 2539–2549, 2004.

14. Y. Christen, "Oxidative stress and Alzheimer disease," American Journal of Clinical Nutrition, vol. 71, no. 2, pp. 621s–629s, 2000.

15. K. Kannan and S. K. Jain, "Oxidative stress and apoptosis," Pathophysiology, vol. 7, no. 3, pp. 153–163, 2000.

16. S. Bostantjopoulou, G. Kyriazis, Z. Katsarou, G. Kiosseoglou, A. Kazis, and G. Mentenopoulos, "Superoxide dismutase activity in early and advanced Parkinson's disease," Functional Neurology, vol. 12, no. 2, pp. 63–68, 1997.

17. Ö. Akyol, H. Herken, E. Uz et al., "The indices of endogenous oxidative and antioxidative processes in plasma from schizophrenic patients: the possible role of oxidant/ antioxidant imbalance," Progress in Neuro-Psychopharmacology and Biological Psychiatry, vol. 26, no. 5, pp. 995–1005, 2002.

18. A. C. Andreazza, M. Kauer-Sant'Anna, B. N. Frey et al., "Oxidative stress markers in bipolar disorder: a meta-analysis," Journal of Affective Disorders, vol. 111, no. 2-3, pp. 135–144, 2008.

19. E. Shohami, E. Beit-Yannai, M. Horowitz, and R. Kohen, "Oxidative stress in closed-head injury: brain antioxidant capacity as an indicator of functional outcome," Journal of Cerebral Blood Flow and Metabolism, vol. 17, no. 10, pp. 1007–1019, 1997.

20. A. El-Ansary, S. Al-Daihan, A. Al-Dbass, and L. Al-Ayadhi, "Measurement of selected ions related to oxidative stress and energy metabolism in Saudi autistic children," Clinical Biochemistry, vol. 43, no. 1-2, pp. 63–70, 2010.

21. S. S. Zoroglu, F. Armutcu, S. Ozen et al., "Increased oxidative stress and altered activities of erythrocyte free radical scavenging enzymes in autism," European Archives of Psychiatry and Clinical Neuroscience, vol. 254, no. 3, pp. 143–147, 2004.

22. A. J. Russo, "Decreased serum Cu/Zn SOD in children with autism," Nutrition and Metabolic Insights, vol. 2, pp. 27–35, 2009.

23. N. A. Meguid, A. A. Dardir, E. R. Abdel-Raouf, and A. Hashish, "Evaluation of oxidative stress in autism: defective antioxidant enzymes and increased lipid peroxidation," Biological Trace Element Research, vol. 143, no. 1, pp. 58–65, 2011.

24. Y. A. Al-Yafee, L. Y. Al-Ayadhi, S. H. Haq, and A. K. El-Ansary, "Novel metabolic biomarkers related to sulfur-dependent detoxification pathways in autistic patients of Saudi Arabia," BMC Neurology, vol. 11, article 139, 2011.

25. O. A. Al-Mosalem, A. El-Ansary, O. Attas, and L. Al-Ayadhi, "Metabolic biomarkers related to energy metabolism in Saudi autistic children," Clinical Biochemistry, vol. 42, no. 10-11, pp. 949–957, 2009.

26. W. R. McGinnis, "Oxidative stress in autism," Integrative Medicine, vol. 3, no. 6, pp. 42–57, 2005.

27. R. P. Agrawal, R. Beniwal, D. K. Kochar et al., "Camel milk as an adjunct to insulin therapy improves long-term glycemic control and reduction in doses of insulin in patients with type-1 diabetes: a 1 year randomized controlled trial," Diabetes Research and Clinical Practice, vol. 68, no. 2, pp. 176–177, 2005.

28. R. P. Agrawal, S. Jain, S. Shah, A. Chopra, and V. Agarwal, "Effect of camel milk on glycemic control and insulin requirement in patients with type 1 diabetes: 2-years randomized controlled trial," European Journal of Clinical Nutrition, vol. 65, no. 9, pp. 1048–1052, 2011.

29. H. Saltanat, H. Li, Y. Xu, J. Wang, F. Liu, and X.-H. Geng, "The influences of camel milk on the immune response of chronic hepatitis B patients," Xi Bao Yu Fen Zi Mian Yi Xue Za Zhi, vol. 25, no. 5, pp. 431–433, 2009.

30. Y. Shabo and R. Yagil, "Etiology of autism and camel milk as therapy," Journal of Endocrine Genetics, vol. 4, no. 2, pp. 67–70, 2005.

31. R. Yagil, "Camel milk and autoimmune diseases: historical medicine," 2004, http://www.camelmilkforhealth.com.

32. H. E. Mohamed, H. M. Mousa, and A. C. Beynen, "Ascorbic acid concentrations in milk from Sudanese camels," Journal of Animal Physiology and Animal Nutrition, vol. 89, no. 1-2, pp. 35–37, 2005.

33. A. I. Al-Humaid, H. M. Mousa, R. A. El-Mergawi, and A. M. Abdel-Salam, "Chemical composition and antioxidant activity of dates and dates-camel-milk mixtures as a protective meal against lipid peroxidation in rats," American Journal of Food Technology, vol. 5, no. 1, pp. 22–30, 2010.

34. Y. Shabo, R. Barzel, M. Margoulis, and R. Yagil, "Camel milk for food allergies in children," Israel Medical Association Journal, vol. 7, no. 12, pp. 796–798, 2005.

35. S. Kappeler, Z. Farah, and Z. Puhan, "Sequence analysis of Camelus dromedarius milk caseins," The Journal of Dairy Research, vol. 65, no. 2, pp. 209–222, 1998.

36. S. Kappeler, Compositional and structural analysis of camel milk proteins with emphasis on protective proteins [Ph.D. thesis], Swiss Federal Institute of Technology, Zurich, Switzerland, 1998.

37. O. Zafra, S. Fraile, C. Gutiérrez et al., "Monitoring biodegradative enzymes with nanobodies raised in Camelus dromedarius with mixtures of catabolic proteins," Environmental Microbiology, vol. 13, no. 4, pp. 960–974, 2011.

38. S. Rose, S. Melnyk, O. Pavliv et al., "Evidence of oxidative damage and inflammation associated with low glutathione redox status in the autism brain," Transl Psychiatry, vol. 2, e134, 2012.

39. W. R. McGinnis, "Oxidative stress in autism," Alternative Therapies in Health and Medicine, vol. 10, no. 6, pp. 22–36, 2004.

40. S. Söğüt, S. S. Zoroğlu, H. Özyurt et al., "Changes in nitric oxide levels and antioxidant enzyme activities may have a role in the pathophysiological mechanisms involved in autism," Clinica Chimica Acta, vol. 331, no. 1-2, pp. 111–117, 2003.

41. O. Yorbik, A. Sayal, C. Akay, D. I. Akbiyik, and T. Sohmen, "Investigation of antioxidant enzymes in children with autistic disorder," Prostaglandins Leukotrienes and Essential Fatty Acids, vol. 67, no. 5, pp. 341–343, 2002.

42. A. Knivsberg, K. L. Reichelt, N. Nodland, and T. Hoien, "Autistic syndromes and diet: a follow-up study," Scandinavian Journal of Educational Research, vol. 39, pp. 223–236, 1995.

43. A. M. Knivsberg, K. L. Reichelt, T. Høien, and M. Nødland, "A randomised, controlled study of dietary intervention in autistic syndromes," Nutritional Neuroscience, vol. 5, no. 4, pp. 251–261, 2002.

44. L. Y. Al-Ayadhi and G. A. Mostafa, "Elevated serum levels of macrophage-derived chemokine and thymus and activation-regulated chemokine in autistic children," Journal of Neuroinflammation, vol. 10, article 72, no. 1, 2013.

45. N. A. Al-wabel, A. Hassan, H. Abbas, and H. Muosa, "Antiulcerogenic effect of camel milk against ethanol induced gastric ulcers in rats," WebmedCentral Veterinary Medicine, vol. 3, no. 3, Article ID WMC002804, 2012.

46. L. Klevay, "Advances in cardiovascular-copper research," in Proceedings of the 1st International Bio-Minerals Symposium: Trace Elements in Nutrition, Health and Disease, G. N. Schrauzer, Ed., Institute Rosell, Montreal, Canada, 2003.

47. S. R. Powell, "The antioxidant properties of zinc," Journal of Nutrition, vol. 130, no. 5, pp. 1447–1454, 2000.

48. S. Faber, G. M. Zinn, J. C. Kern II, and H. M. Skip Kingston, "The plasma zinc/serum copper ratio as a biomarker in children with autism spectrum disorders," Biomarkers, vol. 14, no. 3, pp. 171–180, 2009.

49. E. B. Kurutas, A. Cetinkaya, E. Bulbuloglu, and B. Kantarceken, "Effects of antioxidant therapy on leukocyte myeloperoxidase and Cu/Zn-superoxide dismutase and plasma malondialdehyde levels in experimental colitis," Mediators of Inflammation, vol. 2005, no. 6, pp. 390–394, 2005.

50. P. S. Green, A. J. Mendez, J. S. Jacob et al., "Neuronal expression of myeloperoxidase is increased in Alzheimer's disease," Journal of Neurochemistry, vol. 90, no. 3, pp. 724–733, 2004.

51. D.-K. Choi, S. Pennathur, C. Perier et al., "Ablation of the inflammatory enzyme myeloperoxidase mitigates features of Parkinson's disease in mice," Journal of Neuroscience, vol. 25, no. 28, pp. 6594–6600, 2005.

52. R. M. Nagra, B. Becher, W. W. Tourtellotte et al., "Immunohistochemical and genetic evidence of myeloperoxidase involvement in multiple sclerosis," Journal of Neuroimmunology, vol. 78, no. 1-2, pp. 97–107, 1997.
53. A. K. Anthony, J. Russo, B. Jepson, and A. Wakefield, "Low serum myeloperoxidase in autistic children with gastrointestinal disease," Journal of Clinical and Experimental Gastroenterology, vol. 2, pp. 85–94, 2009.
54. K. Horvath and J. A. Perman, "Autistic disorder and gastrointestinal disease," Current Opinion in Pediatrics, vol. 14, no. 5, pp. 583–587, 2002.
55. I. Rahman, S. K. Biswas, L. A. Jimenez, M. Torres, and H. J. Forman, "Glutathione, stress responses, and redox signaling in lung inflammation," Antioxidants and Redox Signaling, vol. 7, no. 1-2, pp. 42–59, 2005.
56. J. El Heni, S. Sfar, F. Hammouda, M. T. Sfar, and A. Kerkeni, "Interrelationships between cadmium, zinc and antioxidants in the liver of the rat exposed orally to relatively high doses of cadmium and zinc," Ecotoxicology and Environmental Safety, vol. 74, no. 7, pp. 2099–2104, 2011.

CHAPTER 15

ISSUES IN THE TIMING OF INTEGRATED EARLY INTERVENTIONS: CONTRIBUTIONS FROM NUTRITION, NEUROSCIENCE, AND PSYCHOLOGICAL RESEARCH

THEODORE D. WACHS, MICHAEL GEORGIEFF, SARAH CUSICK, AND BRUCE S. MCEWEN

15.1 INTRODUCTION

Evidence documents that children from low-income families in both wealthy[1] and low-income countries[2] have greater exposure to multiple biological and psychosocial risks that can significantly compromise their development. These findings emphasize the importance of integrating and implementing multidimensional biological and psychosocial interventions to compensate for exposure to multiple risks.[3] A critical and long-standing question involves identifying the age period(s) in which such interventions can have the strongest and longest lasting effects. The

Reprinted with permission from Wachs TD, Georgieff M, Cusick S, and McEwen BS. Issues in the Timing of Integrated Early Interventions: Contributions from Nutrition, Neuroscience, and Psychological Research. Annals of the New York Academy of Sciences 1308 (2014), 89-106; doi:10.1111/nyas.12314.

concept that the early years of life are a time when children are particularly sensitive to extrinsic influences has deep-seated roots, dating back to the writings of Plato.[4] In the present era, questions involving timing of events and change over time in relations between contextual elements are central issues in major developmental theories such as developmental systems theory[5] and the bioecological model.[6]

Initial empirical support for the importance of the early years of life came from 20th century embryological research on fetal development and ethological research on imprinting, which culminated in the concepts of critical and sensitive periods of development. While both concepts refer to age periods characterized by plasticity in development, when the effects of exposure to facilitative experiences or developmental risks are particularly strong and lasting, the concepts are not identical.[7] Critical periods are characterized by enhanced sensitivity to exposures that are restricted to a sharply defined time period such that the effects of exposures during this time period are irreversible. In contrast, when sensitive periods occur, the exposure time windows for enhanced sensitivity are broader, and there can be continued, though reduced, plasticity both before and after the sensitive period and exposure during sensitive time windows is not necessarily irreversible.[8]

Evidence from human-level studies favors the operation of sensitive rather than critical periods.[9-12] Research findings also indicate that there may be multiple sensitive periods depending upon the domains of development assessed.[9, 10, 13] Illustrating the operation of multiple sensitive periods is evidence that sensitive periods for neural development may be narrower than sensitive periods for behavioral development[14, 15] and that different sensitive-period windows are seen for cognitive/academic versus social–emotional outcomes.[16, 17] For example, the impact of exposure to poverty (or to interventions designed to reduce poverty) upon later cognitive or academic outcomes appears to be strongest in the period from infancy to early childhood, whereas such exposure appears to adversely affect social–emotional development or behavior problem outcomes across the age span from infancy through adolescence.[18] One implication of this pattern of findings is that different time periods may be needed for biological versus psychosocial interventions or for different psychosocial outcomes.

The primary question addressed by this paper is whether the early years of life are a sensitive time period for implementing integrated biological and psychosocial interventions to promote the development of children living in poverty in low- and middle-income countries? To address this question we will review evidence from nutrition, neuroscience, and developmental psychology on the timing of exposures to biological or psychosocial influences and neural, physiological, and behavioral outcomes. In this paper the early years are defined as the time span between fertilization and the end of the fifth year of life. Our rationale for using the fifth year is based on evidence that lower developmental trajectories during this time period are a significant precursor for poor school readiness and subsequent inadequate school performance as well as later cognitive and social–emotional problems.[2] In addition, although we relate defined time periods to specific outcome dimensions, we recognize the validity of the conclusion drawn by developmental systems theorists that different outcome dimensions are linked in such a way that changes in one outcome can result in changes in other outcomes.[5]

15.2 THE TIMING OF NUTRITION AND BRAIN DEVELOPMENT

Optimal overall brain development in the prenatal period and early years of life depends on providing sufficient quantities of key nutrients during specific sensitive time periods. While all nutrients are important for brain development, certain nutrients (e.g., protein, long-chain polyunsaturated fatty acids (LCPUFAs), iron, copper, zinc, iodine, folate, choline, and vitamins A, B6, and B12) have particularly large effects early in life and exhibit critical or sensitive periods for neurodevelopment (for more details see Table S1). These periods coincide with the times when specific brain regions are developing most rapidly and have their highest nutrient requirements. Because the brain is not a homogeneous organ, there is not a single common growth trajectory or a single sensitive period.[9] Rather, different brain regions (e.g., the hippocampus, striatum, cortex) and brain processes (e.g., myelination) exhibit growth trajectories that span and peak at different times, each with specific nutrient requirements. These periods of peak growth are also those times when the deficiency of a specific nutrient, particularly one that supports basic neuronal/glial metabolic processes (e.g., protein, iron, glucose), is most deleterious. Supplementation of a deficient nutrient after these sensitive windows of development have passed usually results in incomplete correction of the brain insult and thus in an increased risk of long-term neurodevelopmental deficits. Defining the timing of these peak periods of nutrient requirement for certain brain areas is critical for the successful implementation of nutritional interventions to prevent harmful, potentially permanent effects of deficiency on brain development.

Sensitive periods for specific nutrients (Table 1) are typically identified in controlled studies of preclinical models at different stages of early development and subsequently validated with successful nutritional intervention studies in humans that yield beneficial neurobehavioral outcomes in the domains identified in the preclinical models. The literature on early iron nutrition serves as an example of how such multidisciplinary studies work in concert to demonstrate that timing affects a nutrient's relationship with the developing brain.

15.2.1 IRON DEFICIENCY

Iron deficiency is the most common nutritional deficiency worldwide, with an estimated one billion people having iron-deficiency anemia.[19] The developing brain requires iron for enzymes and hemoproteins that regulate cellular processes, including fatty acid production, dopamine neurotransmitter synthesis, and neuronal energy production.[20, 21] The peak periods of brain vulnerability to iron deficiency are those where a high demand for iron coincides with a time period when iron balance is likely to be negative (Table 1). This includes the fetal/neonatal period and infancy/toddlerhood (6 months to 3 years), two time periods when iron deficiency has profound and long-lasting effects and when supplementation has proven to be an effective deterrent of later impairment. It is important to note that while early adulthood is also a period of high risk for negative iron balance, brain development at this time is slower, and thus brain demand for iron is relatively low. Accordingly, iron deficiency in women between 18 and 35 years may cause acute effects, but these effects appear to resolve with restoration of iron status, with no apparent long-term neurobehavioral consequences.[22]

TABLE 1: Brain regions affected by critical nutrients for brain development in the first 1000 days[a]

Nutrient	Period(s) of particularly high brain demand for nutrient	Principal brain region or circuitry affected
Protein	(1) Gestation	(1) Global, hippocampus, striatum, myelin, cerebellum
	(2) 4–12 months postnatal	(2) Cortex (especially prefrontal), myelin
LCPUFAs	Last trimester of gestation: 2–3 months postnatal	Global, retina
Iron	(1) Last trimester of gestation	(1) Myelin, striatum, hippocampus
	(2) 6 months–3 years postnatal	(2) Myelin, frontal cortex, basal ganglia (motor)
Zinc	(1) Last four months of gestation	(1) Autonomic nervous system, cerebellum, hippocampus
	(2) 6 months–10 years	(2) Cortex
Iodine	(1) First trimester of gestation	(1) Global
	(2) Last trimester of gestation	(2) Cortex, striatum, cerebellum, hippocampus
	(3) Infancy–12 years	(3) Myelin, prefrontal cortex
Copper	Last trimester of gestation	Occipital and parietal cortex, striatum, cerebellum, hippocampus

[a]*All nutrients listed are critical in the first 1000 days and have their largest effects on brain development at that time; some nutrient–brain developmental time frames extend into middle childhood with milder effects on different neural systems.*

Newborn infants with iron deficiency from late gestation demonstrate recognition-memory deficits indicative of impaired hippocampal function, slower processing speed potentially indicative of reduced myelination, and altered temperament, characterized by poorer infant–mother interaction and suggestive neurobiologically of altered dopamine metabolism. [23-25] Infants with postnatal iron-deficiency anemia show fewer learning and memory effects, but do display slower speeds of neural transmission in auditory brain stem responses and visual evoked potentials, consistent with hypomyelination.[26, 27] Iron deficiency later in toddlerhood leads to impaired social–emotional behavior, including maintaining closer proximity to caregivers, increased irritability, and decreased positive affect.[28, 29] Iron deficiency at this time appears to particularly affect the brain's monoaminergic system, that is neurochemistry, and these behavioral changes may not be remediable with iron therapy.[20, 30]

Animal studies corroborate the effect that the timing of iron deficiency in infancy versus toddlerhood has on neurobehavioral outcomes. Rodent models of gestational/lactational versus postnatal dietary iron deficiency reveal variable impairments in spatial navigation, trace fear conditioning, and procedural memory, all consistent with functional and structural abnormalities in the hippocampus and striatum, as well as abnormalities in myelin formation and monoamine regulation based on the timing of the deficiency.[31-39] A differential timing effect is also seen in rhesus monkeys, where late gestational iron deficiency results in a less fearful and more impulsive animal, while postnatal iron deficiency results in a more inhibited and anxious one.[40]

15.2.2 IRON SUPPLEMENTATION

Studies of iron supplementation in pregnancy and childhood reinforce these findings and demonstrate that the importance of timing in intervention studies cannot be overstated.[41-44] When the period of high brain demand for iron coincides with a period of high risk for iron deficiency, as in the fetal and toddler periods, neurodevelopmental consequences are more likely to occur. Accordingly, these periods are optimal for iron intervention (for more specific details see Table S2). Prenatal iron supplementation appears to particularly set the stage for postnatal iron and brain health. Iron/folic acid supplementation during pregnancy results in significantly better scores in working memory, inhibitory control, and fine motor functioning in children at 7–9 years of age.[43] In contrast, daily iron/folic acid with or without zinc supplementation of children from age 12 to 35 months, whose mothers do not receive micronutrient supplementation during pregnancy, has no effect on intellectual, executive, or motor function at age 7–9 years.[44] Moreover, supplementation of children from 12 to 36 months whose mothers received iron/folic acid during pregnancy conferred no additional cognitive benefit over prenatal iron/folic acid alone.[42]

While 12–36 months of age is both a period of peak vulnerability to iron deficiency and brain demand for iron (Table S2), the brain system exacting the greatest need for iron at this age is the monoaminergic system. Iron supplementation between 12 and 36 months would thus potentially lead to improvements in socioemotional behavior, but significant improvements in cognitive, intellectual, and motor functioning—the domains tested by the researchers—would necessitate earlier supplementation.

15.2.3 IMPLICATIONS FOR INTERVENTIONS

The established sensitive periods of brain development for each nutrient should guide the timing of implementation of nutrition interventions to ensure optimal brain development (Box 1). Nutritional health of the offspring is related to maternal nutritional health even before the child is conceived. Many important brain systems (e.g., the hippocampus, myelination, synaptogenesis) that are dependent on adequate nutritional supply are maturing in the fetus in the last trimester. Thus, nutritional, medical, and social interventions that ensure a healthy, low-stress pregnancy optimize nutrient delivery to the developing fetal brain. In the postnatal period, earlier screening and identification of nutrient risks/deficits is critical since the preponderance of data show earlier nutritional intervention is more effective in promoting long-term brain health. When developing these interventions, four key principles must also be considered to achieve significant neurobehavioral results: (1) the nutritional intervention must be given concordantly with when the nutrient is most needed (e.g., iron supplementation during pregnancy or early infancy to achieve improved cognitive or motor outcomes in later childhood); (2) the target population must not already be sufficient in the nutrient, as no evidence exists that nutrient delivery greater than that which is needed to ensure sufficiency will provide additional neurobehavioral benefit; (3) the behavioral or cognitive battery used to assess outcomes later in childhood must be appropriately specific (i.e., assess potentially affected neural circuits) and not be too global such that subtle differences will not be detected; and (4) the timing of the assessment battery must also be carefully considered, as a null result in response to intervention may be found if the test is administered too late and the child has outgrown a previous nutritionally induced brain deficit, either by neural plasticity or catch-up growth.

BOX 1. NUTRITION AND BRAIN DEVELOPMENT IN THE FIRST 1000 DAYS

1. Brain growth and development is highly dependent on adequate nutritional substrates for that growth. While all nutrients are necessary for the growth of cells, including those in the brain, certain nutrients appear particularly influential: protein, energy sources including glucose, fats including long-chain polyunsaturated fatty acids (i.e., fish oils), iron, zinc, copper, iodine, folic acid, choline, and vitamin A. Deficits in nutrients can cause the brain to function abnormally during the period of the deficit. These deficits appear to be related to alterations in brain metabolism.

2. Some nutritional deficits confer long-term structural and functional abnormalities well beyond the period of deficit, suggesting that the brain has been permanently altered. These deficits appear to be related to structural changes (i.e., not having built the brain correctly) and genomic (e.g., epigenetic) changes that alter long-term regulation of brain function.

3. The brain is not a homogeneous organ. Rather it is characterized by interconnected regions, each of which has a different developmental trajectory. The times of most rapid development (i.e., cell growth and differentiation) define the time of greatest nutrient needs. Thus, the timing of nutrient provision or deficiency determines how the structure develops and ultimately how it functions. A given nutrient deficit at one age may result in quite different developmental effects than the same nutrient deficit at another age.

These findings imply that critical/sensitive windows exist for many of these systems and that these windows are tightly linked to periods of rapid regional brain growth and differentiation.

4. The majority of brain growth that is nutrient sensitive occurs in the first 1000 days from conception. Ensuring the delivery of specific nutrients coincident with growth spurts that are dependent on those nutrients should shape dietary and nutritional intervention policy. As a blanket approach, overall nutrient sufficiency is most important for the pregnant woman, the newborn infant, and the toddler to ensure long-term brain health in the offspring.

5. Provision of nutrients represents only the supply side of the equation. The metabolic status of the recipient, including the presence of illness and psychological stress, will alter how growth factors are regulated and how nutrients are utilized. Thus, factors that mediate stress (see next section) are also important with respect to the effectiveness of nutritional therapy in promoting brain growth.

15.3 TIMING OF STRESS FOR BRAIN AND NEUROENDOCRINE DEVELOPMENT AND FUNCTION

Stressful experiences throughout the life course and resulting health-promoting or damaging behaviors have effects on metabolism and can be regarded as nutrition sensitive. In response to a changing social and physical environment, the body and brain respond to novelty and potential threats by activating autonomic, neuroendocrine, metabolic, and immune system responses that promote adaptation. As shown in Box 2, this process, called allostasis, helps to maintain homeostasis and is primarily dependent on the brain to perceive and react to novelty and potential threats and activate the coordinated mediators of allostasis. When this mechanism is overused by many stressful events, especially when the balanced responses of the network of allostasis are dysregulated, wear and tear on the body ensues, referred to as allostatic load. This concept has relevance to the intersection between metabolism, stress responsiveness, and malnutrition in the sense of both quality and quantity of food, which are very much involved.

Early life events related to maternal care in animals, as well as parental care in humans, play a powerful role in later mental and physical health, as demonstrated by the adverse childhood experiences (ACE) studies and other recent work. A summary of evidence on findings from animal studies are seen in Box S1. At the human level, one of the consequences of ACE is an increased prevalence of metabolic disorders, obesity, and diabetes that may reflect both quantity and quality of food as well as how the body processes it.[50] Food insecurity may be an added factor[58] along with the stressful nature of an ugly and dangerous'neighborhood living environment influencing obesity and increasing allostatic load.[59, 60] In studies on ACE in human populations, there are reports of increased inflammatory tone, not only in children, but also in young adults related to early-life abuse, that includes chronic harsh language as well as physical and sexual abuse.[61, 62] Chaos in the home is associated with development of poor self-regulatory behaviors, as well as obesity.[63] An ACE study carried out in a middle-class population indicates that poverty is not the only source of early-life stressors.[50]

Nevertheless, low socioeconomic status (SES) does increase the likelihood of stressors in the home and neighborhood, including toxic chemical agents such as lead and air pollution.[63-65] Low-SES children are found to be more likely to be deficient in language skills, as well as self-regulatory behaviors and also in certain types of memory that are likely to be reflections of impaired development of parasylvian gyrus language centers, prefrontal cortical systems, and temporal lobe memory systems.[66, 67] Low SES also correlates with smaller hippocampal volumes.[68] Lower subjective SES, an important index of objective SES, is associated with reduction in prefrontal cortical gray matter.[69] Growing up in a lower-SES environment is accompanied by greater amygdala reactivity to angry and sad faces, which, as noted above, may be a predisposing factor for early cardiovascular disease, which is known to be more prevalent at lower SES levels.[70, 71] Furthermore, depression is often associated with low SES, and children of depressed mothers, followed longitudinally, have shown increased amygdala volume while hippocampal volume was not affected.[72]

BOX 2. ALLOSTASIS AND ALLOSTATIC LOAD

The brain is a target of allostatic load, as is the rest of the body. Depression, anxiety disorders, and substance abuse are expressions of this load, along with cardiovascular disease, type 2 diabetes, and metabolic syndrome, and other disorders that reflect the consequences of chronic stress in terms of poor sleep, overeating, smoking, drinking, and lack of physical activity. [45] Allostatic load changes the architecture of regions of the brain involved in cognition and emotional regulation, including shrinkage of the hippocampus that can be reversed by regular, moderate exercise.[46, 47] In animal models, chronic stress is also associated with shrinkage of dendrites in the medial prefrontal cortex as well as the hippocampus and dendritic growth in the basolateral amygdala and orbitfrontal cortex.[46, 48]

Chronic stress becomes toxic and produces the greatest allostatic load when the individual lacks sufficient control of his or her life owing to inadequate social, emotional, or material resources.[49] Moreover, adverse events in early life predispose the brain and body to greater vulnerability to stress throughout the life course.[49, 50] Prenatal stress of the mother is known to increase anxiety behavior of the offspring and alter brain structure and function, including impaired development of the hippocampus. [51, 52] Prenatal stress in humans is associated with shorter telomeres in offspring, along with behavioral and metabolic dysregulation that includes increased risk for metabolic disorders related to low birthweight.[53-55] There are also possible epigenetic effects that are transmitted from the parents to the offspring.[56, 57]

BOX 3. BRAIN DEVELOPMENT TRANSITIONS IN ADOLESCENCE

Animal models are providing important clues. During adolescence, chronic juvenile stress consisting of 6-h daily restraint from postnatal day 20 to 41 produced depressive-like behavior and significant neuronal remodeling of brain regions likely involved in these behavioral alterations, namely, the hippocampus, prefrontal cortex, and amygdala. Chronically stressed males and females exhibited anhedonia, increased locomotion when exposed to novelty, and altered coping strategies when exposed to acute stress. Coincident with these behavioral changes, there was stress-induced shrinkage of dendrites in the hippocampus and prefrontal cortex and concurrent hypertrophy of dendrites in the amygdala and impaired development of the hippocampus carrying into adult life.[87, 88]

The human prefrontal cortex undergoes a prolonged course of maturation that continues well after puberty and parallels a slowly emerging ability for flexible social behavior.[89, 90] Interestingly, there are differences within the cerebral cortex in heritability. The primary sensory and motor cortices, which develop earlier, show relatively greater genetic effects earlier in childhood, whereas the later-developing dorsal prefrontal cortex and temporal lobes show increasingly prominent genetic effects with maturation.[91]

On the positive side, there are reactive alleles that, in nurturing environments, lead to beneficial outcomes and even better outcomes compared to less reactive alleles, even though those same alleles can enhance adverse outcomes in a stressful early-life environment.[73-75] Regarding adverse outcomes and good and bad environments, it must be recognized, as stated in the active calibration model, that allostatic processes are adjusted via epigenetic influences to optimize the individual's adaptation to, and resulting fitness for, a particular environment, whether more or less threatening or nurturing.[76] Yet, there are trade-offs with reference to physical and mental health that, on the one hand, may increase the likelihood of passing on one's genes by improving coping with adversity and enhancing mental health and overall reproductive success, but, on the other hand, may impair later health, for example by eating of comfort foods.[77] At no time is this more important than during adolescence (Box 3), which is a time of transition in physiology and brain development and maturation.[78, 79]

Adolescents have a propensity for risk taking that is related to the capacity to exert self-control, as can be assessed by tests of delayed gratification, such as the "marshmallow test," that have considerable predictive power for social, cognitive, and mental health outcomes over the life course.[80, 81] The neural basis of self-regulation involves frontal–striatal circuitries that integrate motivational and control processes and appear to be stable for a lifetime, based upon studies of the same individuals over 4 decades.[82] A key feature is an exaggerated ventral striatal representation of appetitive cues in adolescents relative to the ability to exert control. The connectivity within the ventral frontostriatal circuit including the inferior frontal gyrus and dorsal striatum is particularly important to the ability to exert self-regulation.[83] Moreover, adolescents are typically somewhat impaired in both fear learning and fear extinction, which implies that they may take more risks[84] and that, when there is a traumatic event, they may be more affected by this, including the possibility that this carries over into adult life. [85, 86]It is also noteworthy that the prefrontal cortex (PFC) to amygdala connectivity changes from positive to negative between early childhood and adolescence and young adulthood.[70] Indeed, young children are wary of strangers as secure attachment to the mother develops. One index of this sensitive period is that, early in life, ambiguous facial expressions are perceived as conveying negative meaning.[92] However, during adolescence, there is a restriction on extinction of fear learning, suggesting that negative experiences may have greater impact during that developmental period, although it is not yet known whether fearful events during adolescence may be more difficult to extinguish later in adult life.[85]

Finally, it is important to note that early-life adversity in rhesus and humans impairs development of the PFC, among other effects in the brain and body. In rhesus, peer rearing causes changes in 5-HT1A receptor density in a number of brain regions including the PFC and is associated with an enlarged vermis, dorsomedial PFC, and dorsal anterior cingulate cortex without any apparent differences in the corpus callosum and hippocampus.[93, 94] In humans, adverse childhood experiences were associated with smaller PFC, greater activation of the hypothalamic–pituitary–adrenal (HPA) axis, and elevation in inflammation levels compared to nonmaltreated children, while adults with a history of childhood maltreatment showed smaller PFC and hippocampal volume, greater activation of the HPA axis, and elevation in inflammation levels compared to nonmaltreated individuals.[95]

There is also increased risk for obesity and metabolic disorders, including type 2 diabetes. Indeed, the developing as well as adult brain is vulnerable to metabolic dysregulation such as occurs in type 2 diabetes and prediabetes. The brain responds to metabolic hormones such as insulin, leptin, ghrelin, and insulin-like growth factor 1 (IGF-1).[96] In adults both pretype 2 diabetes and diabetes causes the hippocampus, a brain region important for learning and memory and mood regulation, to shrink, resulting in impairment of memory and mood.[97-99] There is also increased risk for later Alzheimer's disease.[100] Moreover, many of these problems begin in childhood, and teenagers with pretype 2 diabetes and diabetes have impaired neural architecture and cognitive function.[101, 102] This has huge potential implications for success in school and acquiring skills for the increasingly technical workforce, with a growing impact on national competitiveness as well as soaring healthcare costs.

15.3.1 MAJOR CONCLUSIONS: STRESS AND ADAPTATION

The brain is the central organ of stress and adaptation to stress and does so through the autonomic, neuroendocrine, immune, and metabolic systems, via the active process of allostasis. The brain is itself a target of the dysregulation and overuse of allostasis resulting in allostatic load and overload, which also is manifested in the body as cardiovascular disease, diabetes, arthritis, and other disorders that commonly increase with age.

Brain architecture is altered by stress so as to weaken brain regions involved in learning, memory, and self-regulation but strengthen brain regions important for anxiety and aggression. However, the brain is normally resilient and able to recover after stress, but this resilience is impaired with aging and also in mood and anxiety disorders.

Adverse experiences in childhood exert lasting effects on physical as well as mental health. Animal models reveal long-lasting changes in brain architecture via epigenetic processes that involve behavioral transmission from the parent to the child as well as modifications of DNA without changing the genetic code that are passed on in the germ cells and in utero in the developing fetus. Early life adversity also increases the level of inflammation in the body that lasts into adulthood and contributes to increased incidence of mood and anxiety disorders, substance abuse, sexual precocity, cardiovascular disease, and diabetes.

Adolescence is a time of major changes in brain architecture, particularly the prefrontal cortex that controls self-regulatory behaviors, and, as a result, adolescence is a time of vulnerability to stress. Childhood obesity and diabetes, which may result, in part, from early life adversity, affect brain development, cognitive function, and learning ability, as well as increasing the risk for dementia later in life.

Metabolic dysregulation related to poor quality of diet and also stress-related patterns of health behaviors, including how ongoing stress and resulting allostatic load alters food consumption and metabolic processing, have profound effects on brain development and function that are only now beginning to be appreciated.

15.3.2 IMPLICATIONS FOR INTERVENTION

Interventions that create a stable, consistent, and nurturing parent–child bond foster the development of vital self-regulatory behaviors in which the late-developing prefrontal cortex plays a key role. The continuing plasticity of the brain offers some hope that behavioral intervention may have some beneficial effect throughout the life course. In addressing the growing problem of obesity and diabetes beginning in childhood, it must be recognized that these disorders take a toll on the brain, affecting the ability of individuals to function in our complex society. A promising strategy to prevent obesity involves teaching self-regulation to Head Start preschoolers,[103] although including parents in such therapy is also important.[104] In addition, programs such as the conditional cash transfer in Oportunidades in Mexico offer some hope in helping poor families rid themselves of infections and adopt healthier lifestyles, with some reported improvements in developmental markers of cognition and improved mental health,[105, 106] although such programs have shown uneven effects on educational learning outcomes.[107]

15.4 TIMING ISSUES IN CONTEXTUAL CONTRIBUTIONS TO COGNITIVE OR SOCIAL–EMOTIONAL DEVELOPMENT

As discussed previously, significant neural development continues after the early years of life, particularly during the adolescent period.[84, 108] Similarly, later neural changes can be influenced by current contextual characteristics.[14, 109, 110] A parallel pattern of findings emerges when we consider the effects of contextual influences on cognitive and social–emotional development. Evidence on contextual influences illustrates that (1) important developmental landmarks or precursors for later development occur both in the early years and at later ages; (2) both early and later contextual influences and interventions can influence subsequent functioning; and (3) in some cases, later influences or interventions may sometimes be necessary to maintain the effects of early influences or interventions. Each of these conclusions is documented in the following sections.

15.4.1 RATES OF BEHAVIORAL DEVELOPMENT

Examples of important developmental landmarks appearing during the first 2 years as well as precursors of later development that emerge over the first 5 years of life are shown in Table 2.

TABLE 2: Ages of emergence of critical developmental landmarks and precursors of critical developmental markers

Early appearing developmental landmarks (birth–24 months):	Normally developing visual function such as visual acuity (primarily first 6 months, with gradual improvement to 4 years) and eye movements following repetitive movement through the visual field (optokinetic nystagmus: 3–24 months).[13]
	Certain domains of language such as phononetic perception (seen in the first 10 months).[111]
	Acquisition of taste preferences (first 3 months).[112]
	Acquisition of basic trust and attachment (primarily seen in the 6- to 12-month period).[113]
Early appearing precursors (preschool and early childhood years) of later developmental landmarks	Internalization of committed compliance to adult requests as a precursor for effortful self-regulation (initially seen in the time period between 14 and 56 months).[114]
	Developing a theory of mind as a precursor for taking another person's perspective (emerges around 4 years of age).[115]
	Understanding of the "wrongness" of moral transgressions as a precursor for later moral reasoning (initially seen in the time period from 2.5–4 years).[116]
	Language-based perceptual categories as a precursor for later word learning (appearing around 18 months).[111]
	Deferred imitative play as a precursor to the development of abstract thinking (appears between 18 and 24 months).[117]
	Development of an internalized conscience or inhibiting aggressive outbursts as a precursor to effortful self-regulation (seen between 4 and 7 years).[118]
Later-appearing developmental functions appearing in middle childhood, adolescence, or adulthood.	Evaluating the comparative values of risks versus rewards as a marker of effortful self-regulation (appears between 12 and 20 years).[84, 108]
	Orientation to future goals and considering long-term consequences (appears between 11 and 17 years).[120]
	Interpersonal competencies such as taking another person's perspective (12–15 years).[117]
	Distinguishing between effort versus ability as primary causes or outcomes of success or failure (9–12 years).[121]
	Cognitive competencies such as working memory (7–15+ years). [122, 123]
	Knowledge-based cognitive dimensions—"crystallized intelligence" (peaks in middle adulthood).[124, 125]

While precursors of later development can be seen in the infancy and toddler periods, early specific skills or behaviors can be lost, expanded or replaced by later-developing skills.[119] For example, experience-dependent brain development in adolescence and early adulthood is thought to mediate the emergence of, and increases in, later appearing social–emotional, communication, and cognitive functions. Developmental characteristics appearing past the early years are also shown in Table 2.

15.4.2 DO EARLY CONTEXTUAL INFLUENCES OR INTERVENTIONS AFFECT CHILDREN'S DEVELOPMENT?

15.4.2.1 EVIDENCE FOR DIRECT EFFECTS

As seen in Table 3, findings from early intervention studies document that the early years of life are a sensitive period for preventing long-term sensory problems, for facilitating social–emotional development, and for promoting child cognitive and academic competence. Results from meta-analytic studies, reviews and randomized control trials also document that interventions involving parents and carried out during the first several years of a child's life can significantly improve parental sensitivity, cognitive stimulation, discipline strategies, and supportive warm parenting. [113, 128, 130, 131, 134] Findings also emphasize the potential importance of intervention quality[130] or parent involvement (for home-based interventions),[135] given that long exposure to a substandard early intervention program may have limited benefits.

While findings from some studies suggest that social–emotional development may be particularly sensitive to interventions or experiences experienced during the first 3 years,[113, 127-129] other studies indicate that there is no specific time window during the first 5–6 years where cognitive or social-emotional intervention effects are uniquely strong.[129, 132, 136, 137] Isolation of unique sensitive time windows during the early years of life are complicated by evidence indicating that significant early intervention effects may not show up until well after the intervention has been completed.[136, 138, 139]

TABLE 3: Impact of early and later interventions or exposures upon children's development

Child outcomes	Early exposures or interventions (infancy–early childhood)	Later exposures or interventions (middle childhood–adolescence)
Perception	Cochlear implants for children with severe hearing deficits can have maximal impact on promoting normal sound reactions if implanted before age 3½ years, with diminishing gains thereafter. [126]	
Social–emotional development	Meta-analytic findings involving previously institutionalized adopted infants document the latter half of the first year as a sensitive period for promoting attachment security.[113, 127]	Adverse long-term consequences associated with exposure in childhood or adolescence to developmental risks, such as societal violence,[149] alcohol,[150] or culturally based socialization for aggressive behavior.[151]
	Findings suggest that the early years of life are a particularly salient time period for preventative interventions to reduce negative emotionality and behavioral problems or promote self-regulation or prosocial behaviors.[128, 129]	Positive consequences associated with exposure in childhood or adolescence to positive developmental influences, such as social support, which facilitates children's resilience after occurrence of a major natural disaster;[152] community acceptance, which supports the adjustment of former child soldiers;[153] treatment programs for abused children;[154] programs to increase child prosocial behavior and reduce aggression;[155] school-based programs to promote better inhibitory control;[144] drug prevention programs;[156] programs for reducing the impact of parental divorce on offspring. [157]
Cognitive/academic competence	Meta-analytic and review findings document that intervention during the early years carried out in either high- or low–medium-income countries can have long-term cognitive–academic benefits.[129-132]	Attending high-quality elementary schools can promote academic achievement for children who did not attend preschool programs.[158]
		Validated programs to reduce learned helplessness or increase self-efficacy beliefs in children with poor academic achievement.[121]
	Meta-analytic findings and results from individual studies show at least partial benefits in cognitive and academic performance for institutionalized children adopted into high-quality homes in the early years of life.[127, 133]	Validated interventions to promote reading skills in elementary school children. [159]
		School feeding programs promote some aspects of educational performance.[160] Evidence supporting indirect effects

Early contextual influences also may have long-term consequences through constraining or enhancing later reactivity either epigenetically or through neural mechanisms.[49, 50, 140] Similarly, developmental researchers have described five behavioral processes through which early exposure to stressors or protective factors can influence later reactivity:[141, 142] (1) facilitation—positive early experiences increase the child's receptivity to positive later experiences; (2) buffering—positive early experiences protect the individual against later stress; (3) sensitization—early risk exposure increases the individual's reactivity to later occurring risks; (4) steeling, which occurs when successfully dealing with early stress increases later stress resistance; and (5) blunting—exposure to early risks also can reduce the ability of the individual to benefit from subsequent positive influences. Examples of each of these processes are found in Table S3. What these five processes illustrate is that we cannot understand the impact of later-occurring contextual influences or interventions without also considering the nature of the child's early context.

15.4.3 ARE EARLY INFLUENCES OR INTERVENTIONS UNIQUELY SUFFICIENT?

While early experiences or early interventions can have direct or indirect long-term consequences, the evidence also shows that experiences or interventions occurring well after the early years of life can also alter subsequent development.[143] For example, interventions such as computer or martial arts training designed to promote children's executive functioning appear to have more benefit when used with 8- to 12-year-old children than when used with 4- to 5-year-olds.[144] Research reviews also document that increased levels of schooling can promote knowledge-based skills (crystallized intelligence), biologically based information processing skills (fluid intelligence), and specific components of intelligence such as reasoning and memory) for children from both high- and low–middle-income countries.[145-148] Additional findings illustrating the effects of later-occurring experiences or interventions are seen in Table 3.

15.4.4 ARE LATER INFLUENCES NECESSARY TO MAINTAIN THE IMPACT OF EARLIER INFLUENCES?

15.4.4.1 EVIDENCE FROM FOLLOW-UP STUDIES

Findings from both meta-analyses and systematic reviews, encompassing both U.S. and non-U.S. small- and large-scale intervention studies, indicate that the stability of long-term cognitive gains, even if still remaining significant, tends to weaken over time.[131, 132, 138] Attenuation of initial cognitive gains following early intervention may result from nonintervention children catching up in cognitive skills once they start attending primary school[131] or, alternatively, from a fadeout of initial gains by intervention children from low-income groups if they attend low-quality primary schools.[138] In either case, primary school influences are implicated as relevant to the stability of intervention-based early cognitive gains. Educational, economic, and behavioral gains or reductions in antisocial behavior resulting from exposure to small-scale high-dosage early interventions are more likely to be maintained over time,[161] whereas gains in these areas associated with large-scale shorter-dosage programs are more likely to attenuate, though still remaining significant for some outcomes.[129, 132, 138]

In addition to program dosage and scale, child characteristics also play a significant role in influencing stability of early intervention gains. While children at higher levels of biological or psychosocial developmental risk have greater need for, and perhaps greater responsivity to, early intervention programs,[130] there also is evidence suggesting that the impact of early intervention programs may be attenuated for children with higher levels of biological or psychosocial risk.[3, 128, 162] The fading of early intervention gains in high-risk populations is consistent with evidence showing that high levels of developmental risk can overwhelm the effects of normally protective influences.[163] One implication of these findings is that it may be necessary to continue interventions or provide follow-up interventions beyond the first 5 years for children with significant levels of cumulative biological or psychosocial risk exposure or children with a history of compromised development.[128, 164-167] For children with high levels of cumulative risk exposure, initial intervention gains are more likely to be lost over time without some type of subsequent high-quality follow-up intervention experience,[158, 168, 169] particularly when such children were enrolled in scaled-up lower-dosage early interventions.[169]

15.4.4.2 THE ROLE OF CAUSAL CHAINS

Whether there is a long-term impact of early interventions also may depend on the degree to which the early intervention initiates causal chains of later-occurring events that serve to maintain the impact of the early event.[142] For example, longitudinal findings show not only how children's participation in a quality preschool program directly enhances cognitive skills at age 6, but also how, over time, intervention children also have a higher probability of subsequently receiving more parental and teacher educational support and involvement, are more likely to attend higher quality schools, and are at lower risk for parent abuse or neglect, repeatedly changing schools, or grade retention.[170] Path analyses illustrate how these later naturally occurring parental and school causal chain links associated with early interventions serve to influence the child's educational attainment through early adulthood.

Other examples of naturally occurring causal chains include evidence that (1) early exposure to developmental risk factors can increase the probability of children encountering other risks later in life;[142, 171] (2) early exposure to developmental risks or protective influences can shut down or open up later opportunities;[128] and (3) children's participation in early enrichment programs can increase the probability of young children being involved in follow-up interventions and can initiate changes in parental rearing styles, such as more reading to their child, or parental life changes, such as getting more education, all of which can in turn promote children's subsequent development.[128, 172] When the long-term impact of early interventions depends upon exposure to later supportive experiences, the concept of a single early time-bounded sensitive period becomes problematic. This is because causal chains mean that the child also must be sensitive to later-occurring events if the impact of the early intervention is to be maintained.

15.4.5 DEVELOPMENTAL CONTRIBUTIONS TO THE QUESTION OF SENSITIVE PERIODS: CONCLUSIONS

Critical aspects of neural and social–emotional development or precursors for later development occur during the first 5 years of life. There are long-term consequences for both concurrent and later cognitive–educational and social–emotional functioning from experiences or interventions occurring during the first 5 years. Such consequences can result from either direct or indirect influences of early experiences or interventions. More intense early interventions during the first 5 years or longer interventions may be necessary to increase the probability that early gains will be maintained over time. This is particularly true for children with a history of high levels of exposure to biological or psychosocial developmental risk factors. There are significant changes in cognitive and social–emotional development occurring at least through adolescence, which are linked to later developing brain regions. There can be significant experience-driven enhancement of cognitive and social–emotional competence in later childhood, adolescence, and adulthood. Some of the long-term impact of early experiences or interventions will depend on subsequent changes in the child's proximal context.

15.4.6 IMPLICATIONS FOR INTERVENTION

The first several years of life may be a sensitive period for promoting social–emotional development and parenting quality. The overall pattern of evidence also suggests that for cognitive/academic outcomes, interventions could start during the preschool years without necessarily influencing their effectiveness. However, when designing interventions to promote positive parenting, cognitive development, or school competence, a wider time window may be necessary to maintain initial gains when dealing with high-risk children or multirisk contexts. For high-risk children or high-risk families, the impact of early psychosocial interventions will be stronger and more durable when there are built-in experiences or follow-up interventions during the early school years as well.

15.5 INTEGRATED CONCLUSIONS AND IMPLICATIONS

Evidence from multiple disciplines documents that there can be unique long-term influences upon human neural growth, health, and cognitive or social–emotional development from early biological or psychosocial interventions and exposure to risk or protective contextual characteristics. The first 3–5 years of life (including the prenatal period) appear to be a sensitive time window for ensuring adequate nutrition to promote brain development, for promoting consistent, responsive, sensitive parenting, for promoting social–emotional competencies and for providing cognitive stimulation to promote school readiness.

However, the evidence does not support the hypothesis that the early years are the sole sensitive time period that has a significant influence upon human development. Adolescence is also a sensitive period for continued growth of the prefrontal cortex, for vulnerability to stress, and for the development of critical dimensions of executive function, perspective taking, and abstract thought. Rather than a single sensitive period the evidence indicates multiple sensitive periods, with the sensitive time windows depending on the rate of development of specific neural regions or behavioral functions, outcomes assessed, and the nature of the experiences encountered or interventions provided. The implication from the findings reviewed here suggests that the choice of age at which to begin interventions should be based on what outcomes are targeted and what interventions are used.[173] For example, for interventions involving iron supplementation or promoting secure attachments,[113] it will be important to start as early as possible, certainly within the first year, whereas starting around age 3 years would not be too late for interventions involving stimulation to promote school readiness.[128]

Further, for children living in high-stress environments, or encountering multiple high-risk events, or receiving lower early-intervention dosages, there may need to be systematic follow-up interventions to maintain the gains resulting from early interventions. For example, the functional consequences of gains in early brain development resulting from early nutritional supplementation may require building in subsequent psychosocial stimulation experiences if the nutritional intervention is to influence the child's school readiness and subsequent school performance. Finally, in evaluating the long-term impact of interventions, it will be critical to look for both main effects and person x intervention interactions, given evidence showing that children with different developmental histories, different genotypes, or different individual characteristics may react in very different ways to the same intervention package.[3]

REFERENCES

1. Evans, G. 2004. The environment of childhood poverty. Am. Psychol. 59: 77–92.
2. Walker, S., T.D. Wachs, S. Grantham-McGregor, et al. 2011. Inequality begins by early childhood: risk and protective factors for early child development. Lancet 378: 1325–1338.
3. Wachs, T.D. & A. Rahman. 2013. "The nature and impact of risk and protective influences on children's development in low income countries." In Handbook of Early Childhood Development Research and Its Impact on Global Policy. P. Britto, P. Engle & C. Super, Eds.: 85–122. New York: Oxford University Press.
4. Plato. 1993. Republic. 377 a-b. R. Waterfield Translator. New York. Oxford University Press.
5. Lerner, R. 2011. Structure and process in relational, developmental systems theories: a commentary on contemporary changes in the understanding of developmental changes across the life span. Hum. Dev. 54: 34–43.
6. Bronfenbrenner, U. & P. Morris. 2006. "The bioecological model of human development." In Theoretical Models of Human Development: Vol 1 of the Handbook of Child Psycholog, 6th ed. R. Lerner, Ed.: 793–828. Hoboken, NJ: Wiley.
7. Bruer, J. 2001. "A critical and sensitive period primer." In Critical Thinking about Critical Periods. D. Bailey, J. Bruer, F. Symons & J. Lichtman, Eds.: 3–26. Baltimore, MD: Brookes Publishing.
8. Bornstein, M.H. 1989. Sensitive periods in development: structural characteristics and causal interpretations. Psychol. Bull. 105: 179–197.
9. Johnson, M. 2005. Sensitive periods in functional brain development: problems and prospects. Dev. Psychobiol. 46: 287–292.
10. Armstrong, V.L., P.M. Brunet, C. He, et al. 2006. What is so critical?: a commentary on the reexamination of critical periods. Dev. Psychobiol. 48: 326–331.
11. Colombo, J. 1982. The critical period concept: research, methodology and theoretical issues. Psychol. Bull. 91: 260–275.

12. Michel, G. & A. Tyler. 2005. Critical period: a history of the transition from questions of when, to what, to how. Dev. Psychobiol. 46: 163–183.
13. Lewis, T.L. & D. Maurer. 2005. Multiple sensitive periods in human visual development: evidence from visually deprived children. Dev. Psychobiol. 46: 163–183.
14. Fox, S.E., P. Levitt & C.A. Nelson III. 2010. How the timing and quality of early experiences influence the development of brain architecture. Child Dev. 81: 28–40.
15. Knudsen, E.I. 2004. Sensitive periods in the development of the brain and behavior. J. Cognitive Neurosci. 16: 1412–1425.
16. Bradley, R.H., B.M. Caldwell & S.L Rock. 1988. Home environment and school performance: a ten-year follow-up and examination of three models of environmental action. Child Dev. 59: 852–867.
17. Landry, S.H., K.E. Smith, P.R. Swank & C. Guttentag. 2008. A responsive parenting intervention: the optimal timing across early childhood for impacting maternal behaviors and child outcomes. Dev. Psychol. 44: 1335–1353.
18. Huston, A. & A. Bentley. 2010. Human development in societal context. Ann. Rev. Psychol. 61: 411–437.
19. World Health Organization. Micronutrient deficiencies. http://www.who.int/nutrition/topics/ida/en/index.html.
20. Lozoff, B., J. Beard, C. Connor, et al. 2006. Long-lasting neural and behavioral effects of iron deficiency in infancy. Nutr. Rev. 64: S34–S43; discussion S72–S91.
21. Fuglestad, A.J., S.E. Ramel & M.K Georgieff. 2010. "Miconutrient needs of the developing brain: priorities and assessment." In Micronutrients and Brain Health, Oxidative Stress and Disease. L. Packer, Ed.: 434. Boca Raton: CRC Press. Xxi.
22. Murray-Kolb, L.E. & J.L. Beard. 2007. Iron treatment normalizes cognitive functioning in young women. Am. J. Clin. Nutr. 85: 778–787.
23. Amin, S.B., M. Orlando, A Eddins, et al. 2010. In utero iron status and auditory neural maturation in premature infants as evaluated by auditory brainstem response. J. Pediatr. 156: 377–381.
24. Wachs, T.D., E. Pollitt, S. Cueto, et al. 2005. Relation of neonatal iron status to individual variability in neonatal temperament. Dev. Psychobiol. 46: 141–153.
25. Burden, M.J., A. Westerlund, R. Armony-Sivan, et al. 2007. An event-related potential study of attention and recognition memory in infants with iron-deficiency anemia. Pediatrics 120: e336–e345.
26. Algarin, C., P. Peirano, M. Garrido, et al. 2003. Iron deficiency anemia in infancy: long-lasting effects on auditory and visual system functioning. Pediatr. Res. 53: 217–223.
27. Roncagliolo, M., M. Garrido, T. Walter, et al. 1998. Evidence of altered central nervous system development in infants with iron deficiency anemia at 6 months: delayed maturation of auditory brainstem responses. Am. J. Clin. Nutr. 68: 683–690.
28. Lozoff, B., K. Clark, Y. Jing, et al. 2008. Dose-response relationships between iron deficiency with or without anemia and infant social-emotional behavior. J. Pediatr. 152: 696–702.
29. Lozoff, B., F. Corapci, M. Burden, et al. 2007. Preschool-aged children with iron deficiency anemia show altered affect and behavior. J. Nutr. 137: 683–689.
30. Beard, J.L. & J.R. Connor. 2003. Iron status and neural functioning. Annu. Rev. Nutr. 23: 41–58.

31. Beard, J.L., B. Felt, T. Schallert, et al. 2006. Moderate iron deficiency in infancy: biology and behavior in young rats. Behav. Brain Res. 170: 224–232.
32. Felt, B.T., J. Beard, T. Schallert, et al. 2006. Persistent neurochemical and behavioral abnormalities in adulthood despite early iron supplementation for perinatal iron deficiency anemia in rats. Behav. Brain Res. 171: 261–270.
33. Felt, B.T. & B. Lozoff. 1996. Brain iron and behavior of rats are not normalized by treatment of iron deficiency anemia during early development. J. Nutr. 126: 693–701.
34. Georgieff, M.K. 2007. Nutrition and the developing brain: nutrient priorities and measurement. Am. J. Clin. Nutr. 85: 614S-620S.
35. McEchron, M.D., A. Cheng, H. Liu, et al. 2005. Perinatal nutritional iron deficiency permanently impairs hippocampus-dependent trace fear conditioning in rats. Nutr. Neurosci. 8: 195–206.
36. McEchron, M.D., C.J. Goletiani & D.N. Alexander. 2010. Perinatal nutritional iron deficiency impairs noradrenergic-mediated synaptic efficacy in the CA1 area of rat hippocampus. J. Nutr. 140: 642–647.
37. Rao, R., I. Tkac, E. Townsend, et al. 2003. Perinatal iron deficiency alters the neurochemical profile of the developing rat hippocampus. J. Nutr. 133: 3215–3221.
38. Connor, J.R. & S.L. Menzies. 1996. Relationship of iron to oligodendrocytes and myelination. Glia 17: 83–93.
39. Ward, K.L., I. Tkac, Y. Jing, et al. 2007. Gestational and lactational iron deficiency alters the developing striatal metabolome and associated behaviors in young rats. J. Nutr. 137: 1043–1049.
40. Golub, M.S., C. Hogrefe, S. Germann, et al. 2006. Behavioral consequences of developmental iron deficiency in infant rhesus monkeys. Neurotoxicol. Teratol. 28: 3–17.
41. Chang, S., L. Zeng, F. Brouwer, et al. 2013. Effect of iron deficiency anemia in pregnancy on child mental development in Rural China. Pediatrics 131: e755–e763.
42. Christian, P., M. Morgan, L. Murray-Kolb, et al. 2011. Preschool iron-folic acid and zinc supplementation in children exposed to iron-folic acid in utero confers no added cognitive benefit in early school-age. J. Nutr. 141: 2042–2048.
43. Christian, P., L. Murray-Kolb, S. Khatry, et al. 2010. Prenatal micronutrient supplementation and intellectual and motor function in early school-aged children in Nepal. JAMA 304: 2716–2723.
44. Murray-Kolb, L.E., S. Khatry, J. Katz, et al. 2012. Preschool micronutrient supplementation effects on intellectual and motor function in school-aged Nepalese children. Arch. Pediatr. Adolesc. Med. 166: 404–410.
45. McEwen, B.S. 2006. Protective and damaging effects of stress mediators: central role of the brain. Dial. Clin. Neurosci. Stress 8: 367–381.
46. McEwen, B.S., P.J. Gianaros. 2011. Stress- and allostasis-induced brain plasticity. Annu. Rev. Med. 62: 431–445.
47. Erickson, K.I., M.W. Voss, R.S. Prakash, et al. 2011. Exercise training increases size of hippocampus and improves memory. Proc. Natl. Acad. Sci. USA 108: 3017–3022.
48. Vyas, A., R. Mitra, B.S.S. Rao & S. Chattarji. 2002. Chronic stress induces contrasting patterns of dendritic remodeling in hippocampal and amygdaloid neurons. J. Neurosci. 22: 6810–6818.

49. Shonkoff, J.P., W.T. Boyce & B.S. McEwen. 2009. Neuroscience, molecular biology, and the childhood roots of health disparities. JAMA 301: 2252–2259.

50. Anda, R.F., A. Butchart, V.J. Felitti & D.W. Brown. 2010. Building a framework for global surveillance of the public health implications of adverse childhood experiences. Am. J. Prev. Med. 39: 93–98.

51. Weinstock, M. 2001. Alterations induced by gestational stress in brain morphology and behaviour of the offspring. Prog. Neurobiol. 65: 427–451.

52. Mairesse, J., A.S. Vercoutter-Edouart, J. Marrocco, et al. 2012. Proteomic characterization in the hippocampus of prenatally stressed rats. J. Proteomics 75: 1764–1770.

53. Entringer, S., E.S. Epel, R. Kumsta, et al. 2011. Stress exposure in intrauterine life is associated with shorter telomere length in young adulthood. Proc. Natl. Acad. Sci. USA 108: E513–E518.

54. Barker, D.J.P. 1997. The fetal origins of coronary heart disease. Acta Paediatr. Suppl. 422: 78–82.

55. Entringer, S., C. Buss & P.D. Wadhwa. 2010. Prenatal stress and developmental programming of human health and disease risk: concepts and integration of empirical findings. Curr. Opin. Endocrinol. Diabetes Obes. 17: 507–516.

56. Pankevich, D.E., B.R. Mueller, B. Brockel & T. L. Bale. 2009. Prenatal stress programming of offspring feeding behavior and energy balance begins early in pregnancy. Physiol. Behav. 98: 94–102.

57. Vucetic, Z., J. Kimmel, K. Totoki, et al. 2010. Maternal high-fat diet alters methylation and gene expression of dopamine and opioid-related genes. Endocrinology 151: 4756–4764.

58. Pan, L., B. Sherry, R. Njai & H.M. Blanck. 2012. Food insecurity is associated with obesity among US adults in 12 states. J. Acad. Nutr. Dietetics 112: 1403–1409.

59. Chang, V.W., A.E. Hillier & N.K. Mehta. 2009. Neighborhood racial isolation, disorder and obesity. Social Forces 87: 2063–2092.

60. Theall, K.P., S.S. Drury & E.A. Shirtcliff. 2012. Cumulative neighborhood risk of psychosocial stress and allostatic load in adolescents. Am. J. Epidemiol. 176(Suppl. 7): S164–S174.

61. Danese, A., T.E. Moffitt, H. Harrington, et al. 2009. Adverse childhood experiences and adult risk factors for age-related disease: depression, inflammation, and clustering of metabolic risk markers. Arch. Pediatr. Adolesc. Med. 163: 1135–114365.

62. Miller, G.E. & E. Chen. 2010. Harsh family climate in early life presages the emergence of a proinflammatory phenotype in adolescence. Psychol. Sci. 21: 848–856.

63. Evans, G.W., C. Gonnella, L.A. Marcynyszyn, et al. 2005. The role of chaos in poverty and children's socioemotional adjustment. Psychol. Sci. 16: 560–565.

64. Diez Roux, A.V. & C. Mair. 2010. Neighborhoods and health. Ann. N. Y. Acad. Sci. 1186: 125–145.

65. McEwen, B.S. & P. Tucker. 2011. Critical biological pathways for chronic psychosocial stress and research opportunities to advance the consideration of stress in chemical risk assessment. Am. J. Public Health 101(Suppl. 1): S131–S139.

66. Farah, M.J., D.M. Shera, J.H. Savage, et al. 2006. Childhood poverty: specific associations with neurocognitive development. Brain Res. 1110: 166–174.

67. Hart, B. & T.R. Risley. 1995. Meaningful Differences in the Everyday Experience of Young American Children. Baltimore, MD: Brookes Publishing Company.

68. Hanson, J.L., A. Chandra, B.L. Wolfe & S. D. Pollak. 2011. Association between income and the hippocampus. PLoS One 6: e18712.
69. Gianaros, P.J., J.A. Horenstein, S. Cohen, et al. 2007. Perigenual anterior cingulate morphology covaries with perceived social standing. Soc. Cogn. Affect. Neurosci. 2: 161–173.
70. Gee, D.G., K.L. Humphreys, J. Flannery, et al. 2013. A developmental shift from positive to negative connectivity in human amygdala-prefrontal circuitry. J. Neurosci. 33: 4584–4593.
71. Adler, N.E., T.W. Boyce, M.A. Chesney, et al. 1993. Socioeconomic inequalities in health. JAMA 269: 3140–3145.
72. Lupien, S.J., S. Parent, A.C. Evans, et al. 2011. Larger amygdala but no change in hippocampal volume in 10-year-old children exposed to maternal depressive symptomatology since birth. Proc. Natl. Acad. Sci. USA 108: 14324–14329.
73. Boyce, W.T. & B.J. Ellis. 2005. Biological sensitivity to context. I: an evolutionary-developmental theory of the origins and functions of stress reactivity. Dev. Psychopathol. 17: 271–301.
74. Caspi, A., K. Sugden, T.E. Moffitt, et al. 2003. Influence of life stress on depression: moderation by a polymorphism in the 5-HTT gene. Science 301: 386–389.
75. Suomi, S.J. 2006. Risk, resilience, and gene x environment interactions in rhesus monkeys. Ann. NY Acad. Sci. 1094: 52–62.
76. Del Giudice, M., B.J. Ellis & E.A. Shirtcliff. 2011. The Adaptive Calibration Model of stress responsivity. Neurosci. Biobehav. R. 35: 1562–1592.
77. Dallman, M.F., N.C. Pecoraro & S.E. la Fleur. 2005. Chronic stress and comfort foods: self-medication and abdominal obesity. Brain Behav. Immunity 19: 275–280.
78. Eiland, L. & R.D. Romeo. 2012. Stress and the developing adolescent brain. Neuroscience 249: 162–171.
79. Sisk, C.L. & D.L. Foster. 2004. The neural basis of puberty and adolescence. Nature Neurosci. 7: 1040–1047.
80. Mischel, W., E.B. Ebbesen & A.R. Zeiss. 1972. Cognitive and attentional mechanisms in delay of gratification. J. Pers. Soc. Psychol. 21: 204–218.
81. Mischel, W., O. Ayduk, M.G. Berman, et al. 2011. 'Willpower' over the life span: decomposing self-regulation. Soc. Cogn. Affect. Neurosci. 6: 252–256.
82. Casey, B.J., L.H. Somerville, I.H. Gotlib, et al. 2011. Behavioral and neural correlates of delay of gratification 40 years later. Proc. Natl. Acad. Sci. USA 108: 14998–15003.
83. Somerville, L.H., T. Hare & B.J. Casey. 2011. Frontostriatal maturation predicts cognitive control failure to appetitive cues in adolescents. J. Cogn. Neurosci. 23: 2123–2134.
84. Steinberg, L. 2005. Cognitive and affective development in adolescence. TRENDS Cogn. Sci. 9: 69–74.
85. Pattwell, S.S., K.G. Bath, B.J. Casey, et al. 2011. Selective early-acquired fear memories undergo temporary suppression during adolescence. Proc. Natl. Acad. Sci. USA 108: 1182–1187.
86. Pattwell, S.S., S. Duhoux, C.A. Hartley, et al. 2012. Altered fear learning across development in both mouse and human. Proc. Natl. Acad. Sc.i USA 109: 16318–16323.

87. Eiland, L., J. Ramroop, M.N. Hill, et al. 2012. Chronic juvenile stress produces corticolimbic dendritic architectural remodeling and modulates emotional behavior in male and female rats. Psychoneuroendocrino 37: 39–47.

88. Isgor, C., M. Kabbaj, H. Akil & S.J. Watson. 2004. Delayed effects of chronic variable stress during peripubertal-juvenile period on hippocampal morphology and on cognitive and stress axis functions in rats. Hippocampus 14: 636–648.

89. Casey, B.J., J.N. Giedd & K.M. Thomas. 2000. Structural and functional brain development and its relation to cognitive development. Biol. Psychol. 54: 241–257.

90. Nelson, E.E. & A. E. Guyer. 2011. The development of the ventral prefrontal cortex and social flexibility. Dev. Cogn. Neurosci. 1: 233–245.

91. Lenroot, R.K., J.E. Schmitt, S.J. Ordaz, et al. 2009. Differences in genetic and environmental influences on the human cerebral cortex associated with development during childhood and adolescence. Hum. Brain Mapp. 30: 163–174.

92. Tottenham, N., J. Phuong, J. Flannery, et al. 2013. A negativity bias for ambiguous facial-expression valence during childhood: converging evidence from behavior and facial corrugator muscle responses. Emotion 13: 92–103.

93. Spinelli, S., S. Chefer, R.E. Carson, et al. 2010. Effects of early-life stress on serotonin(1A) receptors in juvenile Rhesus monkeys measured by positron emission tomography. Biol. Psychiatr. 67: 1146–1153.

94. Spinelli, S., S. Chefer, S.J. Suomi, et al. 2009. Early-life stress induces long-term morphologic changes in primate brain. Arch. Gen. Psychiatr. 66: 658–665.

95. Danese, A. & B.S. McEwen. 2012. Adverse childhood experiences, allostasis, allostatic load, and age-related disease. Physiol. Behav. 106: 29–39.

96. McEwen, B.S. 2007. Physiology and neurobiology of stress and adaptation: central role of the brain. Physiol. Rev. 87: 873–904.

97. Convit, A. 2005. Links between cognitive impairment in insulin resistance: an explanatory model. Neurobiol. Aging 26S: S31–S35.

98. Convit, A., O.T. Wolf, C. Tarshish & M.J. de Leon. 2003. Reduced glucose tolerance is associated with poor memory performance and hippocampal atrophy among normal elderly. Proc. Natl. Acad. Sci. USA 100: 2019–2022.

99. Gold, S.M., I. Dziobek, V. Sweat, et al. 2007. Hippocampal damage and memory impairments as possible early brain complications of type 2 diabetes. Diabetologia 50: 711–719.

100. Rasgon, N.L. & H.A. Kenna. 2005. Insulin resistance in depressive disorders and Alzheimer's disease: revisiting the missing link hypothesis. Neurobiol. Aging 26S: S103–S107.

101. Yates, K.F., V. Sweat, P.L. Yau, et al. 2012. Impact of metabolic syndrome on cognition and brain: a selected review of the literature. Arterioscl. Throm. Vas. 32: 2060–2067.

102. Yau, P.L., M.G. Castro, A. Tagani, et al. 2012. Obesity and metabolic syndrome and functional and structural brain impairments in adolescence. Pediatrics 130: e856–864.

103. Miller, A.L., M.A. Horodynski, H.E. Herb, et al. 2012. Enhancing self-regulation as a strategy for obesity prevention in Head Start preschoolers: the growing healthy study. BMC Public Health 12: 1040.

104. Onnerfalt, J., L.K. Erlandsson, K. Orban, et al. 2012. A family-based intervention targeting parents of preschool children with overweight and obesity: conceptual

framework and study design of LOOPS- Lund overweight and obesity preschool study. BMC Public Health 12: 879.

105. Fernald, L.C., P.J. Gertler & L.M. Neufeld. 2009. 10-year effect of Oportunidades, Mexico's conditional cash transfer programme, on child growth, cognition, language, and behaviour: a longitudinal follow-up study. Lancet 374: 1997–2005.

106. Ozer, E.J., L.C. Fernald, A. Weber, et al. 2011. Does alleviating poverty affect mothers' depressive symptoms? A quasi-experimental investigation of Mexico's Oportunidades programme. Int. J. Epidemiol. 40: 1565–1576.

107. Lomeli, E.V. 2008. Conditional Cash Transfers as Social Policy in Latin America: an assessment of their contributions and limitations. Annu. Rev. Sociol. 34: 475–499.

108. Crews, F., J. He & C. Hodge. 2007. Adolescent cortical development: a critical period of vulnerability for addiction. Pharmacol. Biochem. Behav. 86: 189–199.

109. Feldman, D.E. & E.I. Knudsen. 1998. Experience-dependent plasticity and the maturation of glutamatergic synapses. Neuron 20: 1067–1071.

110. Lupien, S., B. McEwen, M. Gunnar & C. Helm. 2009. Effects of stress throughtout the lifespan on the brain, behavior and cognition. Nat. Rev. Neurosci. 10: 434–445.

111. Werker, J.F. & R.C. Tees. 2005. Speech perception as a window for understanding plasticity and commitment in language systems of the brain. Dev. Psychobiol. 46: 233–251.

112. Trabulsi, J.C. & J.A. Mennella. 2012. Diet, sensitive periods in flavor learning, and growth. Int. Rev. Psychiatr. 24: 219–230.

113. Bakermans-Kranenburg, M.J., M.H. van IJzendoorn & F. Juffer. 2003. Less is more: meta-analyses of sensitivity and attachment interventions in early childhood. Psychol. Bull. 129: 195–215.

114. Kochanska, G., K.C. Coy & K.T. Murray. 2001. The development of self-regulation in the first four years of life. Child Dev. 72: 1091–1111.

115. Barr, R. 2008. "Developing social understanding in a social context." In Blackwell Handbook of Early Childhood Development. K. McCartney & D. Phillips, Eds.: 188–207. Malden, MA: Blackwell.

116. Smetana, J.G., W.M. Rote, M. Jambon, et al. 2012. Developmental changes and individual differences in young children's moral judgments. Child Dev. 83: 683–696.

117. Baird, A.A. 2010. "The terrible twelves." In Developmental Social Cognitive Neuroscience. P.D. Zelazo, M. Chandler & E. Crone, Eds.: 191–207. New York, NY: Psychology Press.

118. Rothbart, M., M. Posner & J. Kieras. 2008. Temperament, attention and the development of self-regulation. In Blackwell Handbook of Early Childhood Development. K. McCartney & D. Phillips, Eds.: 338–357. Malden, MA: Blackwell.

119. Rutter, M. 1996. Transitions and turning points in developmental psychopathology: as applied to the age span between childhood and mid-adulthood. Int. J. Behav. Dev. 19: 603–626.

120. Steinberg, L., S. Graham, L. O'Brien, et al. 2009. Age differences in future orientation and delay discounting. Child Dev. 80: 28–44.

121. Eccles, J., R. Roeser, M. Vida, et al. 2006. "Motivational and achievement pathways through middle childhood." In Child Psychology: A Handbook of Contemporary Issues, 2nd ed. L. Balter & C. Tamis-LeMonda, Eds.: 325–355. New York: Psychology Press.

122. Huizinga, M., C.V. Dolan & M.W. van der Molen. 2006. Age-related change in executive function: developmental trends and a latent variable analysis. Neuropsychologia 44: 2017–2036.

123. Lambek, R. & M. Shevlin. 2011. Working memory and response inhibition in children and adolescents: age and organization issues. Scand. J. Psychol. 52: 427–432.

124. McArdle, J.J., E. Ferrer-Caja, F. Hamagami & R. Woodcock. 2002. Comparative longitudinal structural analyses of the growth and decline of multiple intellectual abilities over the life span. Dev. Psychol. 38: 115–142.

125. Tucker-Drob, E.M. 2009. Differentiation of cognitive abilities across the life span. Dev. Psychol. 45: 1097–1118.

126. Tomblin, J.B., B.A. Barker & S. Hubbs. 2007. Developmental constraints on language development in children with cochlear implants. Int. J. Audiol. 46: 512–523.

127. van IJzendoorn, M.H. & F. Juffer. 2006. The Emanuel Miller Memorial Lectures 2006: adoption as intervention. Meta-analytic evidence for massive catch-up and plasticity in physical, socio-emotional, and cognitive development. J. Child Psychol. Psychiatr. 47: 1228–1245.

128. Love, J., R., R. Chazen-Cohen, H. Raikes & J. Brooks-Gunn. 2013. What makes a difference: Early Head Start evaluation findings in a developmental context. Monogr. Soc. Res. Child Dev. 78: serial # 306.

129. Nores, M. & S. Barnett. 2010. Benefits of early childhood interventions across the world: (under) investing in the very young. Econ. Ed. Rev. 29: 271–282.

130. Engle, P., L. Fernald, H. Alderman, et al. 2011. Strategies for reducing inequalities and improving developmental outcomes for young children in low-income and middle-income countries. Lancet 378: 1339–1353.

131. Barnett, W.S. 2011. Effectiveness of early educational intervention. Science 333: 975–978.

132. Camilli, G., S. Vargas, S. Ryan & W.S. Barnett. 2010. Meta-analysis of the effects of early education interventions on cognitive and social development. Teachers Coll. Rec. 112: 579–620.

133. Kreppner, J.M., M. Rutter, C. Beckett, et al. 2007. Normality and impairment following profound early institutional deprivation: a longitudinal follow-up into early adolescence. Dev. Psychol. 43: 931–946.

134. Van Zeijl, J., J. Mesman, H.M. Koot, et al. 2006. Attachment-based intervention for enhancing sensitive discipline in mothers of 1- to 3-year-old children at risk for externalizing behavior problems: a randomized controlled trial. J. Consult. Psychol. 74: 994–1005.

135. Lagerberg, D. 2000. Secondary prevention in child health: effects of psychological intervention, particularly home visitation, on children's development and other outcome variables. Acta Paediatr. Suppl. 434: 43–52.

136. Zehnah, C., M. Gunnar, R. McCall, et al. 2011. Sensitive periods. Monogr. Soc. Res. Child Dev. 76(serial # 301): 147–162.

137. Duyme, M., A.C. Dumaret & S. Tomkiewica. 1999. How can we boost IQs of "dull children"?: a late adoption study. Proc. Natl. Acad. Sci. USA 96: 8790–8794.

138. Ludwig, J. & D. Miller. 2007. Does Head Start improve children's life chances? Evidence from a regression discontinuity design. Quart. J. Econ. 122: 159–208.

139. Kaminski, R.A., E.A. Stormshak, R.H. Good III & M.R. Goodman. 2002. Prevention of substance abuse with rural Head Start children and families: results of Project STAR. Psychol. Addict. Behav. 16: S11-S26.
140. Roth, T.L. & J.D. Sweatt. 2011. Annual research review: epigenetic mechanisms and environmental shaping of the brain during sensitive periods of development. J. Child Psychol. Psychiat. 52: 398–408.
141. Rutter, M. 2006. Implications of resilience concepts for scientific understanding. In "Resilience in Children." B. Lester, A. Masten & B. McEwen, Eds. Ann. N.Y. Acad. Sci. 1094: 1–12.
142. Wachs, T.D. 2000. Necessary but not Sufficient: The Role of Individual and Multiple Influences on Human Development. Washington, DC: American Psychological Association Press.
143. Werner, E. & R. Smith. 1992. Overcoming the Odds: High Risk Children from Birth to Adulthood. Ithaca, NY: Cornell University Press.
144. Diamond, A. & K. Lee. 2011. Interventions shown to aid executive function development in children 4 to 12 years old. Science 333: 959–964.
145. Ceci, S.J. 1991. How much does schooling influence general intelligence and its cognitive components? A reassessment of the evidence. Dev. Psychol. 27: 703–722.
146. Cliffordson, C. & J.E. Gustafsson. 2008. Effects of age and schooling on intellectual performance: estimates obtained from analysis of continuous variation in age and length of schooling. Intelligence 36: 143–152.
147. Stelzl, I., F. Merz, R. Ehlers & H. Remer. 1995. The effect of schooling on the development of fluid and crystallized intelligence: a quasi-experimental study. Intelligence 21: 279–296.
148. Nisbett, R.E., J. Aronson, C. Blair, et al. 2012. Intelligence: new findings and theoretical developments. Am. Psychol. 67: 130–159.
149. Qouta, S., R.L. Punamäki & E.E. Sarraj. 2008. Child development and family mental health in war and military violence: the Palestinian experience. Int. J. Behav. Dev. 32: 310–321.
150. Guttmannova, K., J.A. Bailey, K.G. Hill, et al. 2011. Sensitive periods for adolescent alcohol use initiation: predicting the lifetime occurrence and chronicity of alcohol problems in adulthood. J. Stud. Alcohol Drugs 72: 221–231.
151. Quinlan, R. & M. Quinlan. 2007. Parenting and cultures of risk: a comparative analysis of infidelity, aggression and witchcraft. Am. Anthropol. 109: 164–179.
152. Ratrin Hestyanti, Y. 2006. Children survivors of the 2004 Tsunami in Aceh, Indonesia: a study of resiliency. In "Resilience in Children." B. Lester, A. Masten & B. McEwen, Eds. Ann. N.Y. Acad. Sci. 1094: 303–307.
153. Betancourt, T., I. Borisova, T. Williams, et al. 2010. Sierra Leone's former child soldiers: a follow-up study of psychosocial adjustment and community integration. Child Dev. 81: 1077–1095.
154. MacLeod, J. & G. Nelson. 2000. Programs for the promotion of family wellness and the prevention of child maltreatment: a meta-analytic review. Child Abuse Neglect 24: 1127–1149.
155. Flannery, D.J., A.T. Vazsonyi, A.K. Liau, et al. 2003. Initial behavior outcomes for the PeaceBuilders Universal School-Based Violence Prevention Program. Dev. Psychol. 39: 292–308.

156. Tobler, N.S., M.R. Roona, P. Ochshorn, et al. 2000. School-based adolescent drug prevention programs: 1998 meta-analysis. J. Primary Prev. 20: 275–336.

157. Pedro-Carroll, J.L., S.E. Sutton & P.A. Wyman. 1999. A two-year follow-up evaluation of a preventive intervention for young children of divorce. School Psychol. Rev. 28: 467–476.

158. Magnuson, K.A., C. Ruhm & J. Waldfogel. 2007. The persistence of preschool effects: do subsequent classroom experiences matter? Early Child Res. Quart. 22: 18–38.

159. Vellutino, F.R., D.M. Scanlon, A. Pratt, et al. 1996. Cognitive profiles of difficult-to-remediate and readily remediated poor readers: early intervention as a vehicle for distinguishing between cognitive and experiential deficits as basic causes of specific reading disability. J. Educ. Psychol. 88: 601–638.

160. Jomaa, L.H., E. McDonnell & C. Probat. 2011. School feeding programs in developing countries: impacts on children's health and educational outcomes. Nutr. Rev. 69: 83–98.

161. Campbell, F.A., C.T. Ramey, E. Pungello, et al. 2002. Early childhood education: young adult outcomes from the Abecedarian Project. Appl. Dev. Sci. 6: 42–57.

162. Hill, J., J. Brooks-Gunn & J. Waldfogel. 2003. Sustained effects of high participation in an early intervention for low-birth-weight premature infants. Devel. Psychol. 39: 730–744.

163. Sameroff, A. & K. Rosenbloom. 2006. "Psychosocial constraints on the development of resilience." In Resilience in Children, Vol. 1094. B. Lester, A. Masten & B. McEwen, Eds.: 116–124. Ann NY Acad Sci.

164. Reynolds, A. & J. Temple. 1998. Extended early childhood intervention and school achievement: age thirteen findings from the Chicago Longitudinal study. Child Dev. 69: 231–246.

165. Temple, J.A., A.J. Reynolds & W.T. Miedel. 2000. Can early intervention prevent high school dropout?: evidence from the Chicago Child-Parent Centers. Urban Educ. 35: 31–56.

166. Currie, J. & D. Thomas. 2000. School quality and the longer-term effects of Head Start. J. Hum. Resour. 35: 755–774.

167. Kagitcibasi, C., D. Sunar, D. Bekman, et al. 2009. Continuing effects of early enrichment in adult life: the Turkish Early Enrichment Project 22 years later. J. Appl. Dev. Psychol. 30: 764–779.

168. Currie, J. & D. Thomas. 1995. Does Head Start make a difference? Am. Econ. Rev. 85: 341–364.

169. Reynolds, A.J., J.A. Temple, D.L. Robertson & E.A. Mann. 2001. Long-term effects of an early childhood intervention on educational achievement and juvenile arrest: a 15-year follow-up of low-income children in public schools. J. Amer. Med. Assoc. 285: 2339–2346.

170. Ou, S.R. 2005. Pathways of long-term effects of an early intervention program on educational attainment: findings from the Chicago longitudinal study. Appl. Dev. Psychol. 26: 578–611.

171. Hertzman, C. & T. Boyce. 2010. How experience gets under the skin to create gradients in developmental health. Ann. Rev. Publ. Health 31: 329–347.

172. Reynolds, A.J. & D.L. Robertson. 2003. School-based early intervention and later child maltreatment in the Chicago Longitudinal Study. Child Dev, 74: 3–26.
173. Bailey, D. 2002. Are critical periods critical for early childhood education? The role of timing in early childhood pedagogy. Early Child Res. Quart. 17: 281–294.

AUTHOR NOTES

CHAPTER 1

Conflict of Interest Statement
Andrew Scholey has received research funding and consultancy from the health supplement industry. The authors declare that the manuscript was prepared in the absence of any commercial or financial relationships that could be construed as a potential conflict of interest.

CHAPTER 2

Acknowledgments
This project was supported by The Urban Child Institute. The funding source had no role in the design, implementation or interpretation of this work or in the manuscript preparation. We gratefully acknowledge the participant recruitment and sample collection by CANDLE staff, and particularly the mothers and children who consented to participate.

Conflict of Interest
The authors declare no conflict of interest.

CHAPTER 3

Conflict of Interest Statement
The authors declare that the research was conducted in the absence of any commercial or financial relationships that could be construed as a potential conflict of interest.

Acknowledgments
Dr. Anett Nyaradi is supported by an Australian Postgraduate Award and a Western Australian Pregnancy (Raine) Cohort Scholarship. Associate

Professor Jianghong Li is supported by a Curtin University Research Fellowship. Dr. Siobhan Hickling is an Assistant Professor at The University of Western Australia. Associate Professor Jonathan Foster is supported by a Curtin University Senior Research Fellowship. Professor Wendy Oddy is funded by a National Health and Medical Research Council Population Health Research Fellowship.

CHAPTER 4

Acknowledgments
A previous version of sections of this paper was published as a technical brief by Alive & Thrive.[59]

Funding and Sponsorship
This publication is based on research funded by a grant to the University of California, Davis from the Bill & Melinda Gates Foundation. The findings and conclusions contained within are those of the authors and do not necessarily reflect positions or policies of the Bill & Melinda Gates Foundation.

Declaration of Interest
The authors have no relevant interests to declare.

CHAPTER 5

Acknowledgments
I thank many colleagues for expert advice and valuable discussion, especially Malcolm Burrows F.R.S., Department of Zoology, University of Cambridge; Dianne Ford, Institute for Cell and Molecular Biosciences and Human Nutrition Research Centre, Institute for Ageing and Health, University of Newcastle; Peter Jones, Head of Department of Psychiatry, School of Clinical Medicine, University of Cambridge; Aarno Palotie, Wellcome Trust Sanger Institute and Genome Campus, Hinxton, Cambridge. The author is a Fellow of Wolfson College, University of Cambridge and thanks the library and computing staff of the College and University for expert advice.

Conflict of Interest
The author declares no conflict of interest.

CHAPTER 6

Conflict of Interest Statement
The authors declare that the research was conducted in the absence of any commercial or financial relationships that could be construed as a potential conflict of interest.

Acknowledgments
This paper is published with the permission of the Director of KEMRI. The study received administrative and financial support through the KEMRI/ Wellcome Trust Research Programme. Penny Holding was supported by a Wellcome Trust Advanced Training Scholarship [grant number OXTREC 024-02]. The authors would like to thank L. Mbonani, J. Gona, R. Kalu, H. Garrashi, E. Obiero, R. Mapenzi, and C. Mapenzi for their role in data collection; and K. Katana and P. Kadii for data entry. We would also like to thank N. Minich for her assistance in statistical analysis. Our sincere gratitude goes to the children and their families who participated in this study and who generously gave their time to make this work possible. We are also grateful to the head teachers of the schools which were involved in the study for permission to recruit pupils from their schools.

CHAPTER 7

Acknowledgments
We thank the mothers and children of the Gestational Iodine Cohort and the Tasmanian Department of Education for their cooperation.
This work was supported by the Royal Hobart Hospital Research Foundation (grant funded the Gestational Iodine Cohort baseline data collection) and the University of Tasmania (Cross Theme Grant funded the salary for K.L.H. and follow-up of the Gestational Iodine Cohort).

Disclosure Summary
The authors have nothing to disclose.

CHAPTER 8

Acknowledgments

This research was supported by a grant from the Korea Food and Drug Administration (13162MFDS892).

Author Contributions

Conceived and designed the experiments: HDW, DWK, YSH, BMC, JHP, JWK, JHY, HWC, JHL, MJK, YMK, JHS, JK. Contributed to the acquisition of data: BMC, JHP, JWK, JHY, HWC, JHL, MJK, YMK, JHS. Analyzed the data: HDW, DWK, JK. Wrote the paper: HDW, JK.

Conflicts of Interest

The authors declare no conflict of interest.

CHAPTER 9

Conflict of Interests

The authors declare that they do not have any conflict of interests.

Authors Contributions

The authors' responsibilities were as follows: Joanna C. Hamlin analyzed data, performed statistical analysis, and contributed to paper writing; Margaret Pauly is certified dietitian who collected dietary data; Stepan Melnyk is a laboratory director who developed metabolic assays; Oleksandra Pavliv conducted metabolic assays; William Starrett conducted metabolic assays; Tina A. Crook analyzed data, performed statistical analysis, and contributed to paper writing; S. Jill James (Principal Investigator) conducted the study, analyzed data, performed statistical analysis, interpreted the data, contributed to paper writing, and had primary responsibility for final content.

Acknowledgments

The authors would like to acknowledge the effort and participation of the mothers of children with autism without whom this study would not have been possible. This research was conducted as part of the Autism Speaks Autism Treatment Network. Further support came from cooperative agreement (UA3 MC 11054) from the U.S. Department of Health and Human Services, Health Resources and Services Administration, Maternal and Child Health Research Program, to the Massachusetts General Hospital. The views expressed in this paper do not necessarily reflect the views of Autism Speaks, Inc. It was also supported by HRSA: Autism Intervention for Physical Health (AIR-P); NICHD: R011HD051873 (SJJ); CTSI: Rochester University.

CHAPTER 10

Competing Interests
The authors declare that they have no competing interest.

Author Contributions
MHC and YMB designed the study, wrote the protocol and manuscripts. YMB, TPS, YSC, JWH, and KLH contributed to the preparation and proof-reading of the manuscript. YMB, TJC, and WHC provided the advices on statistical analysis. All authors read and approved the final manuscript.

Acknowledgements
The study was supported by grant from Taipei Veterans General Hospital (V101D-001-1).

CHAPTER 11

Competing Interests
The authors declare that they have no competing interests.

Author Contributions
BLG conceptualized the study, designed the methodology and implementation, interpreted data, and wrote the report. TLF designed the data collection forms, performed the blinded chart review, and assisted in preparing background information. MCF and MP assisted in collecting data. SM provided statistical analysis. All authors read and approved the final manuscript.

Acknowledgements

This work was supported by the Jeffrey Research Fellowship, Nationwide Children's Hospital/The Ohio State University, and the University of Rochester Clinical Translational Science Institute/Grant Number 1 KL2 RR024136-1 from the National Center for Research Resources (NCRR), a component of the National Institutes of Health (NIH), and the NIH Roadmap for Medical Research. Its contents are the sole responsibility of the authors and do not necessarily represent the official view of NCRR or NIH. Information on NCRR is available at http://www.ncrr.nih.gov/. Information on Re-engineering the Clinical Research Enterprise can be obtained from:http://nihroadmap.nih.gov/clinilcalresearch/overviewtranslational.asp

CHAPTER 12

Conflict of Interest Statement

Katie Adolphus declares that the research was conducted in the absence of any commercial or financial relationships that could be construed as a potential conflict of interest. Louise Dye and Clare L. Lawton have received funding from the food industry to examine the effects of food and food components including breakfast on cognitive function, satiety, glycaemic response, and wellbeing but did not receive any support for this review.

Acknowledgments

Katie Adolphus was supported by an Economic and Social Research Council (ESRC) research studentship and funding from The Schools Partnership Trust Academies (SPTA).

CHAPTER 13

Funding

This research was supported by the Biotechnology and Biological Sciences Research Council (grant BB/F008953/1) and the Fundação para a Ciência e a Tecnologia (FCT) (grant SFRH/BD/69711/2010). The funders had no role in study design, data collection and analysis, decision to publish, or preparation of the manuscript.

Competing Interests

The authors have declared that no competing interests exist.

Author Contributions

Conceived and designed the experiments: CR DV CMW LTB JPES. Performed the experiments: CR. Analyzed the data: CR JPES. Contributed reagents/materials/analysis tools: MR JMM PWT. Wrote the paper: CR CMW JPES. Extraction of anthocyanins from blueberries: PWT JMM. BDNF mRNA probe design and synthesis and assistance in situ hybridization techniques: MR.

INDEX

For Product Safety Concerns and Information please contact our EU
representative GPSR@taylorandfrancis.com
Taylor & Francis Verlag GmbH, Kaufingerstraße 24, 80331 München, Germany

www.ingramcontent.com/pod-product-compliance
Lightning Source LLC
Chambersburg PA
CBHW060745220326
41598CB00022B/2329

* 9 7 8 1 7 7 4 6 3 2 4 1 3 *